T0335724

Applying Business Intelligence to Clinical and Healthcare Organizations

José Machado
University of Minho, Portugal

António Abelha
University of Minho, Portugal

A volume in the Advances in
Bioinformatics and Biomedical
Engineering (ABBE) Book Series

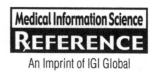

Medical Information Science
REFERENCE
An Imprint of IGI Global

Published in the United States of America by
Medical Information Science Reference (an imprint of IGI Global)
701 E. Chocolate Avenue
Hershey PA 17033
Tel: 717-533-8845
Fax: 717-533-8661
E-mail: cust@igi-global.com
Web site: http://www.igi-global.com

Library of Congress Cataloging-in-Publication Data

Names: Machado, Jos?e Manuel, editor. | Abelha, Antonio, 1964- editor.
Title: Applying business intelligence to clinical and healthcare
  organizations / Jose Machado and Antonio Abelha, editors.
Description: Hershey PA : Medical Information Science Reference, [2016] |
  Includes bibliographical references and index.
Identifiers: LCCN 2015046931| ISBN 9781466698826 (hardcover) | ISBN
  9781466698833 (ebook)
Subjects: LCSH: Health facilities--Business management. | Health services
  administration--Information technology.
Classification: LCC RA971.3 .A67 2016 | DDC 362.1068--dc23 LC record available at http://lccn.
loc.gov/2015046931

This book is published in the IGI Global book series Advances in Bioinformatics and Biomedical
Engineering (ABBE) (ISSN: 2327-7033; eISSN: 2327-7041)

British Cataloguing in Publication Data
A Cataloguing in Publication record for this book is available from the British Library.

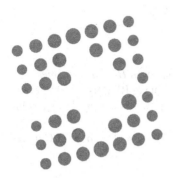

Advances in Bioinformatics and Biomedical Engineering (ABBE) Book Series

ISSN: 2327-7033
EISSN: 2327-7041

Mission

The fields of biology and medicine are constantly changing as research evolves and novel engineering applications and methods of data analysis are developed. Continued research in the areas of bioinformatics and biomedical engineering is essential to continuing to advance the available knowledge and tools available to medical and healthcare professionals.

The **Advances in Bioinformatics and Biomedical Engineering (ABBE) Book Series** publishes research on all areas of bioinformatics and bioengineering including the development and testing of new computational methods, the management and analysis of biological data, and the implementation of novel engineering applications in all areas of medicine and biology. Through showcasing the latest in bioinformatics and biomedical engineering research, ABBE aims to be an essential resource for healthcare and medical professionals.

- Health Monitoring Systems
- Tissue Engineering
- Prosthetic Limbs
- Data Analysis
- Genetic Engineering
- Drug Design
- Therapeutic Engineering
- Computational Biology
- Finite Elements
- DNA Sequencing

IGI Global is currently accepting manuscripts for publication within this series. To submit a proposal for a volume in this series, please contact our Acquisition Editors at Acquisitions@igi-global.com or visit: http://www.igi-global.com/publish/.

Titles in this Series

For a list of additional titles in this series, please visit: www.igi-global.com

Biomedical Image Analysis and Mining Techniques for Improved Health Outcomes
Wahiba Ben Abdessalem Karâa (Taif University, Saudi Arabia & RIADI-GDL Laboratory, ENSI, Tunisia) and Nilanjan Dey (Department of Information Technology, Techno India College of Technology, Kolkata, India)
Medical Information Science Reference • copyright 2016 • 414pp • H/C (ISBN: 9781466688117) • US $225.00 (our price)

Big Data Analytics in Bioinformatics and Healthcare
Baoying Wang (Waynesburg University, USA) Ruowang Li (Pennsylvania State University, USA) and William Perrizo (North Dakota State University, USA)
Medical Information Science Reference • copyright 2015 • 528pp • H/C (ISBN: 9781466666115) • US $255.00 (our price)

Emerging Theory and Practice in Neuroprosthetics
Ganesh R. Naik (University of Technology Sydney (UTS), Australia) and Yina Guo (Taiyuan University of Science and Technology, China)
Medical Information Science Reference • copyright 2014 • 377pp • H/C (ISBN: 9781466660946) • US $265.00 (our price)

Technological Advancements in Biomedicine for Healthcare Applications
Jinglong Wu (Okayama University, Japan)
Medical Information Science Reference • copyright 2013 • 382pp • H/C (ISBN: 9781466621961) • US $245.00 (our price)

Biomedical Engineering and Cognitive Neuroscience for Healthcare Interdisciplinary Applications
Jinglong Wu (Okayama University, Japan)
Medical Information Science Reference • copyright 2013 • 472pp • H/C (ISBN: 9781466621138) • US $245.00 (our price)

Pharmacoinformatics and Drug Discovery Technologies Theories and Applications
Tagelsir Mohamed Gasmelseid (King Faisal University, Kingdom of Saudi Arabia)
Medical Information Science Reference • copyright 2012 • 442pp • H/C (ISBN: 9781466603097) • US $245.00 (our price)

Machine Learning in Computer-Aided Diagnosis Medical Imaging Intelligence and Analysis
Kenji Suzuki (University of Chicago, USA)
Medical Information Science Reference • copyright 2012 • 524pp • H/C (ISBN: 9781466600591) • US $245.00 (our price)

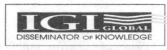

www.igi-global.com

701 E. Chocolate Ave., Hershey, PA 17033
Order online at www.igi-global.com or call 717-533-8845 x100
To place a standing order for titles released in this series,
contact: cust@igi-global.com
Mon-Fri 8:00 am - 5:00 pm (est) or fax 24 hours a day 717-533-8661

Table of Contents

Detailed Table of Contents

Chapter 1

    Hugo Peixoto, Centro Hospitalar do Tâmega e Sousa E.P.E., Portugal
    Andréa Domingues, University of Minho, Portugal
    Bruno Fernandes, University of Minho, Portugal

Information should be accessible everywhere and at any time to help with clinical decision and be available for clinical studies through data computationally interpretable. This work is based on a set of studies performed at Centro Hospitalar do Tâmega e Sousa. An Electronic Semantic Health Record was formalized and implemented which was delivered through a platform named Agency for the Integration, Diffusion and Archive, which is supported by intelligent agents. Furthermore, to strengthen the relation between the patient and the hospital, an appointment alert system was developed, which allowed the reduction of non-programmed misses and a decrease of costs. Finally to promote user's confidence on Information Systems, an open-source tool was developed that enables the scheduling of preventive actions. These tools allowed continuous improvement of systems and are currently well accepted inside the healthcare unit, proving in real clinical situation the effectiveness and usability of the model.

Chapter 2

    José Neves, Universidade do Minho, Portugal
    Eva Silva, Universidade do Minho, Portugal
    João Neves, Drs. Nicolas & Asp, UAE
    Henrique Vicente, Universidade de Évora, Portugal

Nosocomial infections have severe consequences for the patients and the society in general, being one of the causes that increase the length of stay in healthcare facilities. Therefore, it is of utmost importance to be preventive, being aware of how probable is to have that kind of infection, although it is hard to do with traditional methodologies and tools for problem solving. Therefore, this work will focus on the development of a decision support system that will cater for an individual risk evaluation tool with respect to catch nosocomial infections. The Knowledge Representation and Reasoning procedures used will be based on an extension to the Logic Programming language, allowing the handling of incomplete and/or default data. The computational framework in place will be centered on Artificial Neural Networks. It may be emphasized that in addition to the nosocomial infections risk evaluation, it is provided the Degree-of-Confidence that one has on such a happening.

Chapter 3
    Andreia Brandão, University of Minho, Portugal
    Filipe Portela, University of Minho, Portugal & Porto Polytechnic,
        Portugal

With the implementation of Information and Communication Technologies in the health sector, it became possible the existence of an electronic record of information for patients, enabling the storage and the availability of their information in databases. However, without the implementation of a Business Intelligence (BI) system, this information has no value. Thus, the major motivation of this paper is to create a decision support system that allows the transformation of information into knowledge, giving usability to the stored data. The particular case addressed in this chapter is the Centro Materno Infantil do Norte (CMIN), in particular the Voluntary Interruption of Pregnancy (VIP) unit. With the creation of a BI system for this module, it is possible to design an interoperable, pervasive and real-time platform to support the decision-making process of health professionals, based on cases that occurred. Furthermore, this platform enables the automation of the process for obtaining key performance indicators that are presented annually by this health institution. In this chapter, the BI system implemented in the VIP unity in CMIN, some of the indicators (KPIs) evaluated as well as the benefits of this implementation are presented.

Chapter 4
    Eliana Pereira, University of Minho, Portugal
    Filipe Portela, University of Minho, Portugal & Porto Polytechnic,
        Portugal
    António Abelha, University of Minho, Portugal

Nowadays in healthcare, the Clinical Decision Support Systems are used in order to help health professionals to take an evidence-based decision. An example is the Clinical Recommendation Systems. In this sense, a pre-triage system was developed and implemented in Centro Hospitalar do Porto in order to group the patients on two levels (urgent or outpatient). However, although this system is calibrated and specific to the urgency of obstetrics and gynaecology, it does not meet all clinical requirements by the general department of the Portuguese HealthCare (Direção Geral de Saúde). The main requirement is the need of having priority triage system characterized by five levels. Thus some studies have been conducted with the aim of presenting a methodology able to evolve the pre-triage system on a Clinical Recommendation System with five levels. After some tests (using data mining and simulation techniques), it has been validated the possibility of transformation the pre-triage system in a Clinical Recommendation System in the obstetric context. At the end the main indicators achieved with this system are presented in the Business Intelligence Platform already deployed. This paper presents an overview of the Clinical Recommendation System for obstetric triage, the model developed and the main results achieved.

Chapter 5

The healthcare industry generates huge amount of data underused for decision making needs because of the absence of specific design mastered by healthcare actors and the lack of collaboration and information exchange between the institutions. In this work, a new approach is proposed to design the schema of a Hospital Data Warehouse (HDW). It starts by generating the schemas of the Hospital Data Mart (HDM) one for each department taking into consideration the requirements of the healthcare staffs and the existing data sources. Then, it merges them to build the schema of HDW. The bottom-up approach is suitable because the healthcare departments are separately. To merge the schemas, a new schema integration methodology is used. It starts by extracting the similar elements of the schemas and the conflicts and presents them as mapping rules. Then, it transforms the rules into queries and applies them to merge the schemas.

Chapter 6

Well-being is a complex notion of satisfaction towards a human being. There is no doubt that it is not essential but the greater the sense of well-being, the better are living conditions and general happiness. It can be measured and although it is not directly assessed, there are procedures that grasp its value. An example is the act of sensorization of different key related attributes. Sensorization is the ability to gather data which may be used to a plurality of objectives. The greater the number of sensorized attributed, the better evaluation on well-being can be made. But there are more benefits that can be hypothesized such as the construction of community knowledge bases and the search for abnormal relationships between well-being and the attributes sensed. A historical record of our way of life can also present clues to health organizations, both to the creation of regulations and individual diagnosis.

Advancements in Information and Communication Technology (ICT) have led to the development of various forms of electronic records to support general practitioners and healthcare providers in capturing, storing, and retrieving routinely collected medical records and/or clinical information for optimal primary care and translational research. These advancements have resulted in the emergence of interoperable Healthcare Information Systems (HIS) such as Electronic Health Records (EHRs), Electronic Medical Records (EMRs) and Personal Health Records (PHRs). However, even as these systems continue to evolve, the research community is interested in understanding how the use and adoption of HIS can be optimized to support effective and efficient healthcare delivery and translational research. In this chapter, a systematic literature review methodology was used not only to explore the key benefits and technical challenges of HIS, but also to discuss the optimization approaches to maximizing the use and adoption of HIS in healthcare delivery.

The mentality of savings and eliminating any kind of outgoing costs is undermining our society and our way of living. Cutting funds from Education to Health is at best delaying the inevitable "Crash" that is foreshadowed. Regarding Health, a major concern, can be described as jeopardize the health of Patients – Reduce of the Length of Hospital. As we all know, Human Health is very sensitive and prune to drastic changes in short spaces of time. Factors like age, sex, their ambient context – house conditions, daily lives – should all be important when deciding how long a specific patient should remain safe in a hospital. In no way, ought this be decided by the economic politics. Logic Programming was used for knowledge representation and reasoning, letting the modeling of the universe of discourse in terms of defective data, information and knowledge. Artificial Neural Networks and Genetic Algorithms were used in order to evaluate and predict how long should a patient remain in the hospital in order to minimize the collateral damage of our government approaches, not forgetting the use of Degree of Confidence to demonstrate how feasible the assessment is.

Magda Amorim, Universidade do Minho, Portugal
Filipe Miranda, Universidade do Minho, Portugal

The semantic and syntactic interoperability introduces the capability of two machines to communicate and understand each other improving then the quality of Electronic Health Records. In this work, is presented an independent application of the medical record, using a web service (with protocol TCP/IP) capable of provide human interaction with interfaces in different devices (web, android app., browser). SNOMED CT is a comprehensive and scientifically validated health care terminology resulting in an organized computer processable collection of medical terms. This can be mapped into other systems of codes like ICD also used in our application. A data base (SNOMED codes and relations) was created capable of answer to all sort of queries from the users using the browser or the mobile application. The first hospital unit to enjoy this system was the pathological anatomy unit of the CHAA hospital. Here after receiving a "piece" and a task, the responsible performs all kind of procedures with the purpose of performing a report (diagnosis for example). With the implementation of SNOMED CT, to produce reports a physician could search for the name of the "piece" or the code and immediately upload in that patient HER the diagnosis. The usage of this codes leads to report uniformed that could be read and understood around the world. Another important feature of the application is the incorporation within the AIDA, AIDA-PCE and AIDA-BI. Experiments with real user show a successful software implementation judging by the utilization rate and medical personal acceptance. The mobile application should suffer an upgrade allowing the patient usage for example.

Eva Silva, Universidade do Minho, Portugal
Luciana Cardoso, Universidade do Minho, Portugal
Ricardo Faria, Universidade do Minho, Portugal
Manuel Santos, Universidade do Minho, Portugal

The existence of nosocomial infection prediction systems in healthcare environments can contribute to improve the quality of the healthcare institution. Also, can reduce the costs with the treatment of those patients. The analysis of the information available allows to efficiently prevent these infections and to build knowledge that can help to identify the eventual occurrence of nosocomial infections. Good models induced by the DM classification techniques SVM, DT and NB, were achieved (sensitivities higher than 91.90%). Therefore, this system is able to predict these infections consequently, reduce the nosocomial infection incidence. The platform developed presents important information, as well as supports healthcare professionals in their decisions, namely in planning infection prevention measures. So, the system acts as a CDSS capable of reducing nosocomial infections and the associated costs, improving the healthcare and, increasing patient's safety and well-being.

Chapter 11

    Ana Alpuim, University of Minho, Portugal
    Marisa Esteves, University of Minho, Portugal
    Sónia Pereira, University of Minho, Portugal
    Manuel Santos, University of Minho, Portugal

Over the years, information technologies and computer applications have been widespread amongst all fields, including healthcare. The main goal of these organizations is focused on providing quality health services to their patients, ensuring the provision of quality services. Therefore, decisions have to be made quickly and effectively. Thus, the increased use of information technologies in healthcare has been helping the decision-making process, improving the quality of their services. For an example, the insertion of Business Intelligence (BI) tools in healthcare environments has been recently used to improve healthcare delivery. It is based on the analysis of data in order to provide useful information. BI tools assist managers and health professionals through decision-making, since they allow the manipulation and analysis of data in order to extract knowledge. This work aims to study and analyze the time that physicians take to prescribe medical exams in Centro Hospitalar do Porto (CHP), though BI tools. The main concern is to identify the physicians who take more time than average to prescribe complementary means of diagnosis and treatment, making it possible to identify and understand the reason why it occurs. To discover these outliners, a BI platform was developed using the Pentaho Community. This platform presents means to represent information through tables and graphs that facilitate the analysis of information and the knowledge extraction. This information will be useful to represent knowledge concerning not only the prescription system (auditing it) but also its users. The platform evaluates the time prescription, by specialty and physician, which can afterwards be applied in the decision-making process. This platform enables the identification of measures to unravel the time differences that some physicians exhibit, in order to, subsequently, improve the whole process of electronic medical prescription.

# Chapter 12

Stroke is considered the third main cause of death among all population, without distinguishing genders, led by heart diseases in first place. In other hand, despite representing a significant number of mortality, these diseases are the causes for a long-term disability in all countries with a vast recovery time going parallel with its costs. However, leaving aside this facts, stokes and heath diseases can also be easily prevented considering the outcome. This paper presents a new methodology to prevent these events to happen by using segmentation methods, which allows distinguishing and aggregating clusters of historical records, classification methods, such as Artificial Neural Networks, capable of classifying a new record according to its distribution among the clusters. A Multi-Agent Case Based Reasoning system is also proposed to evaluate solutions based in a similar case.

# Chapter 13

This article aims to explain the construction process of the learing systems based on Artificial Neural Networks and Genetic Algorithms. These systems were implemented using R and Python programming languages, in order to compare results and achieve the best solution and it was used Diabetes and Parkinson datasets with the purpose of identifying the carriers of these diseases.

As regards the dosage of drug, children are a much more vulnerable population than the adults. With this in mind it is extremely important the administration of the correct dosage. For this purpose, it was develop a framework, based on a prototype already tested in a real environment, with the main concern to help pediatricians in their daily tasks. Thus, this framework includes tools that can help in the preparation of Total Parenteral Nutrition prescriptions, table pediatric and neonatal emergency drugs, medical scales of morbidity and mortality, anthropometry percentiles (weight, length/height, head circumference and BMI), utilities for supporting medical decision on the treatment of neonatal jaundice and anemia and other calculators. This paper presents the architecture, their functionalities and a SWOT analysis of the solution proposed.

Eliana Pereira, University of Minho, Portugal
Eva Silva, University of Minho, Portugal
Ana Pereira, University of Minho, Portugal
Bruno Fernandes, University of Minho, Portugal
José Neves, University of Minho, Portugal

The strategy of making predictions for a specific case or problem, in particular regarding scenarios with incomplete information, should follow a dynamic and formal model. This chapter presents a specific case concerning the employment of professionals for a health institution, as technicians and physicians, to demonstrate a model that requires the Quality-of-Information and the Degree-of-Confidence of the extensions of the predicates that model the universe of discourse. It is also mentioned a virtual intellect, or computational model, in order to maximize the Degree-of-Confidence that is associated with each term in the extensions of the predicates, according to the approximate representation of the universe of discourse. This model is prepared to be adopted by a Business Intelligence platform in order to increase the Quality-of-Information and the Degree-of-Confidence of the extensions in healthcare.

Preface

INTRODUCTION

The use of Information and Communication Technologies are increasingly occupying an important place in society. The health sector is a particular case, as these Technologies can provide complete and reliable information for healthcare professionals, allowing support their clinical and administrative decisions and consequently decreasing medical errors.

Business Intelligence (BI) is a very popular topic. Scientific business intelligence community has more supporters. BI belongs to the most important current issues. It is related with the so-called democratization of information access when decisions are now based on consistent reasoning process instead of management feelings. This book is a collection of fifteen chapters. It makes a special attention on implementation of BI solutions processes and best practices in hospitals. The problem-solving process is seen with an intelligent vision.

In hospitals, in the clinical domain, the first step to solve problems on the ground is to solve interoperability issues between information systems. The second step is the development of electronic health records. Business Intelligence is the final step. In this book, ETL solutions are presented, data warehouse based on new schema solutions are proposed, BI solutions oriented to monitoring and reporting are addressed and issues related to knowledge discovery using data mining or soft computing are studied. The Knowledge Discovery in Database is a set of ongoing activities that enable the extraction of useful knowledge. The main goal is to discover useful, valid, relevant and new knowledge about a particular activity through algorithms, taking into account the magnitudes of data increasing (Goebel, Siekmann, & Wahlster, 2010). An attempt has been made in order to present valid and sound solutions to particular problems, mostly in real or critical world.

This publication aims to disseminate the Biomedical Informatics concepts, namely the use of Business Intelligence and its newest applications, to the scientific community. Consequently, it may inspire researchers to develop new solutions to healthcare organizations in order to improve the quality of medical care and the patients' quality of life.

BIOMEDICAL INFORMATICS

Biomedical Informatics is an area that is spreading exponentially among several healthcare organizations. This phenomenon is happening due to the need that exists in these organizations to improve the quality of the healthcare. The Biomedical Informatics is fully capable to accomplish this mission. Issues as the BI in healthcare, Clinical Decision Support Systems (CDSS) and the information management are not only reducing the amount of paper in health organizations, but also reducing the occurrence of clinical and administrative errors. The implementation of BI tools in healthcare organizations help the managers and the healthcare professionals in the decision making process. The analysis of data provides relevant information about the activities and processes that happen inside the organization and this information can be essential to the patient diagnosis and problem solving.

BUSINESS INTELLIGENCE

The term Business Intelligence (BI) was introduced by Howard Dresner in 1989. BI is the set of concepts and methods used to improve the decision making process in an organization, using computational methods and tools (Power, 2008; Ghanzanfari, Jafari, & Rouhani 2011). It also includes best practices that transform data into knowledge and enable analysis of information to improve and optimize decisions and performance.

Thus, it promotes a more reasoned decision making and, consequently, better results for the organization (Power, 2008; Prvedllo, Andriole, Hanson, et al., 2010; Glaser, & Stone, 2008). So, the system transforms data into information, that later can generate strategic and relevant knowledge to support the decision making process, allowing better performance (Bonney, 2013; Popovič, Hackney, & Coelho, et al., 2012). BI systems have the ability to timely provide the correct information needed to support the decision making process, resulting in a competitive advantage for the organization.

According to Popovič et al. (Popovič, Hackney, & Coelho, et al., 2012), the implementation of BI systems can contribute to improve the quality of the information used by the organization, through: a faster access; the easiness in querying and exploring data; and the improvements on data consistency as a result of the integration processes performed before data storage on the Data Warehouse.

APPLYING BUSINESS INTELLIGENCE TO CLINICAL AND HEALTHCARE ORGANIZATIONS

The healthcare units have been adopting several informatics and technological solutions in order to contribute to a better functioning of the institutions and to improve the quality of the services provided. However, a healthcare organization is an environment with a large amount of information that is indispensable for the decision making process made by the healthcare professionals. It is necessary to ensure that all this information is available when it is needed and it is fundamental that it be interpreted correctly to avoid errors that can jeopardize the life of a human being. The solution is accomplished through the concept of semantic interoperability that represents the ability of systems to communicate with each other without the change of the meaning of the information, in other words ensure that the information is interpreted likewise by all stakeholders (systems and professionals). Thus, an important procedure to do in healthcare organizations is the semantic mapping of clinical data. Today there are some standard terminologies to represent clinical content, the SNOMED-CT (Systematized Nomenclature of MEDicine - Clinical Terms) is an example. Nevertheless, the semantic interoperability of the Health Information Systems (HIS) is only possible if the clinical data models, like openEHR archetypes, are according the standard terminologies.

Interoperability in HIS is increasingly a requirement rather than an option. Standards and technologies, such as multi-agent systems, have proven to be powerful tools in interoperability issues. In the last few years, we have worked on developing the Agency for Integration, Diffusion and Archive of Medical Information (AIDA), which is an intelligent, agent-based platform to ensure interoperability in healthcare units (Peixoto, Santos, Abelha, et al., 2012). It is increasingly important to ensure the high availability and reliability of systems. The functions provided by the systems that treat interoperability cannot fail and monitoring and controlling intelligent agents is a crucial tool to anticipate problems in HIS. Healthcare systems evolve by adopting more features and solving new problems (Caroso, Marins, Portela, 2014). Interoperability is the first step to provide electronic health records to HIS, and the so-called Paper Free Hospital is not possible without interoperability and Electronic Health Record (EHR). (Salazar, Duarte, Pereira, 2013). With the adoption of the EHR it was possible to acquire the versatility of a device capable of storing a vast sum of data. This was the great advantage obtain with the transition of Paper Clinical Process (PCP) to EHR. The data legibility, the continuous data processing, the ability to detect errors or releasing alarms concerning eventual pathological anomalies can also be considered as positives features acquired with the implementation of EHR. With the inclusion of this advantages, the patient assistance has become more effective, faster and with better quality. Information technology has great potential for transforming the health care system, improving quality of care. With the increasing expansion of health information systems, the Electronic Health Record (EHR) has become one of the finest sources for clinical information aggregators in the context of digital health. The EHR is a core part of a hospital information system, as well as a service on duty of the patient to improve the treatment of patients. It can be considered as a longitudinal electronic record of patient heath information, for example vital signs, medical history or laboratory data, generated by one or more encounters in any care delivery setting. The next step is applying business intelligence to clinical and healthcare organizations.

The implementation of BI in clinical and healthcare organizations is an efficient and adequate method to integrate and explore the clinical data collected by healthcare institutions. Data are collected and stored in databases, and are also used for decision support. BI systems process data, explore them, extract information and discover knowledge. Knowledge representation and reasoning techniques must be capable of covering every possible instance by considering incomplete, contradictory, and even unknown data (Neves, Martins, Vilhena, et al., 2015). These techniques must be very versatile and capable of covering almost every possible instance. This new approach can revolutionize prediction tools in all its variants, making it more complete than the existing methodologies and tools available (Neves, Guimarães, Gomes, 2015). Managing information quality is a continual process but many times, and in particular in clinical and healthcare organizations, it is crucial to know how to take decisions based on incomplete information.

This knowledge can be very relevant to identify, analyse and monitor the activities and processes that happen inside the healthcare institution. With BI, it is possible to discover problems and improvement opportunities in the healthcare environment. Therefore, the implementation of BI systems in healthcare institutions may help to improve the quality and safety of the delivered care; improve the efficiency and the financial performance of the healthcare institution; promote the implementation of evidence-based practices; promote a more efficient resource utilization. These improvements and advantages can occur because BI helps managers and healthcare professionals to make better and faster decisions, through data analysis about the activities and practices of the healthcare unit (Prvedllo, Andriole, Hanson, et. al.; 2010; Foshay & Kuziemsky, 2014). Moreover, the healthcare environment is very complex and dynamic. BI tools are essential to support the decision making process in the healthcare units, providing to the patients better and more affordable healthcare services. It can then be seen as a set of techniques and methods, with the ability to cope with practical solutions, in the same way that humans deal with these solutions either by common sense or intelligence.

BI tools are capable of working with healthcare data in an efficient manner, to generate real-time information and knowledge and this is the reason why they are very attractive to the healthcare sector. The principal benefits of BI technology are the saving of time in the access and in the analysis of data, the flexibility and the improvement in decision making by using information driven from real data. However, a BI system must be able to perform two fundamental tasks: integrate huge amounts of data coming from several different heterogeneous sources and provide the analytical tools for these data analysis. Thus there is a need to build BI tools adapted to the medical field and to the specificity of data that exists in these organizations.

ORGANIZATION OF THE BOOK

The book is organized into fifteen chapters. A brief description of each of the chapters follows:

Chapter 1 reviews issues surrounding interoperability in healthcare. Interoperability is the first step towards building the electronic health record and business intelligence systems, both in the administrative domain as the clinical one. The chapter presents a set of practical case studies carried out in a Portuguese hospital, in particular the use of an interoperability platform supported by intelligent agents.

Chapter 2 establishes the need of developing knowledge representation and reasoning techniques capable of covering every possible instance by considering incomplete, contradictory, and even unknown data. A new paradigm of knowledge representation and reasoning enables the use of the normalized values of the interval boundaries and their degree of confidence values, as inputs to Neural Networks. The output translates the risk prediction for nosocomial infection and the confidence that one has on such a happening.

Chapter 3 addresses the issue of creating a decision support system that allows the transformation of information into knowledge, giving usability to the stored data. A particular case of voluntary interruption of pregnancy study by means of business intelligence is presented in a healthcare unit. The benefits of such an implementation concern are discussed.

Chapter 4 analyses clinical recommendation systems as clinical decision support systems used to help health professionals to take evidence-based decisions. The chapter presents an overview of the clinical recommendation system for obstetric triage, the model developed and the main results achieved.

Chapter 5 proposes contributions to generate the hospital data warehouse schema, an assistant system to facilitate the collection of healthcare staff requirements, a new schema integration methodology to ensure the automatic merging of the schemas and an application of the new approach to build the hospital data warehouse.

Chapter 6 presents the digital concepts under people well-being research through the demonstration of research examples and applications. Health, comfort and well-being are points of concern in smart cities. On the other hand, healthcare organizations have a potential access to individual and grouped electronic records and aggregated records provide a global picture of populations, intervention and where effort should be conducted in order to help public health.

Chapter 7 deploys a systematic literature review methodology not only to explore the key benefits and technical challenges of Healthcare Information Systems (HIS), but also to discuss the optimization approaches to maximizing the use and adoption of HIS in healthcare delivery. The first part of the paper describes the systematic review methodology. In the second part, the focus is on the overview of the system and their associated key benefits and challenges in the healthcare domain. The third part focuses on the optimization techniques and approaches to maximizing the use and adoption of HIS to support effective and efficient healthcare delivery and translational research.

Chapter 8 addresses the problem of keeping a patient in a hospital in order to resolve health problems and the degree of confidence on such a happening despite the increasing of costs. The chapter presents the founding of a computational framework that uses knowledge representation and reasoning techniques to set the structure of the information and the associate inference mechanisms.

Chapter 9 discusses the importance of Electronic Health Records allowing the integration and standardization of clinical information. The problem is the duplication of information or the lack in information availability and reliability. Authors discuss semantic interoperability issues for clinical and business intelligence solutions, proposes SNOMED adoption and presents a case study.

Chapter 10 presents a business intelligence platform for predicting nosocomial infections by means of data mining. The platform supports healthcare professionals in their decisions, namely in planning infection prevention measures. The system acts as a CDSS capable of reducing nosocomial infections and the associated costs, improving healthcare and increasing patient's safety and well-being.

Chapter 11 presents a platform to evaluate the time prescription, which can afterwards be applied in the decision-making process. This platform enables the identification of measures to unravel the time differences that some physicians exhibit, in order to, subsequently, improve the whole process of electronic medical prescription.

Chapter 12 addresses a new methodology to prevent stroke accidents by using segmentation methods, which allows distinguishing and aggregating clusters of historical records, classification methods, such as artificial neural networks, capable of classifying a new record according to its distribution among the clusters.

A multi-agent case cased reasoning system is also proposed to evaluate solutions based in a similar case.

Chapter 13 aims to explain the construction process of learning systems based on soft computing systems, in particular neural networks and genetic algorithms. These systems were implemented using R and Python programming languages, in order to compare results and to achieve the best solution and it was used Diabetes and Parkinson datasets with the purpose of identifying the carriers of these diseases.

Chapter 14 presents a multiplatform decision support tool in Neonatology and Paediatric Care for the daily tasks of paediatricians or even for education and training.

Chapter 15 presents principles to conclude that the real value of Business Intelligence systems lies in their use to support organizations to make better informed decisions that will lead to increased profitability, lowered costs, improved efficiency or whatever the goals of the organization might be. In healthcare institutions, efficiency is a main requisite that makes this tools crucial for a reliable system.

CONCLUSION

This book intends to contribute to the subject matter of BI, in particular in the healthcare sector, when applying to real world problems. The number of BI solutions implemented in hospitals is reduced. In many hospitals, the problem of the lack of semantic interoperability have not been resolved and the electronic health record is still in a late stage. The main aim of this publication is to present some case studies that demonstrate the applicability of BI solutions, pointing out benefits and best practices. The use of appropriate tools by health professionals, can help them to identify causes and more effective treatments focused on patient disease. This book aims to show the importance of developing systems capable of interacting with an intelligent environment system using hybrid methods. It also looks to discuss and address the difficulties and challenges that healthcare organizations have faced in implementing BI technologies and applications. Additionally, the book will explore the impact of such technologies in healthcare organizations.

The target audience is composed by Health Organizations, Hospitals, Health Professionals, Biomedical Engineers, Informatics Engineers, Researchers in the Biomedical Informatics, Artificial Intelligence and Medicine fields.

José Machado
University of Minho, Portuga

António Abelha
University of Minho, Portugal

REFERENCES

Bonney, W. (2013). Applicability of business intelligence in electronic health record. *Procedia: Social and Behavioral Sciences*, *73*, 257–262. doi:10.1016/j. sbspro.2013.02.050

Cardoso, L., Marins, F., Portela, F., Santos, M., Abelha, A., & Machado, J. (2014). The Next Generation of Interoperability Agents in Healthcare. *International Journal of Environmental Research and Public Health*, *11*(5), 5349–5371. doi:10.3390/ijerph110505349 PMID:24840351

Foshay, N., & Kuziemsky, C. (2014). Towards an implementation framework for business intelligence in healthcare. *International Journal of Information Management*, *34*(1), 20–27. doi:10.1016/j.ijinfomgt.2013.09.003

Ghazanfari, M., Jafari, M., & Rouhani, S. (2011). A tool to evaluate the business intelligence of enterprise systems. *Scientia Iranica*, *18*(6), 1579–1590. doi:10.1016/j. scient.2011.11.011

Glaser, J., & Stone, J. (2008). Effective use of business intelligence. *Healthcare Financial Management*, *62*(2), 68–72. PMID:18309596

Goebel, R. Siekmann. J., Wahlster, W. (Eds), (2010). Advances in Knowledge Discovery and Data Mining, Lecture Notes in Computer Science (Vol. 6118). Springer.

Neves, J., Guimarães, T., Gomes, S., Vicente, H., Santos, M., Neves, J., & Novais, P. et al. (2015). Logic Programming and Artificial Neural Networks in Breast Cancer Detection. In I. Rojas, G. Joya, & A. Catala (Eds.), Lecture Notes in Computer Science: Vol. 9095. *Advances in Computational Intelligence* (pp. 211–224). doi:10.1007/978-3-319-19222-2_18

Neves, J., Martins, M. R., Vilhena, J., Neves, J., Gomes, S., Abelha, A., & Vicente, H. et al. (2015). A Soft Computing Approach to Kidney Diseases Evaluation. *Journal of Medical Systems*, *39*(10), 131. doi:10.1007/s10916-015-0313-4 PMID:26310948

Peixoto, H., Santos, M., Abelha, A., & Machado, J. (2012). Intelligence in Interoperability with AIDA. Proceedings of the 20th International Symposium on Methodologies for Intelligent Systems, 2012 World Intelligence Congress, Macau, LNCS (Vol. 7661). Springer. doi:10.1007/978-3-642-34624-8_31

Popovič, A., Hackney, R., Coelho, P. S., & Jaklič, J. (2012). Towards business Intelligence systems success: Effects of maturity and culture on analytical decision making. *Decision Support Systems*, *54*(1), 729–739. doi:10.1016/j.dss.2012.08.017

Power, D. J. (2008). Understanding data-driven decision support systems. *Information Systems Management*, *25*(2), 149–154. doi:10.1080/10580530801941124

Prevedello, L. M., Andriole, K. P., Hanson, R., Kelly, P., & Khorasani, R. (2010). Business intelligence tools for radiology: Creating a prototype using open-source tools. *Journal of Digital Imaging*, *23*(2), 133–141. doi:10.1007/s10278-008-9167-3 PMID:19011943

Salazar, M., Duarte, J., Pereira, R., Portela, F., Santos, M., Abelha, A., & Machado, J. (2013). Step towards Paper Free Hospital through Electronic Health Record. In Á. Rocha, A. M. Correia, T. Wilson, & K. A. Stroetmann (Eds.), *Advances in Information Systems and Technologies, Advances in Intelligent Systems and Computing* (Vol. 206, pp. 685–694). Springer. doi:10.1007/978-3-642-36981-0_63

Chapter 1
Steps towards Interoperability in Healthcare Environment

Hugo Peixoto
Centro Hospitalar do Tâmega e Sousa E.P.E., Portugal

Andréa Domingues
University of Minho, Portugal

Bruno Fernandes
University of Minho, Portugal

ABSTRACT

Information should be accessible everywhere and at any time to help with clinical decision and be available for clinical studies through data computationally interpretable. This work is based on a set of studies performed at Centro Hospitalar do Tâmega e Sousa. An Electronic Semantic Health Record was formalized and implemented which was delivered through a platform named Agency for the Integration, Diffusion and Archive, which is supported by intelligent agents. Furthermore, to strengthen the relation between the patient and the hospital, an appointment alert system was developed, which allowed the reduction of non-programmed misses and a decrease of costs. Finally to promote user's confidence on Information Systems, an open-source tool was developed that enables the scheduling of preventive actions. These tools allowed continuous improvement of systems and are currently well accepted inside the healthcare unit, proving in real clinical situation the effectiveness and usability of the model.

DOI: 10.4018/978-1-4666-9882-6.ch001

INTRODUCTION

Currently, information exchange among people, companies and systems plays an essential role in society. In this paradigm, the organization of society depends upon a method of social and economic development where information, as a means of creating knowledge, plays a fundamental role in the production of wealth and contributes to the wellbeing and quality of life of citizens. A healthcare facility is not exception and has to adapt to constant advances in technologies and systems in order to produce knowledge by data and ensure quality treatment to patient.

Nowadays, exchange and share of clinical information among Information Systems (IS) is becoming one of the main ways to improve the quality in the services provided to patients. Nevertheless, one of the principal obstacles to accomplish this goal is the high number of heterogeneous information sources arising inside a healthcare facility, such as medical applications and software, medical equipment and even clinical staff self-knowledge introduced as needed in the Patient Clinical Record. As defined by Langefors, IS, are a technologically implemented medium for recording, storing, and disseminating linguistic expressions, as well as for drawing conclusions from such expressions (Langefors, 1975). In a healthcare unit it is easy to step into proprietary applications from a wide range of providers, each one talking its own language and its own philosophy and implementation method, treating information according their own thoughts and workflows. This increases complexity to Health Information Systems (HIS), which depends not only on the number of systems but also on the number of providers. Building up all the information and make it readable by physicians has become a high important task. Therefore, HIS are integrated computer-assisted systems to store, manipulate, and retrieve healthcare administrative and clinical data (MeSH, 1987).

Every day in clinical practice, decisions are made that can save human lives. Clinical decisions are taken based on medical records made electronically or by hand in paper, medical examinations, and physical evaluations having the close contact with the patient. Not only the clinical diagnostic is produced taking in consideration all the information available and considered useful by physicians, but also the drug prescription or pathology identification.

Information is spread through healthcare units and it is almost impossible to avoid the creation of information silos. These silos can lead to data loss or even worst can restrict access to important information that could change or interpose clinical diagnosis. Drug allergies or examination reports that the doctor could not have access to may lead to bad patient treatment and medical errors based on incomplete or mistaken information. Interoperability is one of the keys to overlap these constraints and promotes better and easier access to information (Peixoto, Machado, Abelha & Neves, 2010).

On one hand, Interoperability among systems is one common interest within scientific community and several works are being published every day, about the methodologies of implementation and the ways to achieve it. On the other hand, accomplishing such task requires hard work and it is not yet established the best or only way to reach full interoperability.

Healthcare facilities can take advantages from Interoperability, and homogeneity among IS can lead to time reduction in diagnostic and appointments, since physicians have access to relevant information when and where they need it the most. In addition, it also provides better information quality by single patient identification and correct association between all the IS. In the end interoperability may help decreasing medical errors on treatments based on reliable information and results (Miranda, Duarte, Abelha, Machado, & Neves, 2009).

The Health Information Technologies adoption trend by healthcare organizations is unstoppable. However it is expected to be a backlash in view of the current financial crisis. Negative impact on the growth of the Health Information Technology industry is currently underway as hospitals and health systems are taking measured but deliberate action by delaying capital projects, cutting capital and operating budgets, and lying off workers (Sullivan, 2009).

Many of the European guidelines are sustained by Open-source software, which first perceived advantage is the fact that they are made available free or at a low cost, where developers should focus on sharing and complete systems in an open, widely spread and accessible way. Taken globally, several healthcare facilities with the same goals can share information and aims and fight together to improve sustainability for HIS in the Global Economic Crises (Sullivan, 2009).

The main goals behind this work are to evaluate if it is possible to improve HIS in order to improve patient-unity relationship. Furthermore, if an Electronic Semantic Health Record can overwhelm the current Electronic Health Record (EHR). Additionally, can uptimes from servers provide better or even reliable systems and how can IS help improving uptimes according scalable, secure and performance of each institution needs? Finally is all this possible based on Open-source software and can it provide a true alternative to proprietary software.

This work results reports the experiences lived inside a healthcare facility and all the outcomes were produced accordingly to goals and workflows established through meetings and brainstorms of a heterogeneous team composed by physicians, nurses, administrative crew, quality technicians and Information Technology specialists.

One of the main purposes of this work is the analysis and development of Systems based on the Healthcare Information System of the healthcare unity and the main needs of its users. These systems should be interactive and user-friendly, and should become the basis for Decision Support Systems. Providing data source not only to physicians but also to computers and make spread data interpretable by machines and, in the near future, Decision Support Systems it is also an important task to accomplish during this work (Peixoto, Machado, Abelha & Neves, 2010)

BACKGROUND

Over the last decade, the Artificial Intelligence Group, in the Informatics Department at the University of Minho, has dedicated their studies into building a platform for Interoperability, Diffusion and Archive called AIDA (Abelha, Machado, Santos, Allegro, & Paiva, 2002). Their efforts allowed that four major healthcare facilities in Portugal could benefit from an interoperability platform that covers all the main areas and it is becoming an emergent tool in HIS in Portugal.

The adoption of Information and Communication Technologies is essential for modern healthcare delivery systems if they are to gain greater efficiency, reduce overall healthcare costs and improve patient safety. In recent years, the acquisition of computer technologies by healthcare organizations has increased substantially with the spending showing upward tendency placing the industry as one of the major consumer of Information Communication Technology products and services (Sullivan, 2009).

Early in 1984, Hurtubise defined Management Information System as "a system that provides specific information support to the decision making process at each level on an organization" (Hurtubise, 1984). MIS were defined and studied first than HIS; afterwards Helfenbein came up with a global approach which he defined as a "system" (Helfenbein, 1987). Hence, like every other system, HIS has its own agents with organization and structure. HIS are part of a more global framework called Health System which offers curative care, rehabilitative care, disease prevention, and health promotion services.

INTEROPERABILITY IN HEALTHCARE ENVIRONMENT

Healthcare Information Systems

HIS orientation is to combine and use common elements within a healthcare facility in order to produce real resources and ensure information to users when and where they need it the most. HIS was also defined as the socio-technical subsystem of a hospital, which comprises all information processing as well as the associated human or technical actors in their respective information processing roles. One of the main goals this Systems is to contribute to a high-quality and efficient patient treatment. Another of its aims is to simplify administrative workflows, processing of the centralized and distributed healthcare data, and the development of effective system networking. From that moment HIS started to develop from administrative software to cover departments, clinics, and hospitals (Berger & Ciotti, 1993).

Delone and Maclean in 2003 have presented six success dimensions for IS namely (Delone & McLean, 2003):

- System quality;
- Information quality;
- Usage;
- User satisfaction;
- Individual impact; and
- Organizational impact.

For system quality, attributes like system flexibility and accuracy, response time, ease of use and convenience of access should be considered. Information quality can be measured by information system output, meaning information quality, accuracy and usefulness, among others. System and information quality are closely linked and influence each other; but either together or separated both influence use and user satisfaction. Usage refers to the interaction between information products with the user and system and information use. Time, frequency and regularity are examples of attributes to measure this element. User satisfaction can be influenced by the extent of use which leads to a positive or negative effect. Information product on management work and manager's behavior, such as quality of decisions, constitutes the dimension of individual impact (Currie & Procter, 2002). Finally, organizational impact refers to the global impact of HIS on organization performance, e.g. process collaboration, quality or costs (Kivinena & Lammintakanen, 2012). Overall, Kivenen and Lammintakanen enhance that success is a dynamic process and different dimensions relate to it temporally and causally (Kivinena & Lammintakanen, 2012).

Over the last decades several countries have created task forces and assembled teams in order to provide help and guidelines for institutions and users. Several examples can be found in countries over the Americas like Brazil, Canada and United States. Other projects are taking place in Europe in countries like Belgium, Austria, France, and Germany. Asia also has a global planning institution for supporting Medical Informatics. Medical Informatics is the science and art of modeling and recording real-world clinical concepts and events into computable data used to derive actionable information, based on expertise in medicine, information science, information technology, and the scholarly study of issues that impact upon the productive use of IS by clinical personnel (Silverstein, 1999). Though, Medical Informatics has evolved and in the last years a new definition started to be a global accepted concept, Health Informatics. Health Informatics relies not only on IS but most of all in clinical guidelines, which countries start to follow and adopt. Elderly population and health concerns are becoming even more important to governments. Associations around the world have similar focus and goals namely:

- HIS consolidation;
- Collaboration with groups and scientific associations;
- Knowledge management;
- Standards; and
- Information Quality.

Healthcare is a knowledge intensive activity and every department has its own specific language and needs generating a complex web of data spread through the institutions. In the last decades healthcare unities have gain their own independence and even inside healthcare institutions, departments had their own financial independence therefore whenever a new need was pointed from users, administrators and managers easily could buy the appropriate solution. Each service started to have as small database with specific patient data and where users registered pathologies or specific interests. This creates a computational issue that generates development problems. However, these applications are used by people with good satisfaction despite they do not allow a transversal vision of the patient data along different services or specialties, they cannot grow easily and sometimes they do not attend secure and confident procedures. Running applications in distributed environment is a huge problem when applications have not been developed to share knowledge and actions (Peixoto, Machado, Abelha, & Santos, Intelligence in interoperability with AIDA, 2012). Creation of silos of information is easy and access to information is hard and a major concern.

Interoperability

Every day new applications are developed by proprietary companies, in order to assist physicians on their work. Every of these applications is responsible for generating data knowledge and turning healthcare into a science based on information and reputation (Hersh, 2002). Each of these applications has its own language and workflow, besides, together with users known needs have created several boundaries hard to transpose meaning that there is still lack in information quality and easy information access. Actually, the increase number of heterogeneous applications promotes the creation of silos of information, which are constraints to the easy flow of information within a healthcare institution. Interoperability is a key property in enterprise applications, which is hard to achieve due to the large number of inter-operating components and semantic heterogeneity (Peixoto, Machado, Abelha, & Santos, Intelligence in interoperability with AIDA, 2012).

Demands for information handling within the healthcare sector range from clinically valuable patient specific information to a variety of aggregation levels for follow-up and statistical and/or quantifiable reporting.

Furthermore, patients visit several hospital over their life, and every time they are admitted a new episode is registered. Therefore patients have multiple episodes in multiple healthcare units, and this number increases along the time. Most of the times information present in previous episodes is lost and fragmentation occurs. Since healthcare is a science based on information, access to previous data is of extreme need. The need to access patient information grows in parallel with the need to consolidate the patient information across the numerous systems in a healthcare organization.

Regardless the field of study, interoperability can be classified in three distinct ways:

- **Technical Interoperability:** This is a domain-independent approach where the aspect concerning is moving the data from system A to system B, neutral-izing the effects of distance. In this transport layer there is no need to know about meaning of what is exchanged.
- **Semantic Interoperability:** In this approach it is necessary to specify to domain and context. Usually it involves the use of codes and identifiers to ensure that system A and system B understand the set of information without ambiguity. It enables two cooperating systems or components to use and in-terpret the data in the same way.
- **Process Interoperability:** Coordination of work processes that enables the business processes at organization that house system A and system B to work together.

In the last decades, users have understood that the quality of information inside a healthcare institution relies on data interoperability, thus, the enrolling of all the players is extremely necessary. Studies to determine the impact: financial and so-cial, the benefits and constraints and the levels of interoperability are needed and institutions should focus their efforts on this matter in search for the best patient treatment possible.

One of the main challenges for HIS is to represent the semantics of the sector, which are far more complex than in other industries. In order to perform such task, a knowledge-oriented computing framework that includes ontologies, terminology and a semantically enabled health computing platform is needed, in which complex meaning can be represented and shared. At the same time it must support the economically viable construction of maintainable and adaptable health computing systems and patient-centric EHR (OpenEHR, 2007).

The Semantic Web provides a common framework that allows data to be shared and reused across applications, enterprises, and community boundaries. It is a collaborative effort led by W3C with participation from a large number of researchers and industrial partners (W3C, 2010).

Semantic interoperability exists when different systems like computer systems, interacting with each other or with people can cooperate and make effective use of the terms that are used in the interaction (Graybeal, 2009). When two people try to communicate, a lot of redundant information is available for confirming assumptions and refining understanding. Facial expressions, tone of voice, repetition using different words, gestures, actions, and physical objects themselves guide the participants understanding. Also, many terms can be, and really are approximately translated for many purposes, 'friend' and 'colleague', for example, can substitute for each other. The first steps towards semantic interoperability rely on good practices and data management, principally defining data and metadata structure. The appropriate time to execute this is on data creation point, since it is where it is more possible and easy to understand how data are organized (Graybeal, 2009). Once data and metadata structures have been defined, usually by using a content standard to organize metadata, and metadata to describe data structure, it is possible to focus on describing the data in a semantically interoperable way. Where the structural information might recognize the existence of 3 variables in ASCII format separated by tabs, semantic interoperability demands that those variables to be named, and that some correspondence exists between variable names and the names be in a way that other people and computers can recognize them. Making names understandable it can take several forms and be achieved by several means. The easiest in some situations is to choose a vocabulary that can describe all the variables - for example, the SNOMED is one with extensive coverage in the healthcare scenario and declare that all your names will be specified using that vocabulary standards (Graybeal, 2009). Local mapping is available too, in order to do so it is necessary to establish a comparison and mapping between local naming and global defined and accepted standards (Graybeal, 2009). Therefore a vocabulary mapping is needed and other organizations should have access to it (Graybeal, 2009). Not all of these solutions are totally in place for every scenario, but most of the pieces are in place. As more projects need semantic interoperability, and implement the approaches that have been created, the initial cost is considered an increment above the work needed for every institution, and by adapting organizations to this paradigm early results and overcomes are expected (Graybeal, 2009)

Open-Source in Healthcare

Open-source describes practices in production and development that prop up access to the finished source code to users. The basic principles are to provide end-users the code as well as the right to amend it according to the needs. Motivations for using and developing open-source software are mixed, ranging from philosophical and ethical reasons to pure practical issues. Usually, the first perceived advantage of open-source models is the fact that open-source software is made available free or at a low cost. But this characteristic is not exclusive to open-source software, and several proprietary software products are made available in similar way. What really distinguishes open-source software from software available without fee is the combination of effects due to the following characteristics:

- The availability of the source code and the right to modify it, which enables the unlimited tuning and improvement of a software product;
- The right to redistribute modifications and improvements to the code, permits all the advantages due to the modifiability of the software to be shared by large communities;
- The right to use the software in any way. This, combined with redistribution rights, ensures a large population of users, which helps in turn to build up a market for support and customization of the software, which can only attract more and more developers to work in a common project.

The combination of competition and cooperation mechanisms is visible in almost any open source project, where every project is in some sense competing with others for resources and market acceptance, while collaborating with the reuse of the same code base. Usually, this mixture of competition and collaboration is not intentional; in short, everybody is forced to compete by exposing the tools (the source code) they are using, and improvements are quick to spread through the competing projects. Competition and collaboration are probably the ultimate cause of the high efficiency, in terms of quality and quantity of software produced with a given set of resources, which open source projects reach. Open-source models are rapidly being applied in many different fields of endeavor, such as biotechnology and bioinformatics. From a global perspective, healthcare facilities with the same goals and restrictions can improve their IS by sharing source-code and knowledge between them. Besides their above mentioned advantages, open-source applications suffer from several additional barriers to the general Information Technologies implementation issues. They include the lack of professional knowledge, legal and licensing issues, functional gaps and the lack of a road map for sustainability. Krogh and Hippel in 2006 presented the renewed urgency to adopt health and medical informatics applications and how open-source approaches are gaining attention in the healthcare industry (Krogh & Hippel, 2006).

Open-source software can be characterized by collaboration among individuals and organizations with common interests, shared intellectual property, and a commitment to standards. Information technology in the healthcare industry is evolving from an administrative tool for billing and bookkeeping to a clinical tool for improving the quality and efficiency of healthcare, and the scope of information sharing is expanding beyond the walls of individual institutions. Achieving this level of integration will require that software models overcome a host of technical obstacles, and that they are accessible, affordable, and widely supported. While not heralding the end of commercial software vendors, conditions are ripe for open-source solutions to take root in healthcare, and that it will likely become the standard for capturing, sharing, and managing patient information to support quality care. It also notes that healthcare businesses have the opportunity to take the lead and drive the shift to this new model. The main motivations for using open-source software in healthcare are reduced total cost-of-ownership, faster delivery of systems, systems being more secure, elimination of vendor lock-in and control over the software (possibility of adapting to local needs). As Murray describes IS have grown in a structured way and are now considered as being part of good and patient oriented healthcare unities (Murray, Wright, Karopka, Betts, & Orel, 2009). Tools to facilitate the sharing of clinical data are a more recent development in open-source healthcare IT. Healthcare data and interoperability standards, including HL7, CCHIT, and IHE, have all been growing in importance and maturity. Similarly to how standards like HTML, HTTP, and DNS led to the development and adoption of open-source software, a number of open-source software communities have started building tools to implement these healthcare standards. The Mirth project provides an open-source interface engine that can route and transform HL7, NCPDP, and other message formats.

Fundamentally, open-source is about creating a collaborative environment for problem solving. As healthcare technology standards evolve and healthcare IT systems adopt standards-based software technologies that enable greater interoperability, the opportunities for healthcare IT collaboration will only grow (RedHat, 2007).

The compelling economics of open-source and its collaborative development model will continue to improve the affordability of these complex HIS that are crucial to improving the quality of patient care.

SOLUTIONS AND RECOMMENDATIONS

Agency for Diffusion and Archive of Information (AIDA)

Semantic, a key word in this work refers to a computational paradigm that allows for interoperability, enabling intelligent ubiquitous computation and communications in order to increase quality of information and decision support. Indeed, doctors gather dissimilar types of information about patients for clinical practices. Different types of tests are visited in a user-friendly, including physical exams, imaging tests (e.g. XR, CT or MRI), laboratory tests (e.g. blood, urine, fluids or tissues), or pathology and surgical reports, i.e. in Computational Science, the scientific problem must be expressed mathematically, known as the Algorithm. Using semantic web, the algorithm is translated into one or more computer programs and implemented on one or more types of hardware. In our work, the combination of software and hardware is referred to as the Computational Architecture, the AIDA agency. It is shown that user-friendlier interfaces have a high number of visits, reducing costs and increasing the quality-of-care.

The solution is to integrate, diffuse and archive this information under a dynamic framework, in order to share this knowledge with every information system that needs it. Indeed, to build systems for real healthcare environments, the infrastructure must meet a range of basic requirements with respect to security, reliability and scaling. With access granted to Clinical and Historical Databases, agent technology may provide answers to those who give assistance to patients with a maximum of quality and medical evidence. Figure 1 shows the schematic representation of AIDA framework. In this schema, it is possible to understand the workflow of information, as well as integration and interoperability.

AIDA is an agency that provides intelligent electronic workers, here called proactive agents and in charge of tasks such as communicating with the heterogeneous systems, sends and receives information (e.g., medical or clinical reports, images, collections of data, prescriptions), managing and saving the information and answering to requests, with the necessary resources to their correct and an on time accomplishment.

AIDA also supports web-based services to facilitate the direct access to the information and communication facilities set by third parties, i.e., AIDA construction follows the acceptance of simplicity, the conference of the achievement of common goals and the addressing of responsibilities. The main goal is to integrate, diffuse and archive large sets of information from heterogeneous sources (i.e., departments, services, units, computers, medical equipment); AIDA also provides tools in order to implement communication with human beings based on web-based services. Under these presuppositions, a HIS will be addressed in terms of Figure 1:

Figure 1. AIDA: Agency for Integration Diffusion and Archive

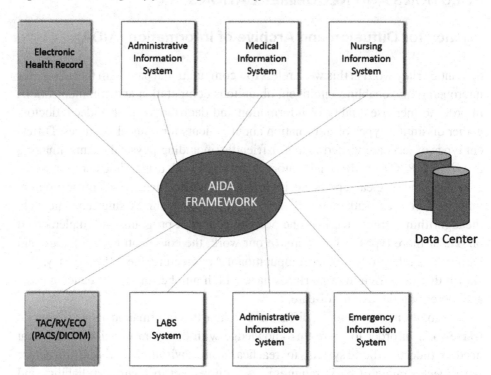

- **Administrative Information System (AIS):** which intends to represent, manage and archive the administrative information during the episode. An episode is a collection of all the operations assigned to the patient since the beginning of the treatment until the end;
- **The Medical Information System (MIS):** which intends to represent, manage and archive the clinical information during the episode;
- **The Nursing Information System (NIS):** which intends to represent manage and archive the nursing information during the episode; and
- **The Electronic Health Record Information System (EMR);** and
- **The Information Systems (DIS):** of all the departments or services, in particular of the laboratories (Labs), Radiological Information System (RIS) and Medical Imaging (PACS - Picture Archive and Communication System), which deals with images in a standard format, the DICOM one.

The architecture presented in Figure 1 was envisaged to support medical applications in terms of AIDA and EHR, a form of web spider of an intelligent information processing system, its major subsystems, their functional roles, and the flow of information and control among them, with adjustable autonomy.

Healthcare staff acquires this information and its value is automatically stored and distributed to where it is needed. Every document created within a specialized service respect this rules, making different and individualized departments closer. The coding and ordering features are very useful to link different data to one specific problem, as coded data is much easier to access and it is recommended for decision support using Artificial Intelligence. The electronic ordering embedded in EHR can be used not only to obtain medical equipment or pharmacological prescriptions, but also for acquiring laboratory and imaging studies outside the service where it is used. Furthermore, it may enable the centralization of exam display, allowing different services to share results concerning the same patient, diminishing costs on unnecessary exams, and above all, improving the quality of service being provided.

There are also different access permissions when dealing with medical data. Although it can only be viewed by the authorized personnel from any terminal inside the healthcare facility or even on its own laptop or PDA, the access must be flexible in order to enable the professionals to access it when needed. In other words, the access to the medical information of the patient is as important in terms of privacy as in terms of significance for medical situations. On the other hand, interfaces must be intuitive and easy to use. Messaging enables one to create, send and retrieve messages online. It may be very useful for handling data, images or even file exchange. Encryption and the right protocols of trading are also paramount. Messaging systems are extremely important not only for the internal workflow in a healthcare institution, but as well as an essential component for the development of group work, namely in the area of diagnostic that is supported by decision support systems.

Adoption of EHR is well known in several countries all over the world. Canada, Australia, England and United States have already started their own way to achieve an infrastructure for national HIS. All of these projects share the main elements and focus on the same important subject, interoperability and integration of HIS in spite of interoperability between healthcare providers being a hard task. Unfortunately, information emerges from an assortment of sources, from informatics applications, medical equipment and physicians' knowledge introduced in the EHR. Decision support systems are enhanced by quality of information and that can only be achieved with good collection of all the data from the patient. With this information overload, it is necessary to infer what information is relevant to be registered in the EHR and decision support systems must allow for reasoning on incomplete, ambiguous and uncertain knowledge. Demands of information handling within the healthcare sector range from clinically valuable patient-specific information to a variety of aggregation levels for follow-up and statistical and/or quantifiable reporting. EHR is a repository of information concerning an individual in an electronic format. It is stored and transmitted securely and may be accessed by multiple users. The main objective is to ensure ubiquity, i.e. information is accessible at anytime and anywhere. The lack of integration between the different HIS is not only an obstacle for a more effective clinical practice, but it may lead to a suboptimal care for the patient.

Appointment Alert System: AASYS

AASYS was implemented in January 2011 and all the results presented bellow correspond to the first semester of 2011. In order to have some comparison the homologue period of 2010 was used. The total number of appointments scheduled from January until May in 2010 was 107.076, while in 2011 the total of appointments was 111.508.Looking at this number is possible to determine an increase of appointments, meaning the effort made to decrease waiting lists. To evaluate the results of the implemented systems was necessary to determine whether the show rate increased or decreased along the first six months of the year 2011 compared to the same period in 2010. Another important issue that was taken in consideration was if the missed appointments were canceled in time to change to other patient that needed that appointment. Table 1 shows the cancellation time of the appointments for the two periods.

As proved by Table 1, the number of cancellations before the appointment day has increased from 13.908 to 16.565. This result lead to new reschedules and helped substantially to reduce waiting lists, since new appointments were scheduled and other patient could take the appointment time instead. Side by side, since no free spaces are available, doctors, nurses and administrative time is monetized leading to better cost control. After appointment day cancellations decreased by 50% and this can already provide the final predicted results to this work and how well AASYS managed to deal with schedule and show rates problem. In 2010 a total of 103.121 appointments were actually performed, while in 2011 the number raised to 109.577.

Figure 2 (a) presents the total number of canceled appointments and Figure 2(b) presents the total of misses to the appointments. As result shows, there was an almost 80% reduction in misses from one year to the other, which is a good indicator of the good performance of the AASYS. Besides this good performance, there are

Table 1. Total of schedule periods

Cancelation Time	2010	2011
Before appointment	13.908	16.565
Same day as appointment	1.077	1.034
After appointment day	1.068	520

Figure 2. Number of (a) canceled and (b) missed appointments

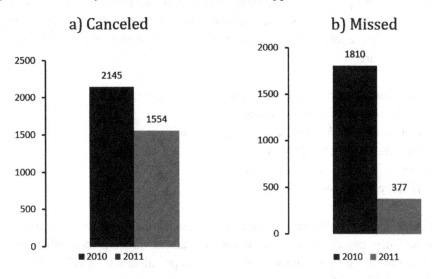

several other aspects to be taken into consideration that could significantly affect the expected results. Indeed a better approach to users should be taken in consideration, since elderly population cannot undertake this changes as well as the younger one. Additionally, AASYS reduced 30% a day, the number of letters sent to post office to be delivered to patients. From a 0,30€ letter cost, just for post office fees, The AASYS platform managed to deliver the same information for patients for just 0,06€ per message. Therefore a faster, safer, law compatible and cheaper system was achieved when AASYS was installed at CHTS appointment department.

Preventive Action Management System: ScheduleIT

One of the major goals of this work was to develop a management platform, called ScheduleIT, to ensure the proper workflow within the healthcare facility, not only in HIS, but also related with patient treatment. Therefore, ScheduleIT has many different area end-users as its main target; yet it does not neglects usability to its main users, namely IT technicians. ScheduleIT uses the healthcare web portal to alert and inform end-users, as well as emails to clinical directors to notify them of the planned actions taking place in the near future. Having these alerts available, it is possible to reduce the impacts of downtimes, since people are already informed of what is expected during stop time. In order to avoid missing an intervention, and since interventions are not yet automatic, notifications for IT technicians are extremely important; ScheduleIT does this by sending notifications to the request tracker and to the global IT mailing list. Designed in PHP, this platform allows users to easily set up a new intervention according to the time interval given by the estimation model. Using these time intervals it is easier to present a preventive action calendar for future interventions. From a global point of view, the main features of this platform are:

- Notifications for clinical and administrative teams;
- Notifications for IT technicians;
- Complete map for Programed Interventions;
- Integration with the IT park software;
- Touch interface compatible; and
- History of interventions.

Figure 3 shows the main interface of ScheduleIT, in which the most important information is presented to IT user, for the current day. Distinct information is presented to the end-user, at the healthcare web portal, and to the IT technician in the ScheduleIT interface.

On one hand, the end-user has access to:

- Main services affected;
- Schedule hour; and
- Estimated downtime.

On the other hand, IT technician has access to the entire previous mentioned, plus:

- IP address;
- Machine name;
- Machine group;
- Physical localization of the system; and
- Previous intervention notes.

Figure 3. ScheduleIT web interface for programed actions for the selected day

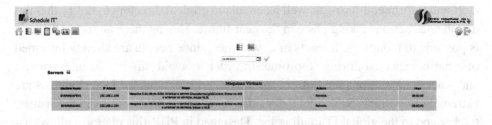

To improve the week interval estimation model, there is a form available to IT technicians in which non-programed interventions are registered. Values collected are presented to initial model and can determine whether changes in week interval are necessary or not. Information provided in Schedule IT forms is always saved and can be used in further studies to increase availability of systems.

One of the main objectives of this work is to demonstrate how IS can provide continuous improvements, not only for healthcare institutions, but also and mainly for the patients. In order to intervene in key areas inside the healthcare institution under study, practical studies were implemented and analyzed. The focus of the studies were to give overall answers for the questions raised at the beginning of this work, taking into account the improvements needed for a better financial, economic and personal management at a healthcare unit.

The quality of the IS department was improved, as well as the relation between the patient and the healthcare facility. In addition, it was noted a better access and quality of the information provided to the users.

The next paragraphs intend to give an overall discussion pointing out the main challenges and difficulties that arise during the implementation, as well as the major outcomes. In the first outcome a diffusion and archive agency was presented that empowered the integration and semantic interoperation of data information present at the healthcare unity. The possibility of exchange information in a structured manner, that can also be recognized and interpreted by machines, will allow in the future for scientific studies, extended researches or even decision support systems which can be based on more and more reliable information. One of the main conclusions of this study is that semantic is an inescapable paradigm that plays, and will continue playing, a fundamental role in research in Health Records. In fact several international projects have been following the lines that are essential for a common final goal, which is totally interoperable systems working and communicating in consonance, despite heterogeneous development sources, in order to improve the patient treatment and well-being. All the projects converge in Semantic Health Records, in which the information is available anywhere and anytime, whether for decision support when diagnosing patients, monitoring their treatment, or for consulting in future appointments.

When facing the question "Can Electronic Semantic Health Record overwhelm the current EHR?", the answer comes demystified: Semantic is indeed the future of IS and can no longer be ignored when dealing with clinical data that arises from heterogeneous data sources with no apparent connection. The next outcome was based in a more practical approach that dealt with patient appointment management. A new platform, named AASYS – Appointment Alert System, was developed in order to narrow the link between patients and healthcare units. By creating an alert system that deals with appointment scheduling, it was possible to act in two important and specific areas of the health system: first, cost reduction due to a decreasing number of missed appointments; and second, a significant improvement in the relation between the patient and the hospital. This study revealed how a simple text message, SMS, or electronic mail was able to improve the appointments management, not only for the hospital but also for the patient itself. On one hand, an alert for the patient could avoid him to miss an appointment that might have taken several months to schedule, depending on the waiting list. On the other hand, by having knowledge about the patient's intention to attend the appointment or not, the hospital can avoid several inconveniences and try to re-schedule a new appointment taking into consideration its own needs and workflow. Thus, the hospital can benefit from an improved management of both staff and physical space. The clinicians can fulfill their work schedule without any blank spaces or interruptions, which allows for a better use of resources that are essential in a healthcare system.

In this manner, by providing a new communication link between the hospital and the patient, IS allow to create a solid relationship between the two entities based on trust. Given the increasing number of cellphones and use of electronic mail in the population, this becomes practically a mandatory procedure within healthcare units. It is then clear that simple and effective procedures conducted by HIS can in fact help redefine the unit/patient dynamics. The usage of Open Source software enables not only the reduction of the total cost-of-ownership, but also increases the security and eliminates the vendor lock-in of systems. Following the guidelines of Open Source software AASYS provided a new level of interoperability and this was achieved having in mind not only the costs of implementation but also patient needs. Finally the last outcome a management and maintenance tool for preventive actions of servers and clients inside the healthcare unit. As mentioned before, the access to information is a crucial aspect and IT experts must paid special attention when dealing with information integrity and availability. A starting point is to make sure that the information is in fact available at any time, everywhere and to any user that needs and has permissions to see it. This is usually guaranteed by systems with high availability, i.e., ensure that information access is not compromised, which can be done by improving uptimes and reducing the number of interventions or non-programmed stops of servers. ScheduleIT is a systems management tool that allows to program preventive actions through an alert interface, available not only for the IT specialists, but also for further users that will be informed about the programmed stops that will take place in specific time intervals. Due to high number of users that will be affected by the stop time of a given server, it is necessary to carefully schedule these programmed stops. It is required to estimate the best time of the day, the best day of the week and the best interval to execute preventive actions on servers in order to guaranteed their optimal performance. ScheduleIT already covers more than 75% of the servers inside CHTS and its usage has been extremely important for the institution, with good results in reducing the number of non-programmed stops. By providing mechanisms that deal with sensitive and complex areas of IS in healthcare and that are aware of IT specialists and user needs, the ScheduleIT platform not only is an effective management tool, but also promotes a self-reliance environment among the existing systems. ScheduleIT is an example of an application module that can be added to AIDA. Showing the scalability, manageability and performance of AIDA, this is maintained when adding application modules.

The main outcome of this work is the improvement of the platform AIDA - Agency for Integration, Diffusion and Archive. The main focus was the necessity for data share and exchange procedures with improved quality. As the need for more information grows it becomes imperative that new implementations are developed, especially in healthcare area. Basically, AIDA intends to serve the main necessities and requirements presented along this thesis. Unlike the previous studies, it does not focus on one single aspect of actuation, but instead it provides formulation of standards and workflows essential to build a healthcare unit with quality and financially viable and sustainable.

The AIDA platform revealed excellent results when dealing and managing the information from different sources, ranging from laboratory results to medical images and even when integrating results from external providers. One of the main challenges was to provide to the clinicians the requested information to help them to decide at the exact moment they need. To do this, the platform uses intelligent agents that deal with requests and ensure the information is provided to the right user, with integrity and when it is asked. This allows reducing the waiting times for results, either when diagnosing or during an appointment, since the information that once was dispersed is now integrated and managed by the platform. Although the concept and principles behind the platform functioning seem trivial, its implementation is in fact more complex, especially when working within a healthcare unit environment. It is necessary to formulate new definitions, introduce user permissions, adequate services so that the global system workflow is not compromised. Through artificial intelligence and web-services it is possible to present the requested information using a web user interface, parameterized, friendly and easy-to-use that allows data visualization as quick as possible. AIDA is a central part of this work. Without AIDA, it will be impossible to have a testing and working platform to enhance this work. AIDA has proved its strength to solve interoperability problems in real world environment and this paper is the most important description of AIDA, being edited by Springer under the well-known series of Lectures Notes in Computer Science.

FUTURE RESEARCH DIRECTIONS

During this work new questions arose and sometimes it can lead to the definition of new paths for research and new states of knowledge that could reveal to be extremely relevant for future work.

It is obvious that there is still a long way to scout before reaching a complete interoperability of Health Information Systems. New methodologies and procedures arise every day, but it urges the formulation of standards so that the investigation does not diverge to less important areas for both users and patients. In this manner, and taking into account the country where this investigation took place, Portugal, it is urgent to adopt new measures, whether by the government authorities or by the healthcare units themselves, working together or individually, in order to pursue solutions for the problems arising every day. HIS specialist should promote the contact between new software tools and the users that will benefit from them. The reality shows that existing procedures are many times confuse or simply inaccessible to the users; it is necessary to create tools, such as websites with forums and blogs or simple white papers distribution, that can stimulate this communion and that boost the pursuit of a healthcare system with higher quality. A simple task that needs to be performed is the elaboration of a document that clearly identifies, resumes and explains the standards followed by healthcare units in agreement with their external partners. In that way, it would be possible to create a national platform that managed standards according to the principles established by the European Union, so that an interaction and cooperation between the healthcare units among the European members could be promoted. The implementation of such a platform could be done in phases, with an increasing number of participating healthcare units.

CONCLUSION

A research work must be seen above all as an important tool to discover new methodologies and techniques to reach pre-determined objectives and to truly bring innovation to improve a service or procedure. Nonetheless, during this work new questions arise and sometimes it can lead to the definition of new paths for research and new states of knowledge that could reveal to be extremely relevant for future work.

Throughout this work, four main questions revealed fundamental as guiding lines for the proposed work, which are related with HIS and its implementation costs, the strategies to achieve interoperability among systems and finally the strengthener of the relation between the patient and the healthcare unit. The exhaustive research on existing projects inside and outside the European Community allowed to better understand the current strategies and methodologies applied at healthcare units to overcome some of the difficulties presented every day. All these projects were supervised by either the European Commission or governmental institutions and indicated that HIS, Quality of Information, Interoperability and EHR are major concerns for world leaders, and that patients and physicians have their needs more exposed than ever. To give answers to the questions mentioned above, four studies were conducted at a regional health care facility. The Electronic Semantic Health Record, showed that semantic is indeed the path to be adopted since it plays a fundamental role for the continuous improvement on HIS. Semantic is a computational paradigm that allows the interoperability, computing and intelligent communication between systems in order to improve the quality of the information available to the users. By promoting a global and intuitive view of the information sources to the user, without the need to skip between applications, the waiting times and the quality of the patient diagnosis can become significantly improved. A better patient-hospital relationship was enhanced by the AASYS system. This system is an alert appointment system based on open-source software that sends to the patient's text messages and electronic mails. AASYS allowed to improve show rates at the healthcare facility, promoting a more effective scheduling of appointments and a better use of human and physical resources, and consequently a reduction of costs. Although it is still on an initial phase of implementation, this system has means to evolve to an end-to-end communication allowing patients to contact the care provider via text message or electronic mail. An open-source platform for preventive actions management was also presented, called ScheduleIT. Preventive actions promote more reliable systems and increase the confidence that users have on the systems that they use every day.

In addition, by using open-source software not only the implementation costs are diminished as also other institutions promoting the sharing and continuously improvement of the software itself can use the platform. ScheduleIT has proved to be an important tool to prevent non-programmed stops. Finally, a platform that manages and integrates the information that emerges from heterogeneous sources inside the hospital was presented. This platform was named AIDA and, as the name says, it is an Agency of Integration, Diffusion and Archive of information that provides the users all the data they need to perform their clinical practice. It is today one of the main tools inside a healthcare unit regarding systems interoperability, artificial and ambient intelligence and intelligent agents. All the implementations mentioned above contribute to make CHTS one of the leading Portuguese hospitals in the area of interoperability and healthcare with quality of services.

REFERENCES

W3C. (2010). *World Wide Web Consortium*. Retrieved from World Wide Web Consortium. Retrieved from http://www.w3.org/

Abelha, A., Machado, J., Santos, M., Allegro, S., & Paiva, M. (2002). Agency for integration, diffusion and archive of medical information. *Proceedings of the Third IASTED International Conference - Artificial Intelligence and Applications*. IASTED International Conference.

Berger, S., & Ciotti, G. (1993). HIS (healthcare information systems) consultants: when are they necessary, and why? *Health Finance Management*, 47(6), 44-49.

Currie, G., & Procter, S. (2002). Impact of MIS/IT upon middle managers: Some evidence from the NHS. *New Technology, Work and Employment*, *17*(2), 102–118. doi:10.1111/1468-005X.00097

Delone, W., & McLean, E. (2003). The DeLone and McLean Model of Information Systems Success: A Ten-Year Update. *Journal of Management Information Systems, 19(4), 9-30*.

Graybeal, J. (2009). *Achieving semantic interoperability*.

Helfenbein, S. (1987). *Technologies for management information systems in primary health care*.

Hersh, W. (2002). Medical informatics: Improving health care through information. *Journal of the American Medical Association*, *288*(16), 1955–1958. doi:10.1001/jama.288.16.1955 PMID:12387634

Hurtubise, R. (1984). *Managing information systems: concepts and tools*.

Kivinena, T., & Lammintakanen, J. (2012). The success of a management information system in health care - a case study from Finland. *International Journal of Medical Informatics*.

von Krogh, G., & vonHippel, E. (2006). The promise of research on open source software. *Management Science*, *52*(7), 975–983. doi:10.1287/mnsc.1060.0560

Langefors, B. (1975). *Information Systems Architecture*.

MeSH. (1987). *Medical subject headings - health information systems*. Retrieved from Medical subject headings - health information systems. Retrieved from http://www.ncbi.nlm.nih.gov/mesh/68006751

Miranda, M., Duarte, J., Abelha, A., Machado, J., & Neves, J. (2009). Interoperability and healthcare. *Proceedings of the European Simulation and Modelling Conference* (pp. 205-212). EUROSIS.

Murray, P., Wright, G., Karopka, T., Betts, H., & Orel, A. (2009). Open source and healthcare in europe - time to put leading edge ideas into practice. Medical Informatics in a United and Healthy Europe (pp. 963-967).

OpenEHR. (2007). *OpenEHR Fundation.* Retrieved from http://www.openehr.org/

Peixoto, H., Machado, J., Abelha, A., & Neves, J. (2010). Semantic Interoperability and Health Records. Em S. Boston, IFIP Advances in Information and Communication Technology (pp. 236-237). Springer Boston. doi:10.1007/978-3-642-15515-4_30

Peixoto, H., Machado, J., Abelha, A., & Santos, M. (2012). *Intelligence in interoperability with AIDA.* Springer. doi:10.1007/978-3-642-34624-8_31

RedHat. (2007). *RedHAT.* Retrieved from Open-Source and Healthcare IT: http://www.redhat.com/f/pdf/OSHealthcareWhitepaper web.pdf

Silverstein, S. (1999). *What is medical informatics, and why is it an important specialty?* Retrieved from http://www.ischool.drexel.edu/faculty/ssilverstein/informaticsmd/infordef1.htm

Sullivan. (2009). *Overview of global economy.*

KEY TERMS AND DEFINITIONS

Electronic Health Record (EHR): Electronic Health Record EHR means a repository of patient data in digital form, stored and exchanged securely, and accessible by multiple authorized users.

Healthcare Information Systems (HIS): Integrated computer-assisted systems to store, manipulate, and retrieve healthcare administrative and clinical data.

Information Systems (IS): A technologically implemented medium for recording, storing, and disseminating linguistic expressions, as well as for drawing conclusions from such expressions.

Interoperability: A mean to achieve a goal, in the case of our industry, to advance the effective delivery of healthcare.

Open-Source Software: Software that can be modified and shared between individuals and institutions without costs.

Chapter 2
Evaluation of Nosocomial Infection Risk Using a Hybrid Approach

José Neves
Universidade do Minho, Portugal

João Neves
Drs. Nicolas & Asp, UAE

Eva Silva
Universidade do Minho, Portugal

Henrique Vicente
Universidade de Évora, Portugal

ABSTRACT

Nosocomial infections have severe consequences for the patients and the society in general, being one of the causes that increase the length of stay in healthcare facilities. Therefore, it is of utmost importance to be preventive, being aware of how probable is to have that kind of infection, although it is hard to do with traditional methodologies and tools for problem solving. Therefore, this work will focus on the development of a decision support system that will cater for an individual risk evaluation tool with respect to catch nosocomial infections. The Knowledge Representation and Reasoning procedures used will be based on an extension to the Logic Programming language, allowing the handling of incomplete and/or default data. The computational framework in place will be centered on Artificial Neural Networks. It may be emphasized that in addition to the nosocomial infections risk evaluation, it is provided the Degree-of-Confidence that one has on such a happening.

DOI: 10.4018/978-1-4666-9882-6.ch002

INTRODUCTION

Nosocomial infections are contagions that have been caught in a hospital and are hypothetically caused by organisms that may be resilient to antibiotics. A nosocomial infection is specifically one that was not present or incubating prior to the patient's being declared to the hospital, but occurring within 72 hours after admittance, 30 days after surgery or for 3 days after discharge (Inweregbu, Dave, & Pittard, 2005; Rigor, Machado, Abelha, Neves, & Alberto, 2008; World Health Organization [WHO], 2011). According to the World Health Organization (2011), in developing countries, 10% of the hospitalized patients contract a nosocomial infection, while for developed countries this rate is about 7%. Moreover, each year more than 4 million patients are affected by nosocomial taints in Europe and 1.7 million in the USA. It must be also stated that inside Intensive Care Units there is a higher probability of occurrence of nosocomial infections, not only owing to the immune status of patients admitted but also due to the invasive procedures in place.

From an economic point of view, a patient with an infection acquired in the hospital stays longer in the healthcare facility, and may need to be readmitted, resulting in additional costs to the organization (Damani, 2003; Inweregbu et al., 2005; Rigor et al., 2008), i.e., on the one hand, nosocomial infections has much impact on mortality and morbidity of patients in a healthcare facility, on the other hand, these infections are a very important indicator to evaluate the quality of care. Consequently, its control and prevention are essential, allowing for cost savings, reducing the risk of infection as well as cutting the discomfort and suffering of patients.

According to Inweregbu et al. (2005), about one third of nosocomial infections can be prevented and controlled through the implementation of appropriate control and prevention procedures. In addition, the healthcare organizations must monitor the results of such programs through the periodic data collection and by the analysis of specific indicators. These indicators are parameters that make possible the characterization of the problem like the rate of nosocomial infection. The analysis of these factors allow the identification of critical activities and/or processes within of the hospital environment, clinical specialties where the implementation of measures is essential to ensure the safety and welfare of patients, priority areas where measures should be implemented urgently. Thus, it is possible to plan and implement targeted and efficient programs to reduce the incidence rate of nosocomial infection and increase the quality of care.

There are several factors that contribute to Nosocomial Infection Predisposing (NIP), namely the age and the immune status of the patient, the length of stay in the healthcare facility, the undergone medical procedures, the use of antibiotics, the diagnostics used, i.e., the hospital also has many infection foci, objects and/or environments in which microorganisms can survive or multiply, such as facilities, invasive devices or equipment used. Indeed, patients, health professionals and visitors can be a vehicle to spread the infectious agents (Damani, 2003; 2005; Rigor et al., 2008). Thus, any inaccuracies in the monitoring and in the prevention of infection combined with a weakened immune status of the patient, can easily lead to a nosocomial infection (Damani, 2003). The factors behind this kind of disease can be grouped in five main generic groups, namely patient information, hospital related factors, treatment related factors, intrinsic risk factors and extrinsic risk factors, as it is illustrated in Figure 1.

The patient information comprises age, gender, admission and discharge dates. The hospital related factors include surveillance methods, prevention strategies and treatment programs. Surveillance is the ongoing, systematic collection, analysis and interpretation of information related to nosocomial infections. It is crucial for the planning, implementation and evaluation of the procedures and also enhance the sharing of knowledge, information and experience between the health professionals. The treatment related factors are associated with blood transfusions, recent antimicrobial therapy, immunosuppressive treatments, recent use of corticosteroids and stress-ulcer prophylaxis. The intrinsic risk factors comprise malnutrition, alcoholism, smoking, chronic liver disease, chronic lung disease, diabetes, transplants, immunodeficiency and dysphasia. Finally, the extrinsic risk factors are linked with the use of invasive devices like endotracheal intubation, central venous catheterization, urinary catheter, extracorporeal renal support, surgical drains, nasogastric tube and tracheotomy.

Figure 1. Relevant aspects in nosocomial infections

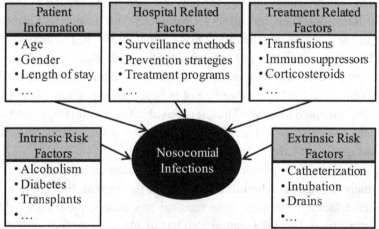

Solving problems related to NIP requires a proactive strategy. However, the stated above shows that the NIP assessment should be correlated with many variables and require a multidisciplinary approach. Thus, it is difficult to assess to the NIP since it needs to consider different conditions with intricate relations among them, where the available data may be incomplete, contradictory and/or unknown. In order to overcome these drawbacks, the present work reports the founding of a computational framework that uses knowledge representation and reasoning techniques to set the structure of the information and the associate inference mechanisms, i.e., we will centre on a Logic Programming (LP) based approach to knowledge representation and reasoning (Neves, 1984; Neves, Machado, Analide, Abelha, & Brito, 2007), and look at a hybrid computing approach to data processing based on Artificial Neural Networks (ANNs) (Cortez, Rocha, & Neves, 2004).

This chapter is organized into five sections. In the former one an introduction to the problem presented is made. Then the proposed approach to knowledge representation and reasoning is introduced. In the third and fourth sections is introduced a case study and presented a solution to the problem. Finally, in the last section the most relevant conclusions are described and the possible directions for future work are outlined.

KNOWLEDGE REPRESENTATION AND REASONING

Many approaches for knowledge representation and reasoning have been proposed using *Logic Programming* (*LP*), namely in the area of Model Theory (Gelfon & Lifschitz, 1988; Kakas, Kowalski, & Toni, 1998; Pereira & Anh, 2009) and Proof Theory (Neves, 1984; Neves et al., 2007). In this work it is followed the proof theoretical approach in terms of an extension to the *LP* language to knowledge representation and reasoning. An *Extended Logic Program* (*ELP*) is a finite set of clauses in the form:

{

$$p \leftarrow p_1, \ldots, p_n, not\ q_1, \ldots, not\ q_m$$

$$?\left(p_1, \ldots, p_n, not\ q_1, \ldots, not\ q_m\right)\ \left(n, m \geq 0\right)$$

$$exception_{p_1}$$

...

$$exception_{p_j} \; (j \leq m, n)$$

$$\} :: scoring_{value}$$

where "*?*" is a domain atom denoting falsity, the p_j, q_j, and p are classical ground literals, i.e., either positive atoms or atoms preceded by the classical negation sign ¬ (Neves, 1984). Under this formalism, every program is associated with a set of abducibles (Kakas et al., 1998; Pereira & Anh, 2009) given here in the form of exceptions to the extensions of the predicates that make the program. The term *scoring*$_{value}$ stands for the relative weight of the extension of a specific *predicate* with respect to the extensions of the peers ones that make the overall program.

In order to evaluate the knowledge that stems from a logic program, an evaluation of the *Quality-of-Information (QoI)* was set in dynamic environments aiming at decision-making purposes (Lucas, 2004; Machado, Abelha, Novais, & Neves, 2010).

The *QoI* with respect to the extension of a *predicate*$_i$ will be given by a truth-value in the interval [0, 1], i.e., if the information is *known* (*positive*) or *false* (*negative*) the *QoI* for the extension of *predicate*$_i$ is 1. For situations where the information is unknown, the *QoI* is given by:

$$QoI_i = \lim_{N \to \infty} \frac{1}{N} = 0 \; (N >> 0)$$

where N denotes the cardinality of the set of terms or clauses of the extension of *predicate*$_i$ that stand for the incompleteness under consideration. For situations where the extension of *predicate*$_i$ is unknown but can be taken from a set of values, the *QoI* is given by:

$$QoI_i = \frac{1}{Card}$$

where *Card* denotes the cardinality of the *abducibles* set for i, if the *abducibles* set is disjoint. If the *abducibles* set is not disjoint, the *QoI* is given by:

$$QoI_i = \frac{1}{C_1^{Card} + \cdots + C_{Card}^{Card}}$$

where C_{Card}^{Card} is a card-combination subset, with *Card* elements.

The next element of the model to be considered is the relative importance that a predicate assigns to each of its attributes under observation, i.e., w_i^k, which stands for the relevance of attribute k in the extension of *predicate$_i$*. It is also assumed that the weights of all the attribute predicates are normalized, i.e.:

$$\sum_{1 \leq k \leq n} w_i^k = 1, \ \forall_i$$

where $\forall$ denotes the universal quantifier. It is now possible to define a predicate's scoring function $V_i(x)$ so that, for a value $x = x_1, \ldots, x_n$, defined in terms of the attributes of *predicate$_i$*, one may have:

$$V_i(x) = \sum_{1 \leq k \leq n} w_i^k * QoI_i(x) / n$$

allowing one to set:

$$predicate_i(x_1, \ldots, x_n) :: V_i(x)$$

that denotes the inclusive quality of *predicate$_i$* with respect to all the predicates that make the program. It is now possible to set a logic program (here understood as the predicates' extensions that make the program) scoring function, in the form:

$$LP_{Scoring \ Function} = \sum_{i=1}^{n} V_i(x) * p_i$$

where p_i stands for the relevance of the *predicate$_i$* in relation to the other predicates whose extensions denote the logic program. It is also assumed that the weights of all the predicates' extensions are normalized, i.e.:

$$\sum_{i=1}^{n} p_i = 1, \ \forall_i$$

It is now possible to engender the universe of discourse, according to the information given in the logic programs that endorse the information about the problem under consideration, according to productions of the type:

$$extensions - of - predicate_i = \bigcup_{1 \le j \le m} clause_j \left(x_1, \ldots, x_n \right) :: QoI :: DoC$$

where $\bigcup$ and m stand, respectively, for set union and the cardinality of the extension of $predicate_i$. DoC_i stands for an assessment of $attribute_i$ with respect to the terms that make the extension of $predicate_i$, i.e., it denotes a measure of one's confidence that the attribute value fits into a given interval, whose boundaries are evaluated in a way that takes into consideration its domain (Neves et al., 2015).

Assuming that a clause denotes a happening, a clause has as argument all the attributes that make the event. The argument values may be of the type unknown or members of a set, or may be in the scope of a given interval, or may qualify a particular observation. Let us consider that the case data is given by the extension of predicate f_1, in the form:

$$f_1 : x_1, x_2, x_3 \rightarrow \{0,1\}$$

where "*{*" and "*}*" is one´s notation for sets, and "0" and "1" denote, respectively, the truth values *false* and *true*.

Taking into account the following clause where the former argument stands for itself, with a domain that ranges in the interval [0, 5], the value of the second one may fit into the interval [5, 7.5] with a domain that ranges in the interval [2.5, 10], and the value of the last one is unknown, being represented by the symbol $\perp$, with a domain that ranges in the interval [0, 8]. Therefore, one may have:

{

$$\neg\, f_1(x_1, x_2, x_3) \leftarrow not\ f_1(x_1, x_2, x_3)$$

$$f_1(\underbrace{2,\quad [5, 7.5],\quad \perp}_{attribute´s\ values\ for\ x_1, x_2, x_3}) :: 1 :: DoC$$

$$\underbrace{[0,\ 5]\ [2.5,\ 10]\ [0,\ 8]}_{attribute´s\ domains\ for\ x_1, x_2, x_3}$$

} :: 1

In this program, the first clause denotes the closure of *predicate* f_1. Once the clauses or terms of the extension of the predicate are established, the next step is to set all the arguments, of each clause, into continuous intervals. In this phase, it is essential to consider the domain of the arguments. As the third argument is unknown, its interval will cover all the possibilities of the domain. The first argument speaks for itself. Therefore, one may have:

{

$$\neg f_1(x_1, x_2, x_3) \leftarrow not\ f_1(x_1, x_2, x_3)$$

$$f_1(\underbrace{[2,\ 2],\quad [5,\ 7.5],\quad [0,\ 8]}_{attribute's\ values\ ranges\ for\ x_1, x_2, x_3}) :: 1 :: DoC$$
$$\underbrace{[0,\ 5]\quad [2.5,\ 10]\quad [0,\ 8]}_{attribute's\ domains\ for\ x_1, x_2, x_3}$$

}::1

It is now achievable to calculate the *Degree of Confidence* (*DoC*) for each attribute that make the term argument (e.g. with respect to the second attribute it denotes one's confidence that the attribute under consideration fits into the interval [5, 7.5]). Next, we set the boundaries of the arguments intervals to be fitted in the interval [0, 1] according to a normalization procedure given by $\left(Y - Y_{min}\right) / \left(Y_{max} - Y_{min}\right)$, where the Y_s stand for themselves. One may have:

{

$$\neg f_1(x_1, x_2, x_3) \leftarrow not\ f_1(x_1, x_2, x_3)$$

$$x_1 = \left[\frac{2-0}{5-0},\ \frac{2-0}{5-0}\right],\ x_2 = \left[\frac{5-2.5}{10-2.5},\ \frac{7.5-2.5}{10-2.5}\right],\ x_3 = \left[\frac{0-0}{8-0},\ \frac{8-0}{8-0}\right]$$
$$f_1(\underbrace{[0.4,\ 0.4],\quad [0.33,\ 0.67],\quad [0,\ 1]}_{attribute's\ values\ ranges\ for\ x_1, x_2, x_3\ once\ normalized}) :: 1 :: DoC$$
$$\underbrace{[0,\ 1]\qquad [0,\ 1]\qquad [0,\ 1]}_{attribute's\ domains\ for\ x_1, x_2, x_3\ once\ normalized}$$

}::1

The *Degree of Confidence (DoC)* is evaluated using the *Pitagoras* theorem, $DoC = \sqrt{1 + \Delta l^2}$, as illustrated in Figure 2. Here Δl stands for the length of the arguments intervals, once normalized.

Below, one has the expected representation of the extensions of the predicates that make the universe of discourse, where all the predicates' arguments are real numbers. They speak for one's confidence that the real values of the arguments fit into the attributes' values ranges referred to above. Therefore, one may have:

{

$$\neg f_1(x_1, x_2, x_3) \leftarrow not\ f_1(x_1, x_2, x_3)$$

$$f_1(\underbrace{1, \qquad\qquad 0.94, \qquad\qquad 0)}_{attribute's\ confidence\ values\ for\ x_1, x_2, x_3} :: 1 :: 0.65$$

$$\underbrace{[0.4,\ 0.4]\quad [0.33,\ 0.67]\quad [0,\ 1]}_{attribute's\ values\ ranges\ for\ x_1, x_2, x_3\ once\ normalized}$$

$$\underbrace{[0,\ 1]\qquad\qquad [0,\ 1]\qquad\qquad [0,\ 1]}_{attribute's\ domains\ for\ x_1, x_2, x_3\ once\ normalized}$$

} :: 1

where the *DoC's* for $f_1(1, 0.94, 0)$ is evaluated as $(1+0.94+0)/3 = 0.65$, assuming that all the argument's attributes have the same weight.

According to what was referred to above, it is possible to point out a normalization algorithm, which takes the form shown in Algorithm 1.

Figure 2. Evaluation of the degree of confidence

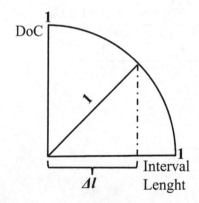

Algorithm 1.

```
Begin,
The predicate's extensions that make the Universe-of-Discourse
are set ←
{
```

$$\neg\, f_1(x_1, x_2, x_3) \leftarrow not\ f_1(x_1, x_2, x_3)$$
$$f_1(\underbrace{2, \quad [5, 7.5], \quad \bot}) :: 1 :: DoC$$
$$\text{\scriptsize attribute's values for } x_1, x_2, x_3$$

$$\underbrace{[0,\ 5]\ [2.5,\ 10]\ [0,\ 8]}$$
$$\text{\scriptsize attribute's domains for } x_1, x_2, x_3$$

```
}  :: 1
The attribute's values ranges are rewritten ←
{
```

$$\neg f_1(x_1, x_2, x_3) \leftarrow not\, f_1(x_1, x_2, x_3)$$
$$f_1(\underbrace{[2,\ 2],\quad [5,\ 7.5],\quad [0,\ 8]}) :: 1 :: DoC$$
$$\text{\scriptsize attribute's values ranges for } x_1, x_2, x_3$$

$$\underbrace{[0,\ 5]\quad [2.5,\ 10]\quad [0,\ 8]}$$
$$\text{\scriptsize attribute's domains for } x_1, x_2, x_3$$

```
}  :: 1
The attribute's boundaries are set to the interval [0, 1] ←
{
```

$$\neg\, f_1(x_1, x_2, x_3) \leftarrow not\ f_1(x_1, x_2, x_3)$$
$$f_1(\underbrace{\ [0.4,\ 0.4],\ [0.33,\ 0.67],\ [0,\ 1]\ }) :: 1 :: DoC$$
$$\text{\scriptsize attribute's values ranges for } x_1, x_2, x_3 \text{ once normalized}$$

$$\underbrace{[0,\ 1]\qquad\quad [0,\ 1]\qquad\quad [0,\ 1]}$$
$$\text{\scriptsize attribute's domains for } x_1, x_2, x_3 \text{ once normalized}$$

```
}  :: 1
The DoC's values are evaluated ←
{
```

$$\neg\, f_1(x_1, x_2, x_3) \leftarrow not\, f_1(x_1, x_2, x_3)$$
$$f_1(\underbrace{1, \qquad\qquad 0.94, \qquad\qquad 0}) :: 1 :: 0.65$$
$$\text{\scriptsize attribute's confidence values for } x_1, x_2, x_3$$

$$\underbrace{[0.4,\ 0.4]\quad [0.33,\ 0.67]\quad [0,\ 1]}$$
$$\text{\scriptsize attribute's values ranges for } x_1, x_2, x_3 \text{ once normalized}$$

$$\underbrace{[0,\ 1]\qquad\quad [0,\ 1]\qquad\quad [0,\ 1]}$$
$$\text{\scriptsize attribute's domains for } x_1, x_2, x_3 \text{ once normalized}$$

```
}  :: 1
End.
```

A CASE STUDY

As a case study, consider a database given in terms of the extensions of the relations (or tables) depicted in Figure 3, which stands for a situation where one has to manage information about nosocomial infection risk detection. Under this scenario some incomplete and/or unknown data is also available. For instance, in case 1, the *Hospital Related Factors* are unknown, while the *Intrinsic Risk Factors* range in the interval [2, 3].

The *Treatment Related Factors* and *Intrinsic/Extrinsic Risk Factors* tables are filled with 0 (zero) and 1 (one) denoting, respectively, *absence/no* or *presence/yes*.

Figure 3. An extension of the relational model

Intrinsic Risk Factors								
#	Alcoholism	Smoking	Malnutrition	Chronic Lung Disease	Chronic Liver Disease	Diabetes	Transplants	Immuno-deficiency	Dysphasia
1	$\perp$	0	0	0	0	1	1	0	0
...	...	...	...	...	...	...	...	...	...
n	0	0	0	0	0	0	0	0	0

Patient Information				
#	Age	Gender	Admission Date	Discharge Date
1	69	M	2013/11/04	2013/12/06
...	...	...	...	...
n	45	F	2013/10/16	2013/11/04

Hospital Related Factors				
#	Surveillance Methods	Prevention Strategies	Treatment Programs	Bed Occupancy Rate
1	$\perp$	$\perp$	$\perp$	$\perp$
...	...	...	...	...
n	$\perp$	$\perp$	$\perp$	2

Nosocomial Infection							
#	Age	Gender	Length of Stay	Hospital Related Factors	Treatment Related Factors	Intrinsic Risk Factors	Extrinsic Risk Factors
1	69	1	32	$\perp$	1	[2, 3]	2
...	...	...	...	...	...	...	...
n	45	0	17	[1, 5]	0	0	2

Treatment Related Factors					
#	Blood Transfusions	Antimicrobial Therapy	Immunosuppressive Treatments	Use of Corticosteroids	Stress-ulcer Prophylaxis
1	1	0	0	0	0
...	...	...	...	...	...
n	0	0	0	0	0

Extrinsic Risk Factors								
#	Endotracheal Intubation	Central Venous Catheter	Peripheral Venous Catheter	Urinary Catheter	Extracorporeal Renal Support	Surgical Drains	Nasogastric Tube	Tracheotomy
1	0	0	1	1	0	0	0	0
...	...	...	...	...	...	...	...	...
n	0	0	1	0	0	1	0	0

The first three columns of the *Hospital Related Factors* tables are also populated with 0 (zero) and 1 (one) denoting, respectively, *absence/no* or *presence/yes*. The last column, in turns, is populated with 0 (zero), one (1) or two (2) according to the Bed Occupancy Rate (BOR). Thus, 0 (zero) denotes BOR < 70%; 1 (one) stands for a BOR ranging in interval [70, 85]; and 2 (two) denotes a BOR > 85%. The values presented in the *Hospital/Treatment Related Factors* and *Intrinsic/Extrinsic Risk Factors* columns of *Nosocomial Infection* table are the sum of the correspondent tables, ranging between [0, 5] [0, 5], [0, 9] and [0, 8], respectively. The *Length of Stay* was computed based on *Admission* and *Discharge Date*, while in the *Gender* column of *Nosocomial Infection* table 0 (zero) and 1 (one) stand, respectively, for *female (F)* and *male (M)*.

Now, we may consider the relations given in Figure 3, in terms of a *noso_infec* predicate, depicted in the form:

$$noso\_infect : Age, \; Gen_{der}, \; L_{enght} \; o_f \; S_{tay}, \; H_{ospital} \; R_{elated} \; F_{actors}, \; T_{reatment} \; R_{elated} \; F_{actors},$$
$$I_{ntrinsic} \; R_{isk} \; F_{actors}, \; E_{xtrinsic} \; R_{isk} \; F_{actors} \rightarrow \{0, \; 1\}$$

where *noso_infect* stands for the *predicate nosocomial infection*, 0 (zero) and 1 (one) denote, respectively, the truth values *false* and *true*. Its extension makes the training and test sets of the Artificial Neural Network given in Figure 4. Then, having a patient that presents the feature vector (76, 0, 56, $\perp$, 2, [4, 5], 2), and applying the procedure referred to above, one may get Algorithm 2.

ARTIFICIAL NEURAL NETWORKS

The previously presented model of nosocomial infection risk works well and demonstrate how all the information comes together to form a diagnosis. In this section, a data mining approach to deal with this information is considered. It was set a hybrid computing approach to model the universe of discourse, based on *Artificial Neural Networks* (*ANNs*), which are used to structure data and capture complex relationships between inputs and outputs (Vicente, Couto, Machado, Abelha, & Neves, 2012; Vicente et al., 2012; Vicente, Roseiro, Arteiro, Neves, & Caldeira, 2013). *ANNs* simulate the structure of the human brain, being populated by multiple layers of neurons, with a valuable set of activation functions. As an example, let us consider the case given above, where one may have a situation in which the assessment to nosocomial infection risk is needed. In Figure 4 it is shown how the normalized values of the interval boundaries and their *DoC* and *QoI* values work as inputs to the *ANN*. The output depicts an assessment of the nosocomial infection risk, plus the confidence that one has on such a happening.

Figure 4. The Artificial Neural Network topology

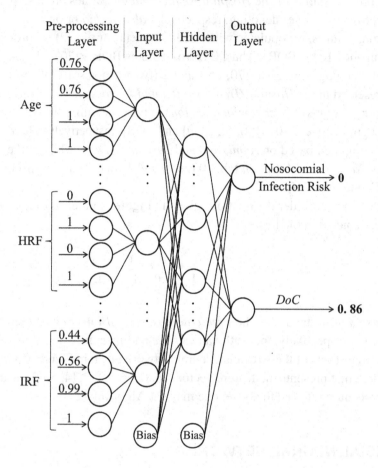

Algorithm 2.

```
Begin,
The predicate's extensions that make the Universe-of-Discourse
are set ←
{
```

$$\neg\, noso\_infect(Age, Gen, LoS, HRF, TRF, IRF, ERF)$$

$$\leftarrow not\; noso\_infect(Age, Gen, LoS, HRF, TRF, IRF, ERF)$$

$$noso\_infect(\underbrace{76,\qquad 0,\qquad 56,\qquad \bot,\qquad 2,\qquad [4,\ 5],\qquad 2}_{attribute's\ values}) :: 1 :: DoC$$

$$\underbrace{[24,\ 92]\ [0,\ 1]\ [2,\ 62]\ [0,\ 5]\ [0,\ 5]\ [0,\ 9]\ [0,\ 8]}_{attribute's\ domains}$$

continued on following page

Algorithm 2. Continued

} :: 1
The attribute's values ranges are rewritten ←
{

$\neg\ noso\_infect(Age, Gen, LoS, HRF, TRF, IRF, ERF)$
        $\leftarrow not\ noso\_infect(Age, Gen, LoS, HRF, TRF, IRF, ERF)$

$noso\_infect(\underbrace{[76,\ 76],\ [0,\ 0],\ [56,\ 56],\ [0,\ 5],\ [2,\ 2],\ [4,\ 5],\ [2,\ 2]}_{attribute's\ values\ ranges}) :: 1 :: DoC$
$\underbrace{[24,\ 92]\quad [0,\ 1]\quad [2,\ 62]\quad [0,\ 5]\quad [0,\ 5]\quad [0,\ 9]\quad [0,\ 8]}_{attribute's\ domains}$

} :: 1
The attribute's boundaries are set to the interval [0, 1] ←
{

$\neg\ noso\_infect(Age, Gen, LoS, HRF, TRF, IRF, ERF)$
        $\leftarrow not\ noso\_infect(Age, Gen, LoS, HRF, TRF, IRF, ERF)$

$noso\_infect(\underbrace{[0.76, 0.76],\ [0,0],\ [0.9, 0.9],\ [0,1],\ [0.4,\ 0.4],\ [0.44, 0.56],\ [0.25, 0.25]}_{attribute's\ values\ ranges\ once\ normalized}) :: 1 :: DoC$
$\underbrace{[0,\ 1]\quad\quad [0,\ 1]\quad\quad [0,\ 1]\quad\quad [0,\ 1]\quad\quad [0,\ 1]\quad\quad\quad [0,\ 1]\quad\quad\quad [0,\ 1]}_{attribute's\ domains\ once\ normalized}$

} :: 1
The DoC's values are evaluated ←
{

$\neg\ noso\_infect(Age, Gen, LoS, HRF, TRF, IRF, ERF)$
        $\leftarrow not\ noso\_infect(Age, Gen, LoS, HRF, TRF, IRF, ERF)$

$noso\_infect(\underbrace{[1,\quad\quad 1,\quad\quad 1,\quad\quad 0,\quad\quad 1,\quad\quad 0.99,\quad\quad 1]}_{attribute's\ confidence\ values}) :: 1 :: 0.86$

$\underbrace{[0.76,\ 0.76]\ [0,\ 0]\ [0.9,\ 0.9]\ [0,\ 1]\ [0.4,\ 0.4]\ [0.44,\ 0.56]\ [0.25,\ 0.25]}_{attribute's\ values\ ranges\ once\ normalized}$

$\underbrace{[0,\ 1]\quad\quad [0,\ 1]\quad [0,\ 1]\quad\quad [0,\ 1]\quad [0,\ 1]\quad\quad [0,\ 1]\quad\quad\quad [0,\ 1]}_{attribute's\ domains\ once\ normalized}$

} :: 1
End.

In this study 1669 patients were considered with an age average of 68.4 years, ranging from 24 to 92 years old. The nosocomial infection was diagnosed in 173 cases, i.e., in 10.4% of the analysed population. The gender distribution was 46.8% and 53.2% for female and male, respectively. The average of length of stay was 19.8 days, ranging between 2 and 62 days.

The dataset holds information about risk factors considered critical in the prediction of nosocomial infection risk. Twenty five variables were selected allowing one to have a multivariable dataset with 1669 records. Figure 5 shows the distribution of the *Treatment Related Factors*, *Intrinsic* and *Extrinsic Risk Factors*.

To ensure statistical significance of the attained results, 30 (thirty) experiments were applied in all tests. In each simulation, the available data was randomly divided into two mutually exclusive partitions, i.e., the training set with 67% of the available data, used during the modeling phase, and the test set with the remaining 33% of the cases, used after training in order to evaluate the model performance and to validate it. The back propagation algorithm was used in the learning process of the ANN. As the output function in the pre-processing layer it was used the identity one. In the other layers we used the sigmoid function.

Figure 5. Distribution of the treatment related factors, intrinsic and extrinsic risk factors

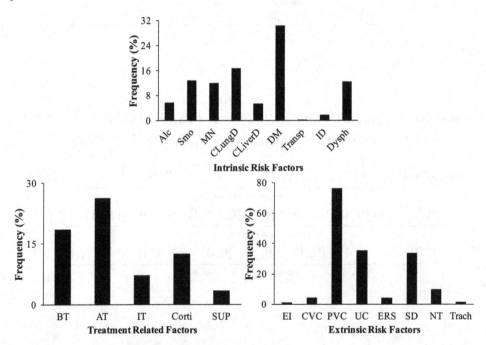

A common tool to evaluate the results presented by the classification models is the coincidence matrix, a matrix of size $L \times L$, where L denotes the number of possible classes. This matrix is created by matching the predicted and target values. L was set to 2 (two) in the present case. Table 1 presents the coincidence matrix (the values denote the average of the 30 experiments).

Table 1 shows that the model accuracy was 90.9% for the training set (1012 correctly classified in 1113) and 88.7% for test set (493 correctly classified in 556). Thus, the predictions made by the ANN model are satisfactory, attaining accuracies close to 90%. Therefore, the generated model is able to predict nosocomial infection risk properly.

In Figure 5 Alc, Sm, MN, CLungD, CLiverD, DM, Transp, ID and Dysph stand, respectively, for Alcoholism, Smoking, Malnutrition, Chronic Lung Disease, Chronic Liver Disease, Diabetes, Transplants, Immunodeficiency and Dysphasia; BT, AT, IT, Corti and SUP denote, respectively, Blood Transfusions, Antimicrobial Therapy, Immunosuppressive Treatments, Use of Corticosteroids , Stress-ulcer Prophylaxis; and EI, CVC, PVC, UC, ERS, SD, NT and Trach stand, respectively, for Endotracheal Intubation, Central Venous Catheter, Peripheral Venous Catheter, Urinary Catheter, Extracorporeal Renal Support, Surgical Drains, Nasogastric Tube and Tracheotomy.

CONCLUSION AND FUTURE WORK

This risk assessment system is able to give an adequate response to the need for a good method of nosocomial infection. To go around the problem, more effectively, much more variables must be studied and considered, thus fulfilling important gaps in the existent risk assessment methods.

Being an area filled with incomplete and unknown data it may be tackled by Artificial Intelligence based methodologies and techniques for problem solving. This work presents the founding of a computational framework that uses powerful knowledge representation and reasoning techniques to set the structure of the

Table 1. The coincidence matrix for ANN model

Target	Predictive			
	Training set		Test set	
	False (0)	True (1)	False (0)	True (1)
False (0)	902	96	437	61
True (1)	5	110	2	56

information and the associate inference mechanisms. Indeed, this method brings a new approach that can revolutionize prediction tools in all its variants, making it more complete than the existing methodologies and tools available.

The knowledge representation and reasoning techniques presented above are very versatile and capable of covering every possible instance by considering incomplete, contradictory, and even unknown data. Indeed, the new paradigm of knowledge representation and reasoning enables the use of the normalized values of the interval boundaries and their *DoC* values, as inputs to the ANN. The output translates the risk prediction for nosocomial infection and the confidence that one has on such a happening.

Future work may recommend that the same problem must be approached using others computational formalisms like Genetic Programming (Neves et al., 2007), Case Based Reasoning (Carneiro, Novais, Andrade, Zeleznikow, & Neves, 2013) or Particle Swarm (Mendes, Kennedy, & Neves, 2004), just to name a few.

REFERENCES

Carneiro, D., Novais, P., Andrade, F., Zeleznikow, J., & Neves, J. (2013). Using case-based reasoning and principled negotiation to provide decision support for dispute resolution. *Knowledge and Information Systems*, *36*(3), 789–826. doi:10.1007/s10115-012-0563-0

Cortez, P., Rocha, M., & Neves, J. (2004). Evolving Time Series Forecasting ARMA Models. *Journal of Heuristics*, *10*(4), 415–429. doi:10.1023/B:HEUR.0000034714.09838.1e

Damani, N. N. (2003). *Manual of infection control procedures* (2nd ed.). New York, NY: Greenwich Medical Media.

Gelfond, M., & Lifschitz, V. (1988). The stable model semantics for logic programming. In R. Kowalski, & K. Bowen (Eds.), *Logic Programming – Proceedings of the Fifth International Conference and Symposium* (pp. 1070-1080).

Inweregbu, K., Dave, J., & Pittard, A. (2005). Nosocomial infection. *Continuing Education in Anaesthesia, Critical Care and Pain*, *5*, 14–17.

Kakas, A., Kowalski, R., & Toni, F. (1998). The role of abduction in logic programming. In D. Gabbay, C. Hogger, & I. Robinson (Eds.), *Handbook of Logic in Artificial Intelligence and Logic Programming* (Vol. 5, pp. 235–324). Oxford, United Kingdom: Oxford University Press.

Lucas, P. (2004). Quality checking of medical guidelines through logical abduction. In F. Coenen, A. Preece, & A. Mackintosh (Eds.), *Research and Developments in Intelligent Systems XX* (pp. 309–321). London, United Kingdom: Springer. doi:10.1007/978-0-85729-412-8_23

Machado, J., Abelha, A., Novais, P., Neves, J., & Neves, J. (2010). Quality of service in healthcare units. *International Journal of Computer Aided Engineering and Technology*, 2(4), 436–449. doi:10.1504/IJCAET.2010.035396

Mendes, R., Kennedy, J., & Neves, J. (2004). The fully informed particle swarm: Simpler, maybe better. *IEEE Transactions on Evolutionary Computation*, 8(3), 204–210. doi:10.1109/TEVC.2004.826074

Neves, J. (1984). A logic interpreter to handle time and negation in logic databases. In R. L. Muller, & J. J. Pottmyer (Eds.), *Proceedings of the Annual Conference of the ACM on the Fifth Generation Challenge* (pp. 50-54). New York, NY: Association for Computing Machinery.

Neves, J., Guimarães, T., Gomes, S., Vicente, H., Santos, M., Neves, J., & Novais, P. et al. (2015). Logic Programming and Artificial Neural Networks in Breast Cancer Detection. In I. Rojas, G. Joya, & A. Catala (Eds.), *Advances in Computational Intelligence – Part II,* LNCS (Vol. 9095, pp. 211–224). Cham, Switzerland: Springer International Publishing. doi:10.1007/978-3-319-19222-2_18

Neves, J., Machado, J., Analide, C., Abelha, A., & Brito, L. (2007, December 3-7). The halt condition in genetic programming. In J. Neves, M. F. Santos, & J. Machado (Eds.), *Progress in Artificial Intelligence: Proceedings of the 13th Portuguese Conference on Artificial Intelligence EPIA 2007*, Guimarães, Portugal, *LNAI* (Vol. 4874, pp. 160-169). Berlin, Germany: Springer. doi:10.1007/978-3-540-77002-2_14

Pereira, L. M., & Anh, H. T. (2009). Evolution prospection. In K. Nakamatsu (Ed.), *New Advances in Intelligent Decision Technologies: Results of the First KES International Symposium IDT 2009 (Studies in Computational Intelligence)* (Vol. 199, pp. 51-64). Berlin, Germany: Springer. doi:10.1007/978-3-642-00909-9_6

Rigor, H., Machado, J., Abelha, A., Neves, J., & Alberto, C. (2008). A web-based system to reduce the nosocomial infection impact in healthcare units. *Proceedings of the International Conference on Web Information Systems – WEBIST 2008* (pp. 264-268). Funchal, Portugal: Scitepress.

Vicente, H., Couto, C., Machado, J., Abelha, A., & Neves, J. (2012). Prediction of Water Quality Parameters in a Reservoir using Artificial Neural Networks. *International Journal of Design & Nature and Ecodynamics*, 7(3), 309–318. doi:10.2495/DNE-V7-N3-309-318

Vicente, H., Dias, S., Fernandes, A., Abelha, A., Machado, J., & Neves, J. (2012). Prediction of the Quality of Public Water Supply using Artificial Neural Networks. *Journal of Water Supply: Research & Technology - Aqua, 61*(7), 446–459. doi:10.2166/aqua.2012.014

Vicente, H., Roseiro, J., Arteiro, J., Neves, J., & Caldeira, A. T. (2013). Prediction of bioactive compound activity against wood contaminant fungi using artificial neural networks. *Canadian Journal of Forest Research, 43*(11), 985–992. doi:10.1139/cjfr-2013-0142

World Health Organization. (2011). *Report on the burden of endemic health care associated infection worldwide: A systematic review of the literature*. Geneva, Switzerland: WHO Press.

Chapter 3
Step towards Improving the Voluntary Interruption of Pregnancy by Means of Business Intelligence

Andreia Brandão
University of Minho, Portugal

Filipe Portela
University of Minho, Portugal & Porto Polytechnic, Portugal

ABSTRACT

With the implementation of Information and Communication Technologies in the health sector, it became possible the existence of an electronic record of information for patients, enabling the storage and the availability of their information in databases. However, without the implementation of a Business Intelligence (BI) system, this information has no value. Thus, the major motivation of this paper is to create a decision support system that allows the transformation of information into knowledge, giving usability to the stored data. The particular case addressed in this chapter is the Centro Materno Infantil do Norte (CMIN), in particular the Voluntary Interruption of Pregnancy (VIP) unit. With the creation of a BI system for this module, it is possible to design an interoperable, pervasive and real-time platform to support the decision-making process of health professionals, based on cases that occurred. Furthermore, this platform enables the automation of the process for obtaining key performance indicators that are presented annually by this health institution. In this chapter, the BI system implemented in the VIP unity in CMIN, some of the indicators (KPIs) evaluated as well as the benefits of this implementation are presented.

DOI: 10.4018/978-1-4666-9882-6.ch003

INTRODUCTION

The use of Information and Communication Technologies (ICT) are increasingly, occupying an important place in society. The health sector is no exception, as these among other things, can provide complete and reliable information for healthcare professionals, allowing to support their clinical and administrative decisions and consequently decreasing medical errors associated to these decisions (Pinto, 2009).

Besides, ICT have a high potential to facilitate information sharing, communication and collaboration between health professionals, increasing the quality and efficiency of the health system as well as the use of Electronic Health Records (EHR) (Abelha et al., 2007; Khodambashi, 2013; Portela et al., 2010) is one of the goals.

In recent times, Business Intelligence (BI) technologies have been the target of interest to health professionals and to the Information Technology (IT) professionals, due to its applicability in EHR (Bonney, 2013). BI is a process that encompasses several methodologies, applications and technologies for collecting, storing, manipulating, analysing and providing access to data in order to help enterprise users making better and faster business decisions. Thus BI has the ability to operationalize the repository content of EHR in supporting evidence-based practice and improving the quality of healthcare delivery (Bonney, 2013; Mettler & Vimarlund, 2009; Portela et al., 2010).

In the case of healthcare organizations, the majority of clinical data documenting their daily activities are stored in a Relational Database Management System (RD-BMS). Because of the extensive amount of information, this information is stored in different ways and therefore highly heterogeneous with each other. On the other hand, a decision-making process, where it is necessary to integrate multiple data provided by clinical, medical, financial and administrative systems and where the sources are quite heterogeneous, large and complex becomes extremely important to meet the data quality that directly interferes in the success of the Knowledge Discovery Database (KDD) process (Mettler & Vimarlund, 2009; Raquel & Oliveira, 2012). So, with this increasing amount of information there is also a corresponding need to apply Data Mining (DM) technologies to extract knowledge from information / data stored in databases and providing real-time decisions (Bonney, 2013). Most clinical data are not structured and the DM techniques work well with structured data. It is inferred another advantage to using BI as a decision support technology since it allows the combination of structured and unstructured data (Bonney, 2013).

Furthermore, it can be stated that the Information Systems interoperability in an institution is one of the key factors in the decision-making process. Interoperability (Cardoso, Marins, Portela, Santos, et al., 2014) ensures systems standardization and allows passing all the inherent complexity of the different data sources ensuring data quality.

Thus, this chapter is focused on presenting the architecture of a global BI platform that can be used in Maternity Care Institution, taking as a case study the Centro Materno Infantil do Norte (CMIN) in Porto, Portugal. It was planned apply BI and DM techniques in order to develop a platform where it is possible generate useful Key Performance Indicators (KPIs) (clinical and management) for healthcare professionals in the context of the Voluntary Interruption of Pregnancy (VIP) module. For the development of this platform, one Data Warehouse (DW) was built using the star schema and a set of DM models were induced. For better accuracy of the solution and validity of information generated, all the work has been pleading with clinicians and specialists.

The solution in development is a pervasive real-time web-based BI application and due to their characteristics allows it to be accessed anywhere and anytime.

Besides the introduction, this chapter includes eight sections. The second section is related to the background knowledge, where a brief look is taken about Maternity Care and Interoperability and it is described the VIP process. Subsequently, section three describes the process of Knowledge Discovery in Databases and section four outlines the BI system that is being implemented in CMIN and some of the indicators to get at the end. Finally, some discussions and conclusions were made and future work was suggested.

BACKGROUND AND RELATED WORK

Maternity Care and Voluntary Interruption of Pregnancy

The Centro Hospitalar do Porto (CHP) results from the union of three hospitals, namely, the Hospital de Santo António (HSA), Hospital Joaquim Urbano (HJU) and Centro Materno Infantil do Norte (CMIN). Each one of these units were separate entities until the creation of the CHP in 2007. With the creation of CHP, women who need urgent care in the specialties of Gynaecological and Obstetrics are directed to MJD, now CMIN, which was not previously checked (Cabral et al., 2013)

CMIN is a health institution, which one of the modules is VIP. In this module, clinically non-surgical methods are used for this purpose. More specifically, World Health Organization (WHO) recommends a drug method that has been proven safe and it is used quite effectively. This method consists of the combination of medication (*mifepristone* and *misoprostol*).

Furthermore, VIP is a procedure, which involves several steps. The first phase consists of a physician appointment followed of a period of three days, where the patient needs to consider its decision. Then, the patient is administered with a dosage of medication, performed at ambulatory in CMIN. A triage is also performed by the nursing staff in order to verify if the patient is capable to make the administration of the second medication dosage at home or if she needs to be monitored by the nursing team in CMIN.

After the medication administration phase, a new medical consultation is performed, where the patient is examined in order to determine whether the procedure was successful. If the opposite occurs, the Interruption of Pregnancy (IoP) was not achieved or the procedure was incomplete (resulting in the patient admission in CMIN) (Valente, Cristina, Rosário, & Alcina, 2012).

In this last phase, two situations may occur: the patient is consulted and he is examined by the physician or the patient does not attend to the consultation. In the first case, the patient is evaluated and it is reported if IoP was successful or not. On the other hand, if ovular remains was verified by ultrasound (incomplete IoP), it is necessary the patient hospitalization, and if IoP was not achieved, it is necessary to repeat the process.

In the second case, the patient was not evaluated, being their condition and the result of the procedure unknown. This situation characterizes the risk patients and can originates some problems, in particular, health risks associated to the patient and their fetus due a lack of medical supervision.

The idea of implementing a BI platform is to provide a follow up able to facilitate the health professional's work and improve the quality of care as is for example the triage system (Abelha et al., 2015). They were responsible for obtaining reports, which should contain indicators related to the information recorded during the proceedings. Nowadays these reports are held annually in paper and are used for evaluation of CMIN, as is the example of VIP module (Valente et al., 2012). This platform can be combined with the Clinical Recommendation Triage System for Obstetric (CTSO) (Eliana Pereira, 2016) in developing in CMIN. In this case the VIP cases found in the triage can have their own indicators in the CRTSO platform.

Interoperability System

At Centro Hospitalar do Porto (CHP), the interoperability between information systems is ensured by Agency for Integration, Archive and Diffusion of Medical Information (AIDA). This system of intelligent agents (Cardoso, Marins, Portela, Abelha, & Machado, 2014) allows communication of the different CHP systems, as well as standardization of clinical systems, overcoming the medical and administrative complexity of the different information sources (Marins et al., 2014). Thus, AIDA ensures Information sending and receiving from the hospital and is able to managing, storing and responding to the requests for information made from third parties (Machado, Alves, Abelha, & Neves, 2007; Peixoto, Santos, Abelha, & Machado,

2012). All information systems of CHP are connected through AIDA, for example, the SAPE (Nursing Support System) and SONHO (Clinical Information System) (Machado et al., 2007; Peixoto et al., 2012).

KNOWLEDGE DISCOVERY IN DATABASES

This section is focused on Knowledge Discovery in Databases (KDD) and DM. In this section all the procedures performed by CRISP-DM methodology, to obtain the DM models associated with VIP unit in CMIN are described.

The Knowledge Discovery in Database (KDD) process is a set of ongoing activities that share the knowledge discovered from databases. According to Fayyad et al. (Fayyad, Piatetsky-shapiro, & Smyth, 1996), KDD process consists in five stages, which were followed in this work:

- **Selection:** Selection of the data needed to perform the Data Mining (DM).
- **Pre-Processing:** This step included cleaning and processing of data in order to make them consistent.
- **Transformation:** In this phase the data were worked out according to the target.
- **Data Mining:** At this stage, the objectives to be achieved and the type of result wanted to achieve were defined. According to the type of desired result, it was defined the type of task being performed (classification, segmentation, summarization, dependency modeling) and identified the technique to be used (decision trees, association rules, linear regression, neuronal networks, among others). Subsequently, it was applied the selected data mining technique to the data set to obtain patterns.
- **Interpretation/Evaluation:** Consisted in the interpretation and evaluation of the patterns obtained. The validity of the results obtained are was verified by applying the patterns found at new dataset (Palaniappan & Awang, 2008).

The KDD process refers to the whole process of discovering useful knowledge in data, while DM refers to the application of algorithms to extract data models. Until 1995, KDD and DM terms were considered interchangeably. Now DM represents a phase of the Knowledge Discovery in Databases process (KDD) and it consists in finding patterns or relationships that may exist in the data stored in data repositories.

The knowledge to be discovered must satisfy three properties: it must be correct (as much as possible), should be understandable by human users, and should be interesting useful/new. Still, the method of knowledge discovery must have the following three characteristics: it must be effective (accurate), generic (applicable to various data types) and flexible (easily modifiable) (Steiner, Soma, & Shimizu, 2006).

Within the VIP unit in CMIN, two DM problems were addressed. The first problem was related to the capability of predicting the most appropriate place for the administration of the second drug dosage (Brandão et al., 2014). With the second problem, it was intended to evaluate the VIP process and consequently identify whether the patient will belong to a risk group - probability of a patient not attend to the revision consultation (Machado et al., 2015).

The methodology addressed for both problems was the Cross Industry Standard Process for Data Mining (CRISP-DM). CRISP-DM divides the DM process into six major phases, as can been seen in Figure 1 (Chapman et al., 2000; Cios, Pedrycz, Swiniarski, & Kurgan, 2007; Gonçalves et al., 2013).

The steps followed were:

- **Business Understanding:** This initial phase of the project DM focused on understanding the objective of the project from a business perspective, defining a preliminary plan to achieve the goal. In this phase, the DM problems can be translated in two questions, namely, "What is the probability of a pregnant woman carrying out the second drug phase with monitoring of nursing staff?" and "What is the probability of a patient belonging to the risk group of patients?".

- **Data Understanding:** Comprised data collection and startup activities for data comprehension, identifying problems or interesting sets. In this phase, for each problem it was extracted data from SAPE and AIDA and it was analyzed the quality of the possible variables to be used in the process. The sample covers the period between 01.01.2012 and 31.12.2012. It corresponds to 1124 VIP cases. Furthermore, a statistical analysis was performed, showing that the data had quality (low number of noise values), however the data needed to be prepared in order to be incorporated into the DM models.

- **Data Preparation:** In the preparation phase, all the tasks involved in creating cases that were used to build the models were included. Data preparation tasks were likely to be performed multiple times, in no particular order. Tasks included building the table of cases, selection of attributes, data cleaning and transformation. Additionally, it was possible add new attributes calculated based on existing ones. The preparation phase of data can significantly improve the information that can be discovered through DM. In these particular cases, the variables that suited the problems were selected. Subsequently, the selected data were subjected to a pre-processing phase where all records containing unfilled or noise fields were eliminated. Some of the procedures

Figure 1. The CRISP-DM process
Source: Chapman et al. (2000)

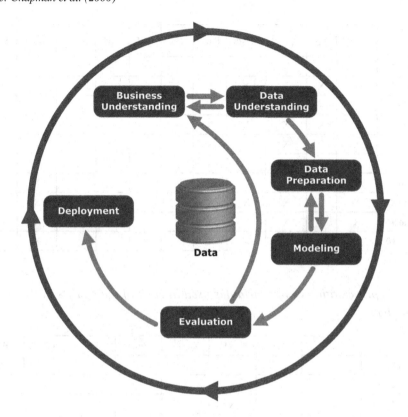

performed to eliminate noise from the data were replacing the comma by point to separate the decimals on numerical variables and also deleting text associated to these variables. After those transformations of the data, it became possible to build the table of cases with some of the scenarios considered most suitable.

- **Modeling:** Several modeling techniques were applied. Thus, it was common return to data preparation during this phase. In this step, for each problem was built a table of cases composed by 10 scenarios that yielded the best results, arising from different combinations of variables, as can be seen in Tables 1 and 2. In each scenario, the target variable was presented, as well as other variables considered crucial to the creation of forecast models. After set the table of cases, the data were submitted to DM techniques, selected in order to be able to identify the best forecasting model for this DM problem. In this case, the DM techniques used were Generalized Linear Model, Support Vector Machine, Naïve Bayes and Decision Tree.

Table 1. Representation of the variables used in each of the models in the first DM problem

	LASD	Age	N_VIP	Gesta	Para	PS	CM	WG	AC_1	AC_2	WGC
Scenario 1	X	X	X	X	X	X	-	-	-	-	-
Scenario 2	X	X	-	X	X	-	-	-	-	-	-
Scenario 3	X	-	-	X	X	-	-	-	-	-	-
Scenario 4	X	X	X	X	X	-	-	-	-	-	-
Scenario 5	X	-	X	X	X	X	-	-	X	-	-
Scenario 6	X	-	X	X	X	X	-	-	-	X	-
Scenario 7	X	-	X	X	X	X	X	-	-	X	-
Scenario 8	X	-	X	X	X	X	-	X	-	X	-
Scenario 9	X	-	X	X	X	X	-	-	-	X	X
Scenario 10	X	-	X	X	X	X	X	-	-	X	X

Table 2. Representation of the variables used in each of the models in the second DM problem

	RC	Age	N_VIP	Gesta	Para	PS	CM	WG
Scenario 1	X	X	X	X	X	X	X	X
Scenario 2	X	X	X	X	X	X	X	-
Scenario 3	X	X	X	X	X	X	-	-
Scenario 4	X	X	X	X	X	-	-	-
Scenario 5	X	X	X	-	-	-	-	-
Scenario 6	X	X	X	X	X	X	-	X
Scenario 7	X	X	X	X	X	-	-	X
Scenario 8	X	X	X	X	X	-	X	X
Scenario 9	X	X	X	X	X	-	X	-
Scenario 10	X	X	X	-	-	-	X	X

The variables used in the first problem were: LASD (Local administration of the second dose), Age, N_VIP (number of previous VIP), Gesta (number of previous pregnancies), Para (number of births), PS (Professional Status), CM (Contraceptive Method), WG (Weeks of Gestation), AC_1 (Age Class 1), AC_2 (Age Class 2), WGC (Weeks of Gestation Class).

In the second problem other variables were used: RC (Revision Consultation), Age, N_VIP (number of previous VIP), Gesta (number of previous pregnancies), Para (number of births), PS (Professional Status), CM (Contraceptive Method), WG (Weeks of Gestation).

- **Evaluation:** There was built models appearing to have great quality from a data analysis perspective. However, it was necessary to check whether the model met the business goals. To evaluate the results achieved by the DM models, statistical metrics were used. In these metrics tree parameters were evaluated: specificity, sensitivity and accuracy.
- **Deployment:** The knowledge gained by the model was organized and presented in a way that the health profession can use. In this particular case, the knowledge gained was organized and presented so that the nurses can use them. These DM processes were integrated in the BI platform, implemented in CMIN.

The next section describes all the steps carried out during the project for the design and implementation of BI platform.

BUSINESS INTELLIGENCE

Currently, a BI platform can be defined as "a set of tools, programmed and integrated technologies and products that are used for the collection, analysis and presentation of data." The BI has the ability to turn the stored information into useful knowledge and provide the right user, in time, to support the decision-making process (Bonney, 2013; Reinschmidt & Francoise, 2000).

With the increase of electronic records and with increasing pressure to have faster and more effective decisions, which are often responsible for the occurrence of medical malpractice, it becomes appropriate to construct a support system to the specific decision making process for the VIP unit in CMIN, using BI technology. Moreover, nursing staff performs annual reports in paper, containing indicators related to the recorded information during the VIP procedures. The work performed by nurses for the creation of the indicators is no longer necessary, by the use BI technologies, the entire process is automatized and executed in real-time.

In the development of BI platform for the VIP unit in CMIN (Brandão et al.; Pereira et al.), it was followed the Kimball approach (El-Sappagh, Hendawi, & El Bastawissy, 2011; Kimball & Ross, 2002). This method identifies a sequence of tasks and highlights activities that must be performed in parallel, entailing the following steps, depicted in Figure 2:

Figure 2. Kimball's Approach Diagram
Source: Kimball & Ross (2002)

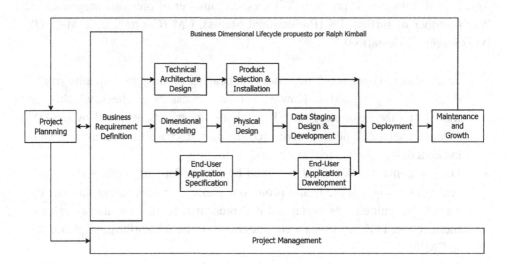

- **Program/Project Planning:** This phase includes project planning, understanding the requirements of organization and the identification of tasks. Thus, at this stage, some tasks were performed: researching important indicators for the IVG unit of CMIN, an initial planning of all stages of the Kimball approach and setting deadlines for these same steps defined.
- **Program/Project Management:** This stage is monitored throughout the project from the initial stage to the end, responsible for strengthening the project plan initially established.
- **Business Requirements Definition:** At this stage, it was performed planning / research all indicators required in the VIP unit with the help of health professionals and professionals of Information Technology (IT) of CMIN in order to obtain a more precise idea of the end requirements of the BI platform.

In the diagram of Figure 2, it can be seen that there are three sets of project activities occurring simultaneously. These sets are associated to the technological part, from the data acquisition until the development and deployment of BI application. The arrows in the diagram indicate the flow of activities within each of parallel paths. Dependencies between tasks are illustrated by vertical alignment of the boxes of the respective task (Kimball & Ross, 2002). These routes are:

- *Technological tasks,* including:
    - **Technical Architecture Design:** A technical scheme of the overall architecture is realized.

- ○ **Product Selection and Installation:** In this step must be selected and installed all of the appropriate Business Intelligence tools in order to be able to build the BI solution. At this stage, some tools were installed and tested, including *Oracle Database*, as applied to the database; *Oracle SQL Developer* as a tool for data extraction and implementation of ETL procedures; and *Pentaho BI Suite* as a tool for OLAP analysis and the creation of dashboards. This last selected tool for the development of BI application was chosen based on a comprehensive study on open-source BI tools.

- *Data tasks,* including:
  - ○ **Dimensional Modeling:** The dimensional model is a DW projection technique, which aims to provide a facilitated support to end users of the consultations. The dimensional model is constituted by the facts table and by the dimensions tables. The facts are typically numerical values, which can be aggregated, while the dimensions are hierarchies and values groups that define events. For the projection of dimensional model can be used various types of architectures. In structuring the DW dimensional model implemented in CMIN, the star schema was used because it was the most appropriate for the intended structure for the provision of data.
  - ○ **Physical Design:** In this phase was defined the data physical structure involving tasks such as setting the database environment and appropriate security setting.
  - ○ **ETL Design and Development:** This phase included extraction, transformation and loading of the data. The extraction consists of two stages, the initial extraction and changed data extraction. In the first stage, extracting the initial data occurs before DW loading, while the second stage is a continuous update of the DW, such as continuous extraction of the inherent data from CMIN databases. The processing corresponds to cleaning, integration and optimization of the data in order to achieve uniform, consistent and accurate data. Finally, there is the loading phase, wherein the data subjected to the above steps wew inserted in a multidimensional structure (DW) targeted to a specific type of end users and applications systems. To carry out this process, procedures and functions have been implemented through SQL Developer. In the ETL procedures, some of the goals were achieve by the elimination of null values, the elimination of redundant data and the processing of information. In addition, procedures were used to standardize the information, such as correcting spelling errors, replacing the comma for the point at values with decimal places, among others.

- The *Practical Application of BI,* includes:
  - ○ **BI Application Design:** At this stage it was necessary to identify the candidates' BI applications and appropriate navigation interfaces to meet the needs of CMIN professionals.
  - ○ **BI Application Development:** At this stage, some tasks were performed, such as construction and validation of specific operational BI applications and navigation portal. Thus, it was used the Pentaho BI Suite for building OLAP cubes and visualization of performance indicators required by the CMIN.
- **Deployment:** In this phase the development of BI application was started. A proper planning of the work was crucial. It was ensured that the paths of technology, data and BI application were tested and they were working correctly together.
- **Maintenance:** Occurs when the system is in production. Includes technical operational tasks that are necessary to maintain the system with optimal performance (monitoring the use, performance tuning, index maintenance, system back-up).
- **Growth:** DW systems tend to expand, if they are successful. In this case, it must be restarted again Kimball cycle and to develop the issues already established, focusing on new requirements. In the case of CMIN, the BI platform can be expanded with new modules of interest in the organization to support the decision-making process (El-Sappagh et al., 2011; Kimball & Ross, 2002).

In the next section, the BI platform developed for the VIP unit of CMIN is presented, where are incorporated the indicators and the DM models developed.

BUSINESS INTELLIGENCE PLATFORM FOR VIP

The BI platform for the VIP unit in CMIN is based on the Web following pervasive characteristics (Filipe Portela, Jorge Aguiar, Manuel Filipe Santos, Álvaro Silva, & Fernado Rua, 2013; C. F. Portela, Santos, Silva, Machado, & Abelha, 2011; F. Portela et al., 2011; F. Portela et al., 2013; F. Portela, Santos, & Vilas-Boas, 2012), which can be accessed anytime and anywhere, according to the access privileges. In this application are represented all the required indicators and also other indicators that can be created by users through the OLAP technology. This platform allows a more detailed analysis at the date level, as it could be viewing the level of the year, the months and days. Some of these indicators are:

- **Characterization of the patient group by number of pregnancies and date**: Identifies the number and percentage of patient by number of previously pregnancies in a selected time period.
- **Characterization of the patient group by number of children and by date:** Identifies the number and percentage of patient by number of children they have, in a selected time period.
- **Characterization of the patient group by number of previous VIP experiences and by date:** Identifies the number and percentage of patient who have previous experience of VIP in a selected time period.
- **Characterization of the patient group concerning the revision consultation for date:** Displays the number and proportion of patient who were present at the revision consultation, corresponding to the appointment made at the end of VIP process for a certain time interval.
- **Characterization of the patient group based on the final outcome of the VIP process and by date:** Identifies the number of patients and the percentage of the three types of possible end results in the VIP process (achieved abortion, incomplete interruption and non-managed abortion) in a selected time period.
- **Characterization of the patient group on the number of failures of VIP process, by year and by month:** Identifies the number of patients whose VIP process has not been successfully achieved.
- **Characterization of the patient group based on contraception early in the process by date:** Identifies the number of patients who already used contraception in the process, which contraception and which faults are associated over a given period of time.
- **Characterization of the patient group based on the end contraception of VIP process by date:** Identifies the number of patients who have adopted contraception at the end of the process and which contraception was chosen over a given period of time.
- **Characterization of the patient group based on gestational age at the time of taking the mifepristone, by year, month and day:** Identifies the number of patients for each of the possible gestational ages, by year, month and day. To this end, it was created an OLAP cube that allows the drill-down and roll-up on the date, providing visualization of the months and days for a given year, as shown in Figure 3.
- **Characterization of the patient group based on the process achievement local, by date:** Identifies the number of patients, based on the achievement local of the process (home or CMIN), by date.

Figure 3. Characterization of the user group based on gestational age at the time of taking the mifepristone, by year, month and day

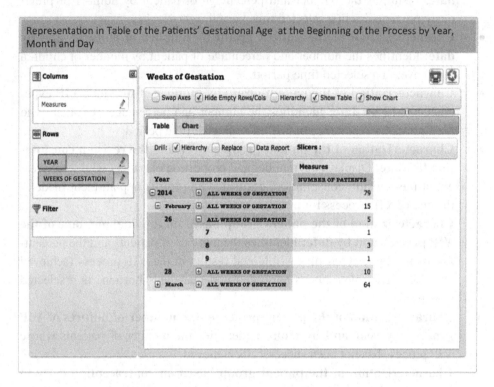

- **Characterization of the patient group by profession and by date:** Identifies the number of patients who are unemployed, students and employees, while setting the respective professions in a given period of time. This indicator is shown as a pie chart and two bar graphs, as can be seen in Figure 4.
- **Characterization of the patients group by age and year:** Identifies the number of patients by age classes in a given year.

Figure 4. Characterization of the user group by profession and by date

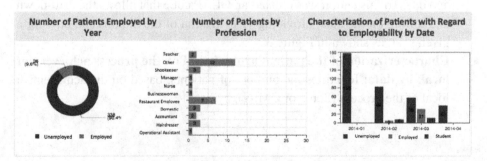

Furthermore, the BI platform in CMIN also incorporates the DM prediction models, discussed above. These models predict where the second dose of the drug should be administered and predict which is the probability of a patient belonging to the group risk. The way that prediction models are represented in BI platform can be seen in Figure 5. For example in the case of group risk a patient with a probability between 60% and 100% (red color) have a higher probability of belonging to the group risk. In the case of this example, the patient probability is 30%.

DISCUSSION

Given the DM models developed for each one of the problems discussed, it can be concluded that the results were quite acceptable based on the assessment carried out for the forecast models. For the first problem, it was obtained sensitivity and acuity values of approximately 91% and 87%, respectively, in model 3, resulting from the application of the technique Decision Trees. Thus, it can be considered that the most important factors for the determination of the second dosage of medication administration place is the number of pregnancies and the number of births that a patient had. The second DM question, gave a maximum of approximately 93% in the model 4, in terms of sensitivity metric, using Support Vector Machine technique. Thus, it appears that the most relevant factors in determining the patients belonging to the risk group are the age, the number of VIPs previously performed, the number of pregnancies and the number of births.

In terms of the development of the BI platform to the VIP unit, there are many benefits of integrating BI technology in CMIN. The main advantage is the autonomy and flexibility that the end users acquire with regard to reporting. It also allows a

Figure 5. Representation of prediction models in BI platform

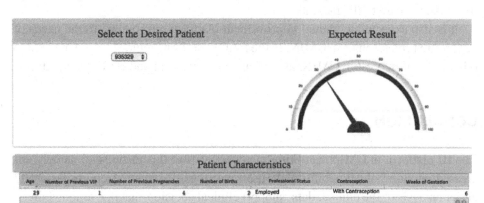

simply and quickly data analysis resulting in an improvement of the decision-making process, a greater operational efficiency and a greater variety of new analytics.

At the scientific level this platform has many advantages. In fact it is a pioneering worldwide project in the VIP area, characterized by obtaining specific indicators to maternity care institutions. Taking into account the results obtained and the accreditation given by health professionals, this platform can provide a starting point for the implementation of improvement measures in the VIP module. Moreover, it may still be useful for the research and development of new modules of interest not only for the VIP module as well as for other health institutions. An example of another module of interest may be the case with non-progressive pregnancy, since they require only a small adaptation of the current system conditions to some new in this procedure.

The implementation of the BI platform in VIP unit is very valuable, since it allows, for example, the interpretation of existing data records, obtaining indicators reflecting the overall operation of this unit, the acquisition of continuous improvement strategies in care based on the results, and the disclosure of the activities carried out in this area.

The main objective of this BI platform is to support the provision of better health care and meet the needs of pregnant women who wish to undergo the VIP process. With this platform, it is aimed to provide personalized care to the patient, enabling an increase in evidence-based clinical practice and providing new knowledge in real-time.

FUTURE RESEARCH DIRECTIONS

In the future can be explored new techniques and create more DM problems. New variables can be selected and new experiments can be performed with new datasets. In terms of BI platform a set of new indicators will be designed in order to provide personalized care to the patients

It is also expected a gradual improvement platform, responding to the needs of healthcare professionals in CMIN. In the future, platform could also be expanded to other units of interest in CMIN, as well as other maternal and child organizations.

CONCLUSION

The BI platform in CMIN can bring many benefits to this institution, namely, increased autonomy and flexibility of the users with regard to creating reports, faster and easier analysis of the clinical data, support clinical decision-making, among others.

With this chapter, it was also demonstrated that it is possible to obtain DM classification models to whether predict where the VIP patient must carry the administration of the second dose of medication, as for predicting whether a patient belongs to the risk group in VIP process. This study was conducted using real data of VIP processes, collected in CMIN, corresponding to a year of operation, namely the year of 2012. It can be concluded then, using data mining classification techniques and the historic data of the patients of the VIP unit CMIN, it is possible provide the most appropriate location for the realization of the second stage of the VIP process, as well as identify patients with greater ability to belong to the risk group in the VIP process. Thus, it was demonstrated the possibility of developing DM models with good predictive ability in order to provide the pregnant woman better treatment under appropriate conditions. These problems of DM described are intended only for VIP, in particular in CMIN however, they can be applied in other hospitals, which has the same problems and use the same procedures in the VIP process.

In addition, this chapter allowed exploring the importance of integrating BI technology in CMIN. The implementation of this technology provides an analysis of the extracted data, while the majority of clinical data are unstructured.

Finally, it can be concluded that the implementation of the BI platform including DM models in CMIN is an innovative idea, as it is the first time that the BI technologies are applied in the VIP area.

ACKNOWLEDGMENT

This work has been supported by FCT - Fundação para a Ciência e Tecnologia within the Project Scope UID/CEC/00319/2013.

REFERENCES

Abelha, A., Analide, C., Machado, J., Neves, J., Santos, M., & Novais, P. (2007). Ambient Intelligence and Simulation in Health Care Virtual Scenarios. In L. M. Camarinha-Matos, H. Afsarmanesh, P. Novais, & C. Analide (Eds.), *Establishing the Foundation of Collaborative Networks* (pp. 461–468). Boston, MA: Springer US. doi:10.1007/978-0-387-73798-0_49

Abelha, A., Pereira, E., Brandão, A., Portela, F., Santos, M. F., Machado, J., & Braga, J. (2015). Improving Quality of Services in Maternity Care Triage System. *International Journal of E-Health and Medical Communications*, 6(2), 10–26. doi:10.4018/IJEHMC.2015040102

Bonney, W. (2013). Applicability of Business Intelligence in Electronic Health Record. *Procedia: Social and Behavioral Sciences, 73*, 257–262. doi:10.1016/j.sbspro.2013.02.050

Brandão, A., Pereira, E., Portela, F., Santos, M., Abelha, A., & Machado, J. (2014). Real-time Business Intelligence platform to maternity care. Proceedings of IECBES 2014 IEEE Conference on Biomedical Engineering and Sciences, Sarawak, Malaysia (pp. 379-384). IEEE.

Brandão, A., Pereira, E., Portela, F., Santos, M. F., Abelha, A., & Machado, J. (2014). Managing Voluntary Interruption of Pregnancy Using Data Mining. *Procedia Technology, 16*, 1297–1306. doi:10.1016/j.protcy.2014.10.146

Cabral, A., Abelha, A., Salazar, M., Quintas, C., Portela, F., Machado, J., . . . Santos, M. F. (2013). *Knowledge acquisition process for intelligent decision support in critical health care*. IGI Global Book. Retrieved from http://repositorium.sdum.uminho.pt/handle/1822/21710

Cardoso, L., Marins, F., Portela, F., Abelha, A., & Machado, J. (2014). Healthcare interoperability through intelligent agent technology. *Procedia Technology, 16*, 1334–1341. doi:10.1016/j.protcy.2014.10.150

Cardoso, L., Marins, F., Portela, F., Santos, M., Abelha, A., & Machado, J. (2014). The Next Generation of Interoperability Agents in Healthcare. *International Journal of Environmental Research and Public Health, 11*(5), 5349–5371. doi:10.3390/ijerph110505349 PMID:24840351

Chapman, P., Clinton, J., Kerber, R., Khabaza, T., Reinartz, T., Shearer, C., & Wirth, R. (2000). *The CRISP-DM User Guide*. NCR Systems Engineering Copenhagen.

Cios, K., Pedrycz, W., Swiniarski, R., & Kurgan, L. (2007). *Data Mining. A knowledge Discovery Approach*. Springer.

El-Sappagh, S. H. A., Hendawi, A. M. A., & El Bastawissy, A. H. (2011). A proposed model for data warehouse ETL processes. *Journal of King Saud University - Computer and Information Sciences, 23*(2), 91–104. doi:10.1016/j.jksuci.2011.05.005

Pereira, E., Portela, F., & Abelha, A. (n. d.). A Clinical Recommendation System to Maternity Care.

Fayyad, U., Piatetsky-shapiro, G., & Smyth, P. (1996). From Data Mining to Knowledge Discovery in Databases. American Association for Artificial Intelligence, 37–54.

Portela, F., Aguiar, J., Santos, M. F., Silva, Á., & Rua, F. (2013). Pervasive Intelligent Decision Support System - Technology Acceptance in Intensive Care Units. In Á Roch, A.M. Correia, T. Wilson, & K.A. Stroetmann (Ed.), Advances in Intelligent Systems and Computing. Springer.

Gonçalves, J., Portela, F., Santos, M. F., Silva, Á., Machado, J., Abelha, A., & Rua, F. (2013). *Real-time Predictive Analytics for Sepsis Level and Therapeutic Plans in Intensive Care Medicine*. International Information Institute.

Khodambashi, S. (2013). Business Process Re-engineering Application in Healthcare in a Relation to Health Information Systems. *Procedia Technology*, *9*, 949–957. doi:10.1016/j.protcy.2013.12.106

Kimball, R., & Ross, M. (2002). *The Data Warehouse Toolkit*. John Wiley and Sons, Inc.

Machado, J., Alves, V., Abelha, A., & Neves, J. (2007). Ambient intelligence via multiagent systems in the medical arena. *Engineering Intelligent Systems for Electrical Engineering and Communications, 15*(3), 151–157. Retrieved from http://www.refdoc.fr/Detailnotice?idarticle=696527

Machado, J. M., Abelha, A., Santos, M., Portela, F., Pereira, E., & Brandão, A. (2015). Predicting the risk associated to pregnancy using data mining.

Marins, F., Cardoso, L., Portela, F., Santos, M. F., Abelha, A., & Machado, J. (2014). Improving High Availability and Reliability of Health Interoperability Systems. *New Perspectives in Information Systems and Technologies* (Vol. 2, pp. 207–216). Springer. doi:10.1007/978-3-319-05948-8_20

Mettler, T., & Vimarlund, V. (2009). Understanding Business Intelligence in the Context of Healthcare. *Health Informatics Journal*, *15*(3), 254–264. doi:10.1177/1460458209337446 PMID:19713399

Palaniappan, S., & Awang, R. (2008). Intelligent Heart Disease Prediction System Using Data Mining Techniques. *Proceedings of the 2008 IEEE/ACS International Conference on Computer Systems and Applications* (pp. 108–115). Washington, DC, USA: IEEE Computer Society. doi:10.1109/AICCSA.2008.4493524

Peixoto, H., Santos, M., Abelha, A., & Machado, J. (2012). Intelligence in Interoperability with AIDA. In L. Chen, A. Felfernig, J. Liu, & Z. Raś (Eds.), *Foundations of Intelligent Systems,* LNCS (Vol. 7661, pp. 264–273). Springer Berlin Heidelberg; doi:10.1007/978-3-642-34624-8_31

Pereira, E., Brandão, A., Portela, C. F., Santos, M. F., Machado, J., & Abelha, A. (2014). Business intelligence in maternity care. *Proceedings of IDEAS 2014 - International Database Engineering & Applications Symposium*, Porto, Portugal. ACM. doi:10.1145/2628194.2628248

Pinto, L. F. B. (2009). *Sistemas de Informação e Profissionais de Enfermagem*. Universidade de Trás-os-Montes e Alto Douro.

Portela, F., Santos, M. F., Silva, A., Machado, J., & Abelha, A. (2011). Enabling a Pervasive Approach for Intelligent Decision Support in Critical Health Care. In M. M. Cruz Cunha, J. Varajao, P. Powell & R. Martinho (Eds.), Enterprise Information Systems, Pt 3 (Vol. 221, pp. 233-243).

Portela, F., Gago, P., Santos, M. F., Silva, A., Rua, F., Machado, J., ... (2011). Knowledge Discovery for Pervasive and Real-Time Intelligent Decision Support in Intensive Care Medicine. *Proceedings of KMIS 2011- International Conference on Knowledge Management and Information Sharing*, Paris, France.

Portela, F., Santos, M. F., & Vilas-Boas, M. (2012). A Pervasive Approach to a Real-Time Intelligent Decision Support System in Intensive Medicine. In A. Fred, J.L.G. Dietz, K. Liu, & J. Filipe (Ed.), Communications in Computer and Information Science, LNCS (Vol. 272, 368-381).

Portela, F., Vilas-Boas, M., Santos, M. F., Abelha, A., Machado, J., Cabral, A., & Aragão, I. (2010). Electronic Health Records in the Emergency Room. *Proceedings of the 2010 IEEE/ACIS 9th International Conference on Computer and Information Science (ICIS)*. doi:10.1109/ICIS.2010.98

Raquel, O., & Oliveira, F. (2012). *Extração de Conhecimento nas Listas de Espera para Consulta e Cirurgia*. Universidade do Minho.

Reinschmidt, J., & Francoise, A. (2000). *Business Intelligence Certification Guide*. IBM.

Steiner, M., Soma, N., & Shimizu, T. (2006). Abordagem de um problema médico por meio do processo de KDD com ênfase à análise exploratória dos dados. *Gest Prod*. Retrieved from http://www.scielo.br/pdf/gp/v13n2/31177.pdf

Valente, C., Cristina, T., Rosário, F., & Alcina, B. (2012). *Acompanhamento de enfermagem na interrupção da gravidez por opção da mulher*. Porto: I.G.O.

ADDITIONAL READING

Peixoto, H., Santos, M., Abelha, A., & Machado, J. (2012). Intelligence in Interoperability with AIDA. In L. Chen, A. Felfernig, J. Liu, & Z. Raś (Eds.), *Foundations of Intelligent Systems SE - 31* (Vol. 7661, pp. 264–273). Springer Berlin Heidelberg; doi:10.1007/978-3-642-34624-8_31

Wang, F., & Hannafin, M. J. (2005). Design-based research and technology-enhanced learning environments. *Educational Technology Research and Development, 53*(4), 5–23. doi:10.1007/BF02504682

KEY TERMS AND DEFINITIONS

AIDA: Platform developed to ensure interoperability among healthcare information systems.

Business Intelligence: A technology that uses data analysis tools and applications to help business users make more informed decision.

Data Mining: Technologies to extract knowledge from information / data stored in databases and providing real-time decisions.

Decision Support System: A computerized information system used to support decision-making process in an organization or business.

Interoperability: Autonomous ability to interact and communicate.

Maternity Care: Health institution where patients of gynaecology and obstetrics specialties are admitted.

Voluntary Interruption of Pregnancy: This is the process of a woman voluntary interrupt their pregnancy. Clinically non-surgical methods are used for this purpose. More specifically, World Health Organization (WHO) recommends a drug method that has been proven safe and it is used quite effectively. This method consists of the combination of medication (*mifepristone* and *misoprostol*).

Chapter 4
A Clinical Recommendation System to Maternity Care

Eliana Pereira
University of Minho, Portugal

Filipe Portela
University of Minho, Portugal & Porto Polytechnic, Portugal

António Abelha
University of Minho, Portugal

ABSTRACT

Nowadays in healthcare, the Clinical Decision Support Systems are used in order to help health professionals to take an evidence-based decision. An example is the Clinical Recommendation Systems. In this sense, a pre-triage system was developed and implemented in Centro Hospitalar do Porto in order to group the patients on two levels (urgent or outpatient). However, although this system is calibrated and specific to the urgency of obstetrics and gynaecology, it does not meet all clinical requirements by the general department of the Portuguese HealthCare (Direção Geral de Saúde). The main requirement is the need of having priority triage system characterized by five levels. Thus some studies have been conducted with the aim of presenting a methodology able to evolve the pre-triage system on a Clinical Recommendation System with five levels. After some tests (using data mining and simulation techniques), it has been validated the possibility of transformation the pre-triage system in a Clinical Recommendation System in the obstetric context. At the end the main indicators achieved with this system are presented in the Business Intelligence Platform already deployed. This paper presents an overview of the Clinical Recommendation System for obstetric triage, the model developed and the main results achieved.

DOI: 10.4018/978-1-4666-9882-6.ch004

INTRODUCTION

Currently, in health institutions, there is an increasing amount of information. The need of making decisions the most correct as possible, emerges the Decision Support Systems (DSS) as a way of supporting the decisions of healthcare professionals based on evidences. In this context are inserted the Clinical Recommendation Systems, whose objective is the use of various computational techniques to achieve a particular purpose (Mackway-Jones K., 1997) (Filipe Portela César Quintas, José Machado, José Neves, & Santos, 2013) and recommending a clinical action.

Furthermore, the triage systems used in hospital emergency units may be considered a Clinical Recommendation System. In the case of *Centro Hospitalar do Porto (CHP)*, the triage system aims to select the type of patients in terms of clinical urgency, prioritizing the treatment response speed, the type of assistance and response resources to the level of urgency. So patients with a higher level of urgency and with increased risk of worsening of the disease, are attended as soon as possible. The most commonly used triage systems are those with five levels of severity, such as the Emergency Severity Index (ESI), the Manchester Triage System (MTS) and the Canadian Triage Acuity Scale (CTAS). The main limitation of this type of scales is the lack of flexibility, since usually they are used only in general emergency units and they are not specific for other units (Murray, Bullard, & Grafstein, 2004) (Portela et al., 2013). Due to this lack of flexibility for specific specialties, particularly for the obstetrics specialty, a pre-triage system was developed in 2010 in order to categorize the patients on two levels: Urgent (URG) and Consultation (ARGO) (Portela et al., 2013). It should be mentioned that this system only performs a routing triage. This system can forward the patient to the urgency (URG) - if the clinical features justify it, or for consultation - in the less urgent cases.

On the other hand, it is currently recommended by the general department of the Portuguese HealthCare (*Direção Geral de Saúde (DGS)*), more specifically by the *Comissão Nacional da Saúde Materna, da Criança e do Adolescente (CNSMCA)*, the use of the priority triage system with five priority levels in the obstetric emergency units (Infantil, 2013).

Having in consideration these two factors a set of studies was developed (Pereira, Brandão, Salazar, et al., 2014) (Abelha, Pereira, Brandão, Portela, Santos, & Machado, 2014) involving Data Mining and Simulation techniques in order to evaluate if it would be possible transforming the existing pre-triage system in a Clinical Recommendation Triage System for Obstetric (CRTSO). The Business Intelligence Platform (Brandão et al., 2014; Pereira et al., 2014) will contains several indicators about triage process (% usage room, type of patient, waiting time (expected, real, average, by level, among others). Additionally the own CRTSO also can be considered a Business Intelligence system due the way of how it was developed and their main goals as is improving the decision making process by providing useful information in real-time (S. O. Filipe Portela, Manuel Filipe Santos, António Abelha, José Machado, 2015; F. Portela et al., 2011). Using CRTSO as a BI platform is also possible create indicators related with the waiting triage time and patient priorities. This information will be available in the emergency room in situated devices, being it updated in real-time.

In this article the proposed CRTSO is exposed, as well as all the methodology used in its construction.

Apart from the introduction this article consists of five section. The second section presents the Background and Related Work. In the third section is presented the research methodology used and the methods used for the development of CRTSO. In the fourth section is presented the CRTSO developed as well as some adjustments that are necessary to perform the same be functional. In the fifth section are discussed some crucial points and presented the main conclusions. Finally, the sixth section are presented the future research directions.

BACKGROUND AND RELATED WORK

In this section is presented the project background and the theoretical aspects of the main triage systems existing in the world.

Case Study Contextualization and the Pre-Triage System

This project designed as CRTSO was developed in partnership with the *Centro Hospitalar do Porto* (CHP), more specifically with the *Centro Materno Infantil do Norte* (CMIN), old *Maternidade Júlio Dinis* (MJD). CMIN was inaugurated in 2014 and covers the needs associated with the care of paediatrics, neonatology, gynaecology and obstetrics (GO). The CMIN is responsible for the inpatient unit, intensive and intermediate care, diagnostic areas, day hospital, births block and has a GO emergency department (Portela et al., 2013).

Due to the inefficiency of the Manchester Triage System (MTS) to triage specific cases, most concretely GO, a specific pre-triage system (Cabral et al., 2011; Filipe Portela, Alexandra Cabral, et al., 2013; Filipe Portela et al., 2010) for obstetrics emergency department was implemented in 2010. This system is characterized by a set of discriminators for the obstetrics urgency allowing a patients triage in two levels: Urgent Consultation (ARGO) and Urgent (URG) (Abelha, Pereira, Brandão, Portela, Santos, Silva, et al., 2014). In addition, this system is also characterized by six specific flowcharts (Pregnant ("Yes"), Postpartum Women ("No", "Yes"); Not Women ("No," No"); Pregnant Maybe ("Maybe"); Voluntary Interruption of Pregnancy

(VIP) ("To IGO"); Cardiotocography (CTG) ("To CTG")). This measure allowed a significant reduction (7%) of women at the obstetric emergency department as can be seen in *Improving Quality of Services in Maternity Care Triage System* (Abelha, Pereira, Brandão, Portela, Santos, Silva, et al., 2014). This pre-triage system is supported by the Agency for Integration, Diffusion and Archive Clinic and Medical Information (AIDA), the interoperability platform of CHP (Peixoto, Santos, Abelha, & Machado, 2012). This interoperability platform (Marins et al., 2014) is based on the use of intelligent agents (Cardoso, Marins, Portela, Santos, et al., 2014) to enable communication among different systems. This multi-agent system (Cardoso, Marins, Portela, Abelha, & Machado, 2014) allows the standardization of clinical systems and overcomes medical and administrative complexity inherent to different sources of information (Pereira, Brandão, Portela, et al., 2014).

Triage Systems

As mentioned there are several triage systems currently implemented in healthcare institutions. However, the main limitation of this type of triage systems is the lack of flexibility, i.e., they are not able to respond to the requirements of specific emergency departments (Smithson et al., 2013). One such instance, are the patients that fall in the gynaecology and obstetrics specialties. They are characterized by specific symptoms and signs that are not evaluated by the general triage systems available today.

A literature review was carried out about the triage systems most used in the GO Units. In this case highlights the Manchester Triage System (MTS) and Obstetric Triage Accuracy Scale (OTAS). Manchester Triage System (MTS) is a general priorities triage system implemented in the majority of Portuguese and European institutions and Obstetric Triage Accuracy Scale (OTAS) is an obstetric priorities triage system.

Manchester Triage System

The Manchester Triage System (MTS) was introduced in the United Kingdom (UK) in 1996 and quickly became widespread in Europe. In mid of 2000 it was implemented in the United States of America (Portela et al., 2013). This system, as most of the triages systems, aims to identify in a practical and systematic way the severity criteria indicating the clinical priority of a patient should be treated as well as the respective maximum waiting time that each patient should be subject. MTS includes a set of fifty two flowcharts, containing a specific set of discriminators associating the patients to a given urgency class, as can be seen in table 1.

Table 1. MTS Nomenclature (adapted from (Grupo Português de Triagem, 2002))

Number	Name	Colour	Target Time
1	Emergent	Red	0
2	Very Urgent	Orange	15
3	Urgent	Yellow	30
4	Less Urgent	Green	60
5	Non- Urgent	Blue	120

According to the *Comissão Nacional de Saúde Materna da Criança e do Abolescente* (CNSMCA) evaluating the advantages and disadvantages of MTS in relation to obstetrics proved to be a difficult task. However, it can be identified that the flowchart 34 ("Pregnancy") is inappropriate for obstetric triage. Furthermore, some advantages was identified like the fact that the MTS be valid and universally accepted. The patients are triage into five levels of clinical priorities, and the focus is in the speed and in the objectivity. MTS also enables the monitoring of the implementation and development of quality and efficiency indicators (triage time, waiting time, managed care, list of priorities with the high and hospitalizations, etc.). It should be noted the fact of this system is being adopted in Portugal and it is currently linked to the Medical Support System (SAM) (Infantil, 2013).

Obstetrical Triage Acuity Scale

The Obstetrical Triage Acuity Scale (OTAS) has been shaped by the Canadian Triage and Acuity Scale (CTAS). It was introduced in 1999 and has undergone revisions in years 2006 and 2008 (Murray et al., 2004). The CTAS has a high degree of reliability and validity, however, this only includes a limited number of parameters obstetric which, in turn, does not reflect the diversity of women that go to obstetric triage units. Thus, in order to allow the creation of a tool encompassing a wide variety of patients in the obstetric units it was developed the OTAS. The parameters evaluated are shown in Table 2.

Thus, OTAS revised five specific parameters of pregnant women: Working Labour and Fluid, Haemorrhage, Hypertension, Fetal Assessment, other (Smithson et al., 2013). In this follow-up it was formed an expert group of physicians and nurses and it was analysed the classification system in order to safeguard the accuracy and integrity of the obstetric discriminators defined.

OTAS is the first comprehensive obstetric tool with an accurate classification, establishing reliability and validity in terms of obstetric triage. It is a renowned

Table 2. OTAS Nomenclature (adapted from (Smithson et al., 2013))

Number	Name	Colour	Target Time	Reassessment
OTAS 1	Recursive	Red	0	Immediate
OTAS 2	Emergent	Orange	15	All 10 min
OTAS 3	Urgent	Yellow	30	All 15 min
OTAS 4	Less Urgent	Green	60	All 15 min
OTAS 5	Non-Urgent	Blue	120	All 60 min

scale and already has a wide application in various obstetric triage units and general emergencies. OTAS provides care to a significant number of women in the obstetrics specialty (Smithson et al., 2013).

In general, this system has the advantage of considering separately the maternal and fetal reviews and separating the pregnancy labour from the pathology. This system is also well-structured for obstetrics in the definition of signs, symptoms and timing of care.

However, this system is not implemented in Portugal and it is not allowed a practice assessment, so it is unknown the OTAS compatibility with the existing systems in the Portugal GO Emergency Department (Infantil, 2013).

MATERIALS, METHODS, AND METHODOLOGIES

Being this project based in scientific studies, a research methodology was followed and a set of materials and methods were used in order to achieve the best model.

Research Methodology

The project presented throughout this chapter was developed using the research methodology *Design Research* (DR). The DR purpose is to guide and validate the construction of artefacts. This presupposes the action of a particular study based in a real problem. In this case, there is a problem requiring a solution being necessary design a solution (artefact) to the problem and assess it. In this sense, the researcher is not a mere observer but an individual who acts in the research context. He seeking to understand a given reality by using their creative potential to create solutions to real problems or needs (Wang & Hannafin, 2005). So this methodology is divided into five sequential steps: Awareness of Problem, Suggestion, Development, Evaluation and Conclusion. In this sense and following this methodologies CRTSO was developed.

Development Methodology of the Clinical Recommendation Triage System for Obstetric

To develop the CRTSO, several steps to assess (technically and scientifically) the feasibility of the proposal were carried out and they are presented in section entitled by *Triage Systems*.

The procedures performed are shown below.

Literature Review: Initially a survey was conducted about the existing triage systems in the Portuguese and World hospitals. In this context it was concluded that MTS are the most used in the Portuguese reality, and therefore, more suitable for analysis (Infantil, 2013). Specifically, the OTAS System constitutes a world reference for obstetric triage (Smithson et al., 2013).

Development of a CRTSO Proposal: In practical terms it was evaluated the evolution possibility of the pre-triage system into a CRTSO. First in the article entitled as *Improving Quality of Services in Maternity Care Triage System* (Abelha, Pereira, Brandão, Portela, Santos, Silva, et al., 2014) was presented the pre-triage system, their specific flowcharts and discriminators. Subsequently the process of evolution to a CRTSO it was evaluated by Data Mining (DM) techniques. In the article entitled as *Pre-Triage Decision Support Improvement in Maternity Care by means of Data Mining* (Pereira, Brandão, Salazar, et al., 2014) it was proven that the pre-triage system is calibrated for the patients triage on two levels (URG and ARGO), however it was found that the pre-triage system needs for some improvements. That said, it was developed a simulation algorithm intending to simulate a triage system with five priority levels. This algorithm was developed having as base the pre-triage system. In general as shown in the article entitled *Simulating A Multi-Level Priority Tri- age System For Maternity Emergency* (Abelha, Pereira, Brandão, Portela, Santos, & Machado, 2014) it was concluded that the transformation of the pre-triage system in to a CRTSO is viable. After the application of the algorithm developed to the data provided by the existing pre-triage system it was found that there are patients who fall into all levels of the priorities designed. This conclusion can also be withdrawn by observing the graph presented in the Figure 1.

Figure 1 presents the results obtained by the pre-triage System and the simulated system. By analysing figure 1 is possible observing that much of the URG pregnant is in level 3 and ARGO pregnant is in level 5. This analysis gives some confidence in concluding the viability assessment study of turning the pre-triage system into a CRTSO.

After these preliminaries studies, the proposal was developed using:

- OTAS system, because it already is a specific system of obstetric triage (Smithson et al., 2013).

Figure 1. Results of pre-triage system and the simulated system grouped by number of patients, for maximum waiting time and time average waiting (adapted from (Abelha, Pereira, Brandão, Portela, Santos, & Machado, 2014))

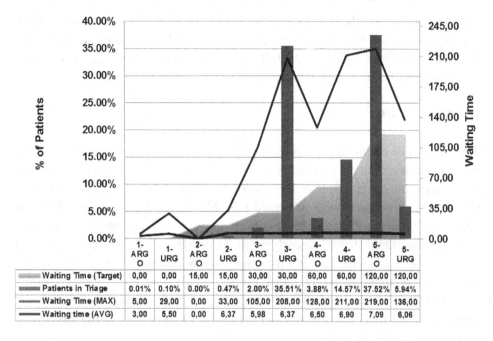

	1-ARGO	1-URG	2-ARGO	2-URG	3-ARGO	3-URG	4-ARGO	4-URG	5-ARGO	5-URG
Waiting Time (Target)	0,00	0,00	15,00	15,00	30,00	30,00	60,00	60,00	120,00	120,00
Patients in Triage	0.01%	0.10%	0.00%	0.47%	2.00%	35.51%	3.88%	14.57%	37.52%	5.94%
Waiting Time (MAX)	5,00	29,00	0,00	33,00	105,00	208,00	128,00	211,00	219,00	136,00
Waiting time (AVG)	3,00	5,50	0,00	6,37	5,98	6,37	6,50	6,90	7,09	6,06

- MTS system, because it is a standard Triage System for general emergency departments.
- Empirical knowledge of health specialists in obstetric area that currently work, or have already exercised triage activities.

Model Evaluation: In the evaluation process and after being designed the proposal of clinical CRTSO, three joint meetings were performed with all the professionals involved, with the following order of work:

- At the first meeting the system proposal was presented to all members.
- At the second meeting and after everybody involved in the work be framed on the subject, there was made an analysis of all flowcharts in order to proceed to their medical and scientific evaluation;
- At the third meeting, an agreement on the proposal made was achieved.

This process was time consuming but rewarding, since after the interaction made between the information system professionals and the healthcare professionals it was possible to obtain a final model sensitive and adapted to a specific reality: gynaecology service.

CLINICAL RECOMMENDATION SYSTEM FOR OBSTETRIC TRIAGE

This section presents the transformation model of pre-triage system into a CRTSO. Initially it is shown the nomenclature chosen for the CRTSO. Then the CRTSO developed is presented. Finally in the last topic of this section the overall adjustments to the proposal be functional are presented.

Nomenclature

The analysis of the nomenclature and definitions currently in use by the existing triage systems revealed the existence of some similarities but also some differences between the pre-triage systems. Two of the systems in analysis were the MTS and OTAS. The terms used were presented in Tables 1 and 2 respectively. With the analysis of these two systems was possible to quickly reach an agreement on a new nomenclature. In this regard, to each one of the new triage categories was assigned a level, a name, a colour, a target time (maximum wait time for the admission) and a re-evaluation time, as presented in Table 3.

This initial nomenclature will be re-calibrated in the future after testing the model by using real data. The main changes can be essentially in the target time and in the reassessment time.

Model

Three different models have been developed taking into account the types of users: Pregnant ("Yes"), Postpartum, ("No", "Yes"), Not Postpartum Women ("No", "No") and Maybe Pregnant ("Maybe"), as described in the article entitled *Improving Quality of Services in Maternity Care Triage System* (Abelha, Pereira, Brandão, Portela, Santos, Silva, et al., 2014).

Table 3. Clinical recommendation triage system for obstetrics nomenclature

Level	Name	Colour	Target Time	Reassessment
1	Emergent	Red	0	Immediate
2	Very Urgent	Orange	15	All 10 min
3	Urgent	Yellow	30	All 15 min
4	Less Urgent	Green	60	All 15 min
5	Non- Urgent	Blue	120	All 60 min

Due to similarities between issues/discriminators the six flowcharts were grouped in three different flowcharts, and the flowcharts "To VIP" and "To CTG" were extinguished of the triage system as is explained below.

As part of this work and due to confidentiality duties, only it is presented the model for the flowchart Pregnant ("Yes"). Although this fact the other two models also have been developed.

In Table 4, is represented the model developed for the flowchart of patients identified as Pregnant ("Yes").

Table 4. Model of the Clinical Recommendation Triage System for Obstetrics, Flowchart Pregnant patients ("Yes")

Triage GO (Pregnant)	1 (Emergent)	2 (Very Urgent)	3 (Urgent)	4 (Less Urgent)	5 (Non-Urgent)
Target Time	Immediate care	<=15 min	<= 30 min	<= 60 min	<=120 min
Re-assessment	Continuous Nursing Care	Every 15 min	Every 15 min	Every 30 min	Every 60 min
Labor/Fluid	Imminent birth	Loss of amniotic fluid. Rhythmic and painful uterine contractions and week of pregnancy <35?	Loss of amniotic fluid and Rhythmic and painful uterine contractions		
Vaginal bleeding	Hemorrhage (Severe)?	Hemorrhage (Moderate)?	Hemorrhage (Scarce)?		
Blood Pressure	(Systolic> 160 and diastolic> 110) and / or (headache, visual changes or epigastric pain / right upper quadrant Pain)?		Systolic> 140 and diastolic> 90) and (headache or visual changes or epigastric pain / right upper quadrant)?	Ref. Tension Rise? Systolic> 140 and diastolic> 90?	
Fetal Assessment			Absence of fetal movements?	Decreased of fetal movements?	
Glasgow Coma Scale	Glasgow (3)?	Glasgow (4-5)?	Glasgow (6-8)?	Glasgow (9-12)?	Glasgow (13-15)?
Pain scale (local, intensity, duration)	Pain (10) and (abdominal pain or low back pain or pain in the lower abdomen)?	Pain (7-9 and (abdominal pain or low back pain or pain in the lower abdomen)?	Pain (4-6) and (abdominal pain or low back pain or pain in the lower abdomen)?	Pain (1-3) and (abdominal pain or low back pain or pain in the lower abdomen)?	Pain (0)?

continued on following page

Table 4. Continued

Triage GO (Pregnant)	1 (Emergent)	2 (Very Urgent)	3 (Urgent)	4 (Less Urgent)	5 (Non-Urgent)
Fever		>= 41, 0 °C	38,5 – 40,9 °C	37,5 °C – 38,4 °C	<37,4 °C?
Umbilical cord prolapse	Umbilical cord prolapse?				
Other	• Dyspnoea • Seizures?	• Lipothymy • Trauma in pregnant	• Uncontrollable vomiting? • Epigastric pain / right upper quadrant and weeks of gestation> 20? • Higher pain 1 week? • Jaundice and gestational weeks> 20? • General condition (Bad)?	• Epigastric pain / right upper quadrant and weeks of gestation <20? • Jaundice and weeks gestation <20 • Urinary symptoms? • General condition (Average)?	• General condition (Good) • To IGO or not Evolutionary Pregnancy • Combur? • Other situations (contact with chickenpox and rubella)?

In this system some relevant parameters are evaluated in order to distinguish the priority of pregnant woman ("Yes") taking into account the clinical characteristics at the triage time: labour, haemorrhage, hypertension, fetal assessment, the Glasgow Coma Scale (GCS), pain scale, fever and others variables as can be seen in Table 4.

In order to changing the pre-triage system to a CRTSO with five priority levels, the existing pre-triage system requires some changes:

Change in nomenclature of the existing discriminators:

- Uterine contractions > Rhythmic and Painful Contractions;
- Nausea / Vomiting > Uncontrollable Vomiting;
- Change the Colour of the skin > Jaundice;
- In general, the categorization of the other parameters evaluated in Table 4 was trivial between the pre-triage system and OTAS.

Add new discriminators:

- Discharge;
- Itching;
- Other conditions (contact with varicella and rubella);

- To IGO or Not Evolutionary Pregnancy: Women for IGO should be included in the type of pregnant patients. If this is not associated with a medical condition should be inserted in less urgent level (level 5);
- Dyspnoea;
- Imminent birth;

Changing the type of variable:

- The parameters "Weeks of Pregnancy", "Blood Pressure" and "Fever" should become numeric (permit the choice of a value or enter a numerical value only).

General Adaptations

After the models development, a set of overall adjustments were designed to the three proposed models (one for each flowchart).

The first adjustment is in the fact of the flow discriminators described in the previous subsection (model) are not performed sequentially in the pre-triage system. Thus, it is suggested that during the implementation of this model should be imposed a condition, preventing the priority reduction by the system, or a recast where first it is asked the main discriminator and so forth, as can be seen in Figure 2.

In Figure 2 is defined a set of priority questions, that must be doing to the patients when they are admitted to the emergency department. First should be asked to patient the reason for the visit the emergency department. In the case of bean emergent situation the patient is attended immediately, i.e., he is not submitted to the triage process.

Then the clinical professional should try to see what type of patient she is. She can be a Pregnant Woman ("Yes"), Postpartum Women ("Yes", "No") or not Pregnant Women ("No", "No") / Pregnant Maybe ("Maybe"). That said, should be carried out a set of priority questions, according to the chosen flowchart. Finally should be recommended the priority level.

The second adjustment is to the patients identified as Urgent Consultation (ARGO) in the pre-triage system. They should be distinguished with the Blue priority (level 5) and sent for urgent consultations as happen actually with pre-triage system. On the other hand, patients assigned to category Urgent (URG) in the pre-triage system must be distributed among the remaining four levels of priorities proposed (Red (level 1), Orange (level 2), Yellow (level 3) and Green (level 4)) being then referred to the obstetric emergency room according to their clinical condition (priority).

Figure 2. Proposal for general clinical recommendation system for obstetric triage

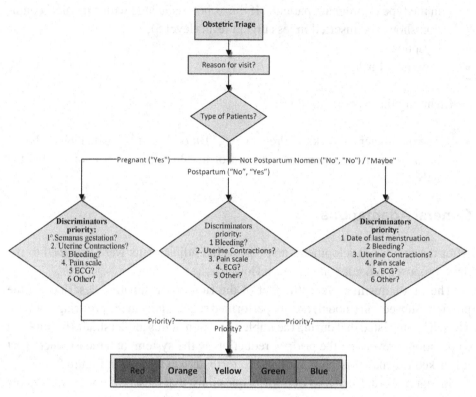

With this condition it can be can recommended a referral of the patients in more detail and more effectively, especially for urgent patients. They are now divided by different levels of clinical care.

Finally the classes of patients "To CTG" and "To IGO" were removed from the CMIN obstetric emergency. The patients "To CTG" are not considered urgent once the exams and pregnancy monitoring process are not an urgent situation. Relatively to the patients "To IGO", they are not also considered urgent cases, unless exceptions where the patients present situations inspiring urgent care (e.g. vaginal bleeding). In these situations the women should be placed on pregnant woman ("Yes") flowchart.

DISCUSSION AND CONCLUSION

The possible implementation of a CRTSO will provide significant benefits for CMIN while health institution as well as to the patients who use this health institution. It allows a patient categorization in five levels according to the level of clinical needs, prioritizing their care according their condition.

For the development of this proposal it was required an extensive work of literature review, planning, development and evaluation of the proposed CRTSO. Throughout this section it is made an analysis between the work developed and guidelines suggested by the CNSMCA regarding to the obstetric triage.

They were evaluated four points:

1. **Scientific gathering information on the various existing systems:** for this process it was conducted a scientific review on the existing triage systems in worldwide. In sub section *Triage System* were described the theoretical aspects of MTS and OTAS Systems and in the article entitled *by Improving Quality of Services in Maternity Care Triage System* (Abelha, Pereira, Brandão, Portela, Santos, Silva, et al., 2014) is described the pre-triage system implemented in CMIN.

2. **Knowledge criteria of the Portuguese reality through contact with triage systems in use**: on this topic, according to the study done by CNSMCA where a survey was conducted at 38 institutions Portuguese about the obstetric triage, it was identified that 34 of these institutions has the obstetric urgency and the general urgency separated. Of these, only 12 performed the obstetric triage. Usually it turns out the existence of these systems in hospitals where the flow of patients in obstetric emergency is high. It was also detected that there is a wide variety software with adaptations made as is the ALERT software with MTS, or very simplistic triage systems that only differentiate between urgent and non-urgent patients (Portela et al., 2013) (Infantil, 2013) (Abelha, Pereira, Brandão, Portela, Santos, Silva, et al., 2014).

3. **Defining criteria for the CRTSO developed:**

    a. *The most scientific and consensually internationally valid:* in this context the two systems valid at international level are: the OTAS and MTS. The first was developed for triage in obstetric emergency. The second is recognized at international level and it is in the Portuguese healthcare institutions. Then there is also the pre-triage system, which although it is not a global system, their efficiency has been demonstrated in the articles *Improving Quality of Services in Maternity Care Triage System* (Abelha, Pereira, Brandão, Portela, Santos, Silva, et al., 2014), *Pre-Triage Decision Support Improvement in Maternity Care by means of Data Mining* (Pereira, Brandão, Salazar, et al., 2014) and *Simulating Multi-Level Priority Triage System For Emergency Maternity* (Abelha, Pereira, Brandão, Portela, Santos, & Machado, 2014). It is characterized by a set of discriminators adapted to the CMIN and the reality of an obstetric emergency.

    b. *Must be compatible with the software applications of the Ministry of Health, i.e. interconnection to existing software level hospitals:* Given that the starting point is that the pre-triage system should be supported by AIDA which interlinks with other National Health systems (Medical Support System (SAM) Nursing Practice Support System (SAPE), etc.). In the future the CRTSO proposed will take up these features too.

c. *Easy to learn and intuitive as possible:* The pre-triage system was already implemented in the MJD, since 2010 and it was subsequently transferred to the CMIN. Being the CRTSO an adaptation of the pre-triage system, the healthcare professionals at CMIN are much familiarized with the system.

d. *Adapted or the ability to adapt to obstetric specialty, i.e., flowchart and discriminated specific for obstetrics:* The pre-triage system is characterized by having specific discriminators to obstetrics therefore the developed model also has this valence. In addition to the specific discriminators already used in pre-triage system this CRTSO has new discriminators. The existing discriminators, such as those added to the model went through a process of natural discussion to assess their viability.

4. **Defining the criteria for who does obstetric:** Usually this pre-triage process should be performed by health professionals: Nurse Specialist in maternal and child health or Physician specialist in obstetric. Once the triage process currently is carried out by experts in Obstetric, this feature also will be present in the new CRTSO.

It is important to note that although this CRTSO have been designed based on the MTS, OTAS and pre-triage system of CMIN, should not be classified as a priority triage system but as a Clinical Recommendation System (CRS). CRTSO only allows a recommend forwarding and a service order taking into account a range of clinical aspects of patients, however the final decision is always taken by the health professional responsible for this process.

It is therefore concluded that the proposed transformation of the pre-triage system into a CRTSO is a pioneer project with great potentialities. The main goal is not replace the MST but create an alternative to most specific departments as is GO emergency units.

FUTURE RESEARCH DIRECTIONS

In view of the project success, as future work is suggested one set of sequential steps:

1. Presenting of the this CRTSO in the CMIN to discuss its possible implementation and testing;

2. Contact the Portuguese Group of Triage (Grupo Português de Triagem, 2014), responsible institution for the implementation of triage systems in Portugal, in order to approve the CRTSO developed;

3. If approved by those two institutions should proceed to the implementation of the flowcharts associated to the respective discriminators and conditions specified for the transformation considered in the article. If the project is not approved, should be made the necessary changes in order to approve the project, after the changes should be executed again the point 1 of this sequence.

4. Preparation of documents and specific protocols supporting the use of the system implemented, for example, a manual to support the healthcare professional in the triage process.

5. Performing periodic evaluations in order to make timeout adjustments to optimize the speed of attending patients in critical condition. One of the methodology to be followed it was focused in article entitled by *Pre-Triage Decision Support Improvement in Maternity Care by means of Data Mining* (Pereira, Brandão, Salazar, et al., 2014). This article used DM techniques to obtain prediction models. At same time it was developed a Business Intelligence platform to manage pre-triage indicators. This platform also can incorporate indicators from the CRTSO developed. This Business Intelligence platform can be consulted in the articles entitled by *Business Intelligence to Maternity Care* (Pereira, Brandão, Portela, et al., 2014) and it allows obtaining Key Indicator Performance (KPI) about the performance of the pre-triage system.

6. Developing data mining models (Filipe Portela, Filipe Pinto, & Santos, 2012; Santos & Portela, 2011) to improve the CRTSO models

7. Assessing the CRTSO using as example earlier studies (Filipe Portela, Jorge Aguiar, Manuel Filipe Santos, Álvaro Silva, & Fernado Rua, 2013)

The proposal CRTSO presented in this article aims the implementation in CMIN as a testing phase. However the objective is that in the future may be used by other health institutions that contemplate the obstetric emergency department.

ACKNOWLEDGMENT

This work is funded by National Funds through the FCT - Fundação para a Ciência e a Tecnologia (Portuguese Foundation for Science and Technology) within projects PEst-OE/EEI/UI0752/2014 and PEst-OE/EEI/UI0319/2014. The work of Filipe Portela was supported by a postdoctoral grant associated to FCT project INTCare II - PTDC/EEI-SII/1302/2012.

REFERENCES

Abelha, A., Pereira, E., Brandão, A., Portela, C. F., Santos, M. F., & Machado, J. (2014). Simulating a multi-level priority triage system for Maternity Emergency. *Proceedings of ESM - 28th European Simulation and Modelling Conference*, Porto, Portugal. EUROSIS.

Abelha, A., Pereira, E., Brandão, A., Portela, F., Santos, M. F., Silva, Á., & Braga, J. (2014). Improving Quality of Services in Maternity Care Triage System. *International Journal of E-Health and Medical Communications, 6(2), 10-26.*

Brandão, A., Pereira, E., Portela, F., Santos, M., Abelha, A., & Machado, J. (2014). Real-time Business Intelligence platform to maternity care. *Proceedings of IECBES 2014 - IEEE Conference on Biomedical Engineering and Sciences*, Sarawak, Malaysia (pp. 379-384). IEEE.

Cabral, A., Pina, C., Machado, H., Abelha, A., Salazar, M., & Quintas, C. et al.. (2011). Data Acquisition Process for an Intelligent Decision Support in Gynecology and Obstetrics Emergency Triage. In M. M. Cruz-Cunha, J. Varajão, P. Powell, & R. Martinho (Eds.), *Enterprise Information Systems* (Vol. 221, pp. 223–232). CCIS.

Cardoso, L., Marins, F., Portela, F., Abelha, A., & Machado, J. (2014). Healthcare interoperability through intelligent agent technology. *Procedia Technology, 16,* 1334–1341.

Cardoso, L., Marins, F., Portela, F., Santos, M., Abelha, A., & Machado, J. (2014). The Next Generation of Interoperability Agents in Healthcare. *International Journal of Environmental Research and Public Health, 11*(5), 5349–5371. doi:10.3390/ijerph110505349 PMID:24840351

Comissão Nacional de Saúde Materna da Criança e do Abolescente. (2013). *Triagem Obstétrica- modelo de Triagem.* Lisboa: Direção Geral de Saúde.

Grupo Português de Triagem. (2002). *Triagem no serviço de Urgência – Manual do Formador* (2nd ed.). Lisboa: BMJ Publishing Group.

Grupo Português de Triagem. (2014). Grupo Português de Triagem. Retrieved from http://www.grupoportuguestriagem.pt/jm/

Mackway-Jones, K., M. J. & W. J. (1997). Emergency triage: Manchester triage group. *BMJ (Clinical Research Ed.).*

Marins, F., Cardoso, L., Portela, F., Santos, M. F., Abelha, A., & Machado, J. (2014). Improving High Availability and Reliability of Health Interoperability Systems. In *New Perspectives in Information Systems and Technologies* (Vol. 2, pp. 207–216). Springer. doi:10.1007/978-3-319-05948-8_20

Murray, M., Bullard, M., & Grafstein, E. (2004). Revisions to the Canadian Emergency Department Triage and Acuity Scale implementation guidelines. *Cjem, 6*(6), 421–7. Retrieved from http://www.ncbi.nlm.nih.gov/pubmed/17378961

Peixoto, H., Santos, M., Abelha, A., & Machado, J. (2012). Intelligence in Interoperability with AIDA. In L. Chen, A. Felfernig, J. Liu, & Z. Raś (Eds.), *Foundations of Intelligent Systems SE - 31* (Vol. 7661, pp. 264–273). Springer Berlin Heidelberg; doi:10.1007/978-3-642-34624-8_31

Pereira, E., Brandão, A., Portela, C. F., Santos, M. F., Machado, J., & Abelha, A. (2014). Business Intelligence in Maternity Care. *Proceedings of the 18th International Database Engineering & Applications Symposium* (pp. 352–355). New York, NY, USA: ACM. doi:10.1145/2628194.2628248

Pereira, E., Brandão, A., Salazar, M., Portela, C. F., Santos, M. F., & Machado, J. … Jorge, B. (2014). Pre-Triage Decision Support Improvement in Maternity Care by means of Data Mining. In A. Azevedo, & M. F. Santos (Eds.), Integration of Data Mining in Business Intelligence Systems. Hershey, PA, USA: IGI Global Book.

Portela, F., Santos, M.F., & Abelha, A., Machado, J. (2015). A Real-Time Intelligent System for tracking patient condition.

Portela, F., Aguiar, J., Santos, M. F., Silva, Á., & Rua, F. (2013). Pervasive Intelligent Decision Support System - Technology Acceptance in Intensive Care Units. In Á. Rocha, A.M. Correia, T. Wilson, & K.A. Stroetmann (Ed.), Advances in Intelligent Systems and Computing, CCIS (Vol. 206, pp. 279-292). Springer.

Portela, F., Pinto, F., & Santos, M. F. (2012). Data Mining Predictive Models For Pervasive Intelligent Decision Support. *Intensive Care Medicine*.

Portela, F., Santos, M. F., Gago, P., Silva, Á., Rua, F., Abelha, A., … . (2011). Enabling real-time intelligent decision support in intensive care. *Paper presented at the 25th European Simulation and Modelling Conference ESM'2011*, Guimarães, Portugal.

Portela, F., Vilas-Boas, M., Santos, M. F., Abelha, A., Machado, J., Cabral, A., … .. (2010). Electronic Health Records in the Emergency Room. *Proceedings of the 9th IEEE/ACIS International Conference on Computer and Information Science* (pp. 195-200). doi:10.1109/ICIS.2010.98

Portela, F., Cabral, A., Abelha, A., Salazar, M., Quintas, C., Machado, J., Neves, J., & Santos, M. F. (2013). Knowledge Acquisition Process for Intelligent Decision Support in Critical Health Care. In R. Martinho, R. Rijo, M.M. Cruz-Cunha, & J. Verajao (Eds.), Information Systems and Technologies for Enhancing Health and Social Care (Ch. 4, pp. 55-68). Hershey, PA, USA: IGI Global.

Santos, M. F., & Portela, F. (2011). Enabling Ubiquitous Data Mining in Intensive Care - Features selection and data pre-processing. *Proceedings of the 13th International Conference on Enterprise Information Systems*, Beijing, China.

Smithson, D. S., Twohey, R., Rice, T., Watts, N., Fernandes, C. M., & Gratton, R. J. (2013). Implementing an obstetric triage acuity scale: Interrater reliability and patient flow analysis. *American Journal of Obstetrics and Gynecology, 209*(4), 287–293. doi:10.1016/j.ajog.2013.03.031 PMID:23535239

Wang, F., & Hannafin, M. J. (2005). Design-based research and technology-enhanced learning environments. *Educational Technology Research and Development, 53*(4), 5–23. doi:10.1007/BF02504682

ADDITIONAL READING

Murray, M., Bullard, M., & Grafstein, E. (2004). Revisions to the Canadian Emergency Department Triage and Acuity Scale implementation guidelines. *Canadian Journal of Emergency Medical Care, 6*(6), 421–427. Retrieved from http://www.ncbi.nlm.nih.gov/pubmed/17378961 PMID:17378961

Peixoto, H., Santos, M., Abelha, A., & Machado, J. (2012). Intelligence in Interoperability with AIDA. In L. Chen, A. Felfernig, J. Liu, & Z. Raś (Eds.), *Foundations of Intelligent Systems SE - 31* (Vol. 7661, pp. 264–273). Springer Berlin Heidelberg. doi:10.1007/978-3-642-34624-8_31

Smithson, D. S., Twohey, R., Rice, T., Watts, N., Fernandes, C. M., & Gratton, R. J. (2013). Implementing an obstetric triage acuity scale: Interrater reliability and patient flow analysis. *American Journal of Obstetrics and Gynecology, 209*(4), 287–293. doi:10.1016/j.ajog.2013.03.031 PMID:23535239

Wang, F., & Hannafin, M. J. (2005). Design-based research and technology-enhanced learning environments. *Educational Technology Research and Development, 53*(4), 5–23. doi:10.1007/BF02504682

KEY TERMS AND DEFINITIONS

AIDA: Platform developed to ensure interoperability among healthcare information systems.

Business Intelligence: A technology that uses data analysis tools and applications to help business users make more informed decision.

Clinical Recommendation System: Combines several computational techniques to select custom items based on user interests and as the context in which they live.

Decision Support System: A computerized information system used to support decision-making process in an organization or business.

Gynaecology and Obstetrics: The medical specialty dealing with fields of through only one postgraduate training programmer. This combined training prepares the practicing Gynaecology and Obstetrics to be adept at the care of female reproductive organs' health and at the management of obstetric complications, even though surgery.

Interoperability: Autonomous ability to interact and communicate.

Maternity Care: Health institution where patients of gynaecology and obstetrics specialties are admitted.

Pre-Triage System: A triage system has as main aim to improve the quality of care in that it provides a service based on clinical characteristics and the target time.

Triage: The sorting of patients (as in an emergency room) according to the urgency of their need for care.

Chapter 5
A New Approach to Generate Hospital Data Warehouse Schema

Nouha Arfaoui
Institut Supérieur de Gestion de Tunis, Tunisia

Jalel Akaichi
Institut Supérieur de Gestion de Tunis, Tunisia

ABSTRACT

The healthcare industry generates huge amount of data underused for decision making needs because of the absence of specific design mastered by healthcare actors and the lack of collaboration and information exchange between the institutions. In this work, a new approach is proposed to design the schema of a Hospital Data Warehouse (HDW). It starts by generating the schemas of the Hospital Data Mart (HDM) one for each department taking into consideration the requirements of the healthcare staffs and the existing data sources. Then, it merges them to build the schema of HDW. The bottom-up approach is suitable because the healthcare departments are separately. To merge the schemas, a new schema integration methodology is used. It starts by extracting the similar elements of the schemas and the conflicts and presents them as mapping rules. Then, it transforms the rules into queries and applies them to merge the schemas.

DOI: 10.4018/978-1-4666-9882-6.ch005

INTRODUCTION

The healthcare industry is considered as one of the world's largest, fastest-developing and most information-rich industries (Foundation, 2006). It generates huge amount of data related to patients, drugs, doctors, etc. The collected data plays a crucial role to ensure complex statistical analysis. It is used to calculate the measurement and key performance indicators that are vital for the organization to be more agile, flexible and fluent (Mike, 2014).

The continuous development, the difficulties related to the collection of the data in the healthcare organization for the analysis, the reduction of the computing cost and the explosion of the healthcare data make the use of Hospital Data Warehouse (HDW) an efficient solution to well exploit the collected data to make good decisions.

The DW is defined as *a subject-oriented, integrated, non-volatile and time-variant collection of data in support of management's decisions* (Inmon, 2005). It allows the end-users to self-service their needs (Inmon, 2005). It may provide information to users in areas ranging from research to management (Sen and Jacob, 1998). It facilitates the storage, enhances timely analysis and increases the quality of area time decision making processes (Sahama and Croll, 2007). It offers one space to store the global truth to enable healthcare analysis such as identifying quickly the causal relationship of diseases. It aggregates, then, the data from clinical and financial systems into one repository.

The top-down starts from the description of the needs of all the users to construct the schema corresponding to the entire DW (Malinowski and Zimanyi, 2008). The bottom-up constructs the global schema of DW starting from the different schemas of Data Mart (DM) (Malinowski and Zimanyi, 2008). The hybrid approach takes advantages of the two previous approaches (Malinowski and Zimanyi, 2008). It has the speed and the user-orientation of the top-down and the integration enforced by a DW of the bottom-up.

The healthcare centers are composed by different departments such as accident and emergency, anesthetics, cardiology, diagnostic imaging, general surgery, maternity departments, neurology, Pharmacy, etc. The departments record their own data, they are still stand along, they do not communicate with other health care centers and they do not share their documents with others (Dutta, 2013). Starting by designing the schemas of the Hospital Data Mart (HDM) one for each healthcare department, then, generating the HDW schema using the bottom-up approach is very suitable and profitable in such case.

The DM is defined *as a flexible set of data, ideally based on the most atomic (granular) data possible to extract from an operational source, and presented in a symmetric (dimensional) model that is most resilient when faced with unexpected user queries* (Kimball and Ross, 2002). It is accessed directly by end users, and its data is structured in a way that is easy for users to understand and use (Moody and Kortink, 2000).

In this work, we mix two approaches: hybrid and bottom-up. The first one is used to generate the HDM taking into consideration the healthcare staffs' requirements and the existing data sources. An assistant system is introduced, at this level, to facilitate to the users the specification of their needs. The second approach is applied to build the HDW from HDM schemas. In the two steps, we use a new schema integration methodology to ensure the automatic generation of the schemas.

Starting by generating HDM helps to resolve the different problems that arise within each department because of the various care practices, data types and definitions, the perceived incompleteness of clinical information systems, the type of information that the medicine and healthcare need (Mul et al., 2012) which make the creation of the HDW in one step a very hard task.

As working hypothesis, it is proposed to present the schemas as star or snowflake because they are the most used models and they are easy to understand (Lee and Ling, 1997), (Levene and Loizou, 2003). Concerning the data sources, it is proposed to deal with Entity-Relationship (ER) database because it adopts the more natural view that the real world consists of entities and relationships; it incorporates some of the important semantic information and it can achieve a high degree of data independence (Chen, 1976).

BACKGROUND

In this section, we start by presenting some DW design methodologies to move next to summarize some work proposing the use of DW in healthcare domain.

Data Warehouse Design Methodologies

Several methodologies, in literature, have been proposed to design the DW. The following table (Table 1) presents some of them.

Data Warehouse and Healthcare

According to our knowledge, few works propose the use of the DW in the medical field. In the following, some of them are described. In (Bennett et al., 2009), the authors propose the implementation of the DW because it offers opportunities when

Table 1. Example of DW methodologies

	Step	Input	Output
[Golfarelli and Rizzi, 2009]	Requirement analysis	Requirements collected from users	Glossaries or Goal-oriented diagrams
	Analysis and reconciliation	Data sources	Reconciled schema
	Conceptual design	User requirements and data extracted from the reconciled schema.	Conceptual schema (the form of a set of fact schemata)
	Workload refinement	Preliminary workload	UML use case diagrams
	Logical design	Conceptual schema	Logical schema
	Data staging design	Source schemata, reconciled schema and the DM logical schema.	ETL procedures
	Physical design	Workload and user profiles, logical schema	Physical schema
	Implement	Workload and user profiles, physical schema, logical schema, and ETL procedures	Implementation
[Peralta et al., 2003]	Conceptual level	Non-functional user requirements	multidimensional conceptual schema
	Logical level	multidimensional conceptual schema, mappings, guideline	Logical relational schema
	Physical level	Logical relational schema	The implementation
[Bizarro and Madeira, 2002]	Logical level	Business view, operational data, design rules, predicated usage profile, meta-data	Optimized star scheme
	Physical level	Optimized star scheme	Optimized physical star scheme
	Preliminary administrative tasks	Optimized physical star scheme	Final star scheme
[Hüsemann et al., 2000]	Requirement analysis and specifications	Operational database schema	Semiformal business concept
	Conceptual design	Semiformal business concept	Formal conceptual schema
	Logical design	Formal conceptual schema	Formal logical schema
	Physical design	Formal logical schema	Physical database schema
[Malinowski and Zimanyi, 2008]	Requirements specification	Source systems, users	Document requirements specification
	Conceptual design	Initial schema	Final schema and mapping
	Logical design	Developed schema	Definition of ETL processes
	Physical des	Developed schema	Implementation of ETL processes and staging area

it is used in the healthcare domain. It aggregates the data from clinical and financial systems into one repository. It identifies quickly the causal relationship of diseases. It allows the end-users to self-service their needs.

In (Sheta and Eldeen, 2012), the authors develop and implement a prototype healthcare DW specific for cancer diseases. They employ the DW to incorporate large quantity of analysis information needed for healthcare decision-making.

The author introduces, in (Dutta, 2013), DW architecture for the Influenza (Flu) diseases. The developed DW is used by database administrator or executive manager, doctors, nurses, other staff members of the health care. It helps to store all information about the patients to facilitate making decisions. The authors, in (Banek et al., 2006), suggest a multidimensional conceptual model of a federated DW. The conceptual model of the component warehouses offers a traditional view on financial measures, yet it does not enable the processing of time-segmented medicine administration data, whose grain level is even lower than the basic grain level of the model.

In (Berndt et al., 2003), the authors construct a comprehensive healthcare DW that provides automated support for CATCH (Comprehensive Assessment for Tracking Community Health). The innovation is about combining the extensive field experience with CATCH and the application of the DW technology. According to the authors the implementation of this type of DW and its use in monitoring, as well as improving health status, will become a primary role of public health agencies in the future. Darmont in (Darmont, 2008) introduce a DW model of complex DW for the health of elite athletes. This tool allows the storage of complex medical data from various fields of medicine and biology. It allows two types of analysis; the first one supports the personalized medicine of anticipation for well-identified patients. The second one is related the statistical analysis of patients.

In (Berndt et al., 2001), the authors implement the DW to support health assessments of communities throughout the state. It is used to explore the relationship between surgical volume and successful outcomes. The healthcare DW includes fine-grained data, such as hospital discharges, births, deaths, and specific disease registries. It includes also demographic, economic, and marketing data to derive many health status indicators. A large collection of stored procedures calculates the health status indicators, propagating the data from fine-grained structures to higher-level reporting components. In (Einbinder et al., 2001), the authors create clinical data repository CDR. The purpose is to support the research and education functions of the academic medical center, also to provide the data for the managers and administrators.

Discussion

Compared to the previous works, we suggest focusing on each department separately because of the lack of communication and documents exchange. We propose, also, the use of an assistant system to help the healthcare staffs to specify their requirements.

Our approach is composed by the following steps:

- It starts by collecting the requirements of the different healthcare staffs. It uses an assistant system HDwADS (Hospital Data warehouse Assistant Design System) to facilitate the specification of the multidimensional components (fact, measures, dimensions and attributes) basing on the stored traces of the previous users. The collected requirements are represented as star schemas.
- Next, it generates the global schema corresponding to HDM conceptual schema from uses' requirements. It uses the schema integration methodology that extracts the semantically closest elements as well as the conflicts and presents them as mapping rules. Then, it merges the different schemas to get at the end the global schema by generating the queries from the mapping rules and executing them.
- Then, the conceptual schemas are mapped to logical ones. This is done in two steps. In the first one, it extracts all possible multidimensional schemas from the databases. In the second step, it generates the logical schemas. Indeed, it updates the conceptual schemas by adding the necessary information extracted from the multidimensional schemas using the mapping rules.
- Finally, using the schema integration technique, the set of logical schemas of HDM are merged to build the final schema of the HDW.

MAIN FOCUS OF THE CHAPTER

This chapter proposes four contributions:

- A new approach to generate the schema of the HDW by mixing the bottom-up approach and the hybrid approach. The different proposed solutions use one approach bottom-up, top-down or hybrid. Because of the specificity of our case (generating HDM for each healthcare center and then merging them to build the DW), we need to mix two approaches the hybrid and the bottom-up. Indeed, each department has its own database and its own requirements, so we apply the mixed approach to generate HDM i.e. taking into consideration both the needs and the available data sources. Then, using the bottom-up approach the HDW is constructed from the set of HDM schemas.

- An assistant system to facilitate the collect of healthcare staffs' requirements. The healthcare staffs are not experienced with the DW technologies and they can find difficulties to express their requirements. To facilitate this task, we use a system that assists the user during this task by proposing the possible next elements to use basing on the previous experiences that are already stored.

- A new schema integration methodology to ensure the automatic merging of the schemas. Different schema integration (SI) methodologies have been proposed to construct the global schema from a set of local schemas. They are applied mainly with the databases. In this work, we propose its use to automate the bottom-up approach. The new methodology is composed by few steps to deal with specificities structure of DW/DM schemas that they are different compared to the databases schemas.

- Appling the new approach to build HDW. The proposed approach facilitates the construction of HDW faster by taking into account the needs of each department and its available information. The share of information between different departments/centers becomes easier and the communication between them becomes possible. Having a global view of the existing information facilitates the process of making decisions.

COLLECTION OF USERS' REQUIREMENTS

In order to ensure a good design of HDM, it is crucial to start by collecting the requirements that specify *what data should be available and how it should be organized as well as what queries are of interest* (Malinowski and Zimanyi, 2008). We extract, then, the important elements related to the multidimensional schema: facts, measures, dimensions, and attributes that reflect the users' needs.

Hospital Data Warehouse Assistant Design System (HDwADS)

The healthcare staffs find difficulties to specify their needs using the SQL queries especially when they apply the GROUP BY and/or HAVING clauses (Annoni et al., 2006) and (Gyssens and Lakshmanan, 1997). Also, they have difficulties to cooperate with the designers since there is not a common language for sufficiently unambiguous communication between them (Börger, 1998).

In order to facilitate this task, we propose the use of an assistant system named Hospital Data warehouse Assistant Design System (HDwADS) (Figure1) that offers helps basing on previous experiences stored as traces (this latter will be explained later). It compares the current manipulation to the stored traces to propose the new

Figure 1. The composition of HDwADS

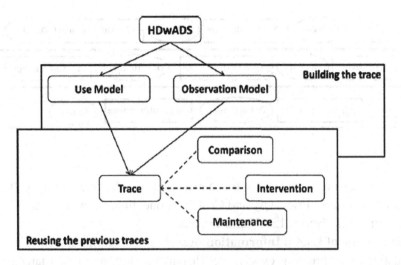

possible object(s). It extracts, then, the objects using the use model and the actions using the observation model. The two models build the traces that are stored into "Trace" database. We have then for each user the information related to his manipulation.

- **Use Model:** It extracts the objects from the current manipulation in order to facilitate their comparison to the objects of the previous experiences. The objects belong to the following categories (C): "C: Fact", "C: Dimension", "C: Attribute", and "C: Measure". These various categories are linked into single schema as presented in Figure 2.
- **Observation Model:** It extracts the actions (‖A: ‖) handled by a single user during his session. It gives a vision on the use and the manipulation of the application and more precisely on how to deal with the existing objects of the use model.
- **Trace:** It is the basis of HDwADS. It is built using the use model and the observation model as consequence it is a secession of objects and actions over the time. It keeps for each user its own trace. Figure 3 presents a portion

Figure 2. The Use Model schema

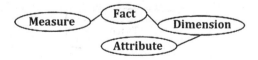

Figure 3. Example of trace

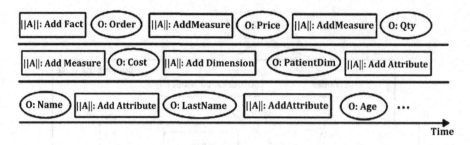

of a trace where there is a star schema composed by one fact table "Order", three measures "Price, Qty and Cost" and one dimension "PatientDim" with its attributes "Name, LastName and Age".

- **Extraction of Useful Information**: It is about comparing the current manipulation to the previous experiences that are already stored into database. The comparison task helps to locate the user to suggest the possible next objects to manipulate. The detection of similar cases is automatically and in parallel with the use of the system, and the intervention is done in real time i.e. the research of the cases and the proposal of solution are made in parallel with the specification of the requirements.

The comparison: There are two cases of comparison:

- HDwADS takes into consideration the last manipulated object (Figure 4).
- HDwADS takes into consideration all the manipulation respecting the order of the objects over the time (Figure 5).

In the both cases, if there is the corresponding object(s) in the database "Trace" this implies that there are at least one experience that can be used in the next step,

Figure 4. Comparing the last manipulated object

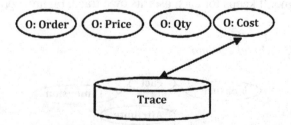

Figure 5. Comparing all the objects of the current manipulation

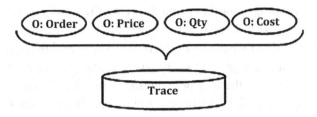

else, the system keeps the new objects until the validation of the final schema, then, it saves them as new trace. In the case of no validation of the final schema, the objects are neglected.

The intervention: It is done in three different ways:

- If the system finds traces from the base that can be used to assist the user in the next step, it intervenes by proposed the next object to manipulate (Figure 6).
- If the system finds traces from the base that can be used to assist the user in the next step, it intervenes by proposed the rest of the trace respecting the order of the existing objects (Figure 7).
- If the system does not find any trace from the base, it proposes the closest objects (by using the degree of similarities and choose the objects with the highest values).

Figure 6. Intervention by proposing the next object extracted from the existing traces

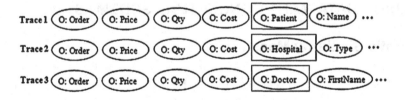

Figure 7. Intervention by proposing the rest of object extracted from the existing traces

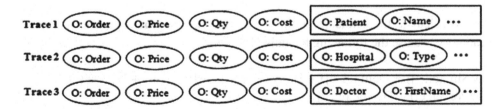

The maintenance: The purpose of the maintenance of the base of the trace is to keep a database running smoothly through saving the most pertinent traces for a reuse. Indeed, we need to keep a reasonable number of trace so that it will not saturate the base, and reduce the response time (to keep real time aspect).

We propose then to assign with each trace its frequency (the number of times that is used i.e. created by the user or exploited in the intervention phase), and we keep the traces with the highest frequency numbers. We give the freedom to the user to specify the threshold.

The Structure of the Generated Schemas

To well exploit the users' requirements, HDwADS presents them as conceptual star schemas having the following structure:

- Fact table corresponds to the subject of analysis. It is defined by: FN and MF{} with:
    - ○ FN: represents the name of the fact.
    - ○ MF {m1, m2, m3, m4, ...}: corresponds to the set of measures related to the fact.
- Dimension tables represent the axis of analysis. Each one is composed by: DN, A{} with:
    - ○ DN: corresponds to the name of the dimension.
    - ○ A {a1, a2, a3, a4, ...}: presents the set of attributes describing the current dimension.

BUILDING DATA MART CONCEPTUAL SCHEMAS

Semantic Similarity Measure

Let Sch1 and Sch2 be two schemas. Let Cp be the categories of elements existing in the schema with Cp = {fact, dimension, measure, attribute}

$\forall e_i \in$ Sch1, $\exists e_j \in$ Sch2, so that e_i and e_j belong to the same category Cp.

To calculate the semantic similarity of two elements belonging to the same category, we use the following formula (1):

DeSim (ei, ej) = DeId (ei, ej) + DeSy (ei, ej) + SeTy (ei, ej) + DePost (ei, ej) + DePre (ei, ej) + DeAbb (ei, ej)   (1)

With:

- DeId (e_i, e_j) = 1 if e_i and e_j are identical i.e. they have the same name, and 0 if not.
  Example: Sch1.fact = "Order" and Sch2.fact= "Order".

- DeSy (ei, ej) = 1 if ei and ej are synonymous i.e. they have two different names with the same meaning, and 0 if not.
  Example: Sch1.dimension = "Medication" and Sch2.dimension = "Drug".

- DeTy (ei, ej) =1 if e_i and e_j are the same with the existence of typos.
  Example: Sch1.measure = "Price" and Sch2.measure = "Prace".

- DePost (ei, ej) = 1 if one is the postfix of the other and 0 if not.
  Example: Sch1.attribute = "Name" and Sch2.attribute = "FirstName".

- DePre (ei, ej) = 1 if one is the prefix of the other, and 0 if not.
  Example: Sch1.dimension = "PatientDim" and Sch2.dimension = "Patient".

- DeAbb (ei, ej) = 1 if one is the abbreviation of the other, 0 if not.
  Example: Sch1.measure = "Qty" and Sch2.measure = "Quantity".

The New Schema Integration Methodology

At this level, we have a set of conceptual HDM schemas. We propose their gathering using schema integration technique that starts by generating the necessary rules and then applying those rules to ensure the merging of the schemas. To facilitate this task, we specify a common interface structure, so we are sure that the different schemas have the same data model, and each element of the schema belongs to a specific category (fact, dimension, measure or attribute).

To achieve our task, the new schema integration methodology is composed by the following steps:

- Categorization: It is to specify the category of each element.
- Construction of the similarity matrix: It is to use the similarity matrix as a way to find the closest elements. The cells contain the coefficient of similarity of the different elements belonging to the same category. It is calculated using the formula (1).

- Generation of the mapping rules: The rules visualize the relationships between the instances of the elements belonging to the same category. They are expressed as: "If Similar (X, Y) then Action (X, Y) and Save (X, Y)", with:
  - ○ X and Y: two elements belong to the same category.
  - ○ Similar (): it is a function that specifies if the two inputs are similar or not. It uses the similarity matrix determined in the previous step.
  - ○ Action (): it specifies the action to perform. It can be union, or intersection.
    - ▪ Union: R = union (ei, ej) implies that R contains all the components of ei and all components of ej.
    - ▪ Intersection: R= intersection (ei, ej) implies that R contains the components that exist in ei and ej.
  - ○ Save (): it saves the two elements.
- Merging the schemas: It is about transforming the previous mapping rules to queries and executing them.

Let us apply the previous steps on Figure 8.

Figure 8. (a) (b). Example of schemas corresponding to the users' requirements

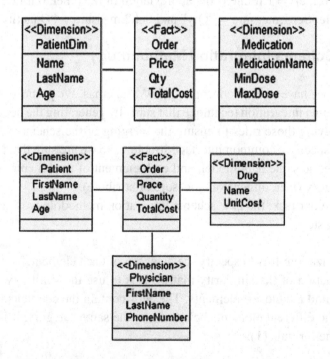

- Categorization:
  - Fact: In Figure 8 (a), the fact is "Order", and in Figure 8 (b) is "Order".
  - Measure: In Figure 8 (a), the measures are "Price, Qty, TotalCost", and in Figure 8 (b), they are "Prace, Quantity, TotalCost".
  - Dimension: In Figure 8 (a), the dimensions are "PatientDim and Medication", and in Figure 8 (b), they are "Patient, Drug and Physician".
  - Attribute: In Figure 8 (a) the attributes are "Name, LastName, Age, MedicationName MinDose, MaxDose". In Figure 8 (b), they are "FirstName, LastName, Age, Name, UnitCost, FirstName LastName, PhoneNumber".
- Construction of the similarity matrix: In the following, we give some examples of similarity matrix.

Figure 9 presents the similarity matrix used to compare the two facts. The value of "Max" is 1 so that they are similar.

Figure 10 presents the similarity matrix used to compare the measures. Basing on the values of Max, we have as similar pairs of measures: {{Price, Prace}; {Qty, Quantity}; {TotalCost, TotalCost}}.

Figure 11 presents the similarity matrix used to compare the dimensions. The similar ones are: {PatientDim, Patient} and {Medication, Drug}

Figure 9. Similarity matrix to compare the facts

Fact	Order	Max
Order	1	1

Figure 10. Similarity matrix to compare the measures

Measure	Prace	Quantity	TotalCost	Max
Price	1	0	0	1
Qty	0	1	0	1
TotalCost	0	0	1	1

Figure 11. Similarity matrix to compare the dimensions

Dimension	Patient	Drug	Physician	Max
PatientDim	1	0	0	1
Medication	0	1	0	1

Figure 12 presents the similarity matrix used to compare the attributes of the two dimension tables "PatientDim/Patient" existing in the two schemas. According to the matrix, we have the following similar pairs of attributes {Name, FirstName}, {LastName, LastName} and {Age, Age}.

Figure 13 presents the similarity matrix used to compare the attributes of the two dimension tables "Medication/Drug" existing in the two schemas. According to the matrix, we have the following similar pair of attributes {MedicationName, Name}.

- Generation of the mapping rules: As example of mapping rules, we can present:
  - ○ If Similar (Order, Order) then Union (Order, Order) and Save (Order, Order)
  - ○ If Similar (Drug, Medication) then Intersection (Drug, Medication) and Save (Drug, Medication)
  - ○ If Similar (PatientDim, Patient) then Intersection (PatientDim, Patient) and Save (PatientDim, Patient)
- Merging the schemas: As example of queries, we can present:
  - ○ Query1 = "Insert into Fact (FactName, idSchema) values ('Order',"+ schemaId +")" ;
  - ○ Query2 = "Insert into Measure (MeasureName, idFact) values (Price',"+ factId +")" ;

Figure 12. Similarity matrix to compare the attributes of the dimension tables "PatientDim/Patient"

Attributes of the dimensions "PatientDim/Patient"	FirstName	LastName	Age	Max
Name	1	0	0	1
LastName	0	1	0	1
Age	0	0	1	1

Figure 13. Similarity matrix to compare the attributes of the dimension tables "Medication/Drug"

Attributes of the dimensions "Medication/Drug"	Name	UnitCost	Max
MedicationName	1	0	1
MinDose	0	0	0
MaxDose	0	0	0

    ○   Query3 = "Insert into Dimension (DimensionName, idSchema) values ('Patient'," +schemaId + ") ";

    ○   Query4 = "Insert into Attribute (AttributeName, idDimension) values ('FirstName'," +dimensionId +")";

With:

- schemaId: is the identifier of the new schema.
- factId: is the identifier of the new fact table.
- dimensionId: is the identifier of the new dimension table.

The result of executing the queries is stored into specific database composed by the following tables:

- The table "Schema" contains the set of schemas to be merged. Each schema is identified through a unique numeric identifier automatically incremented. At the end of the integration process, "Schema" contains only one element corresponding to the identifier of the final schema.
- The table "Fact" stores the names of the facts. It has one primary key and a foreign key connected to the table "Schema".
- The table "Measure" contains the set of measures. It is defined by a primary key and a foreign key connected to the table "Fact".
- The table "Dimension" contains the set of dimensions for each schema. It is described by a primary key, and a foreign key connected to the table "Schema".
- The table "Attribute" is used to store the attributes of each dimension. This table is defined by one primary key, the name of the attributes, their types, and a foreign key connected to the table "Dimension".

At the end of this step, we obtain the following schema (Figure 14) corresponding to the merging of the two previous schemas (Figure 8). It has one fact "Order" with three measures "Price, Quantity and TotalCost", surrounded by three dimensions "Patient, Drug and Physician". Each dimension contains a set of attributes.

GENERATING MULTIDIMENSIONAL SCHEMAS

In this part, we propose the generation of multidimensional schemas from Entity-Relationship (ER) databases. This choice is because ER adopts the more natural view that the real world consists of entities and relationships, it incorporates some of the

Figure 14. The HDM Conceptual schema

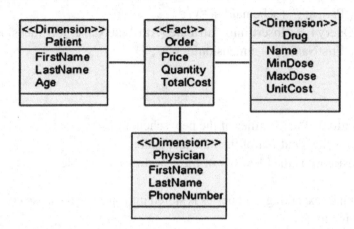

important semantic information about the real world; it can achieve a high degree of data independence (Chen, 1976). The generated schemas can be star or snowflake.

To achieve this task, we propose the following algorithm that is composed by three steps:

Step 1: *Normalize the ER model.* Apply the 1NF, 2NF and 3NF to construct the ER normalized:

- ○ **First Normal Form (1NF):** It should be no nesting or repeating groups in a table.
- ○ **Second Normal Form (2NF):** The key attributes determine all non-key attributes.
- ○ **Third Normal Form (3NF):** The non-key attributes should be independent.

Step 2: *Build the tree from ER model.* From the ER model, we extract the entities (Ef) having n-ary relationships with other entities and those having numerical attributes. They represent the potential facts. Every Ef becomes the root of the tree. The number of trees corresponds to the number of Ef entities. From the ER we extract the entities (E) that are directly linked to Ef corresponding to the potential dimensions.

Step 3: *Transform the tree to multidimensional model.*

- ○ The fact is created having as name "Fact_N" with N is an incremental number.
- ○ The existing numeric attributes become the potential measures.
- ○ The nodes that are directly linked to the roots are transformed to dimensions keeping their attributes and their identifiers.

    ◦   The primary keys of the children nodes become foreign keys in the parents' nodes.

Figure 15 corresponds to a multidimensional schema presented as snowflake with one fact table "Fact_1" having as primary key the set of primary keys of the dimensions. The measures are "NbPatient", "AvailabilityDoctor", "Price", "Quantity" and "TotalCost". Concerning the dimensions, we have "Patient", "Drug", "Doctor", "Date" and "Hospital" that is connected to the parameter "Address". Each table has its primary key and its attributes. The keys and the type of attributes are specified.

GENERATING HOSPITAL DATA MART LOGICAL SCHEMAS

The Structure of the Logical Schemas

The logical HDM schemas can be star or snowflake.

The star schema has the following structure:

- The fact table is defined by FN, FP and MF{ } with:
  - ◦   FN represents the name of the fact.
  - ◦   FP represents the primary key of the fact table.

Figure 15. Example of multidimensional schema

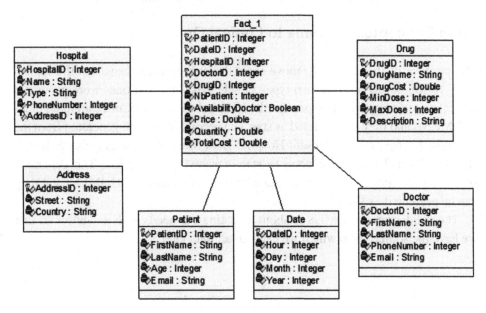

- ○ MF {m1(Tym1), m2 (Tym2), m3 (Tym3), m4 (Tym4), ...} corresponds to the set of measures related to the fact. Each measure has its type.
- Each dimension table is composed by DN, DK and A{ }, with:
  - ○ DN corresponds to the dimension name.
  - ○ DK corresponds to the primary key of the dimension table.
  - ○ A {a1 (Tya1), a2 (Tya2), a3 (Tya3), a4 (Tya4), ...} presents the set of attributes describing the current dimension. Each attribute has a type.

The structure of a snowflake schema is as following:

- The fact table is defined by FN, FP, and MF{ } with:
  - ○ FN represents the name of the fact.
  - ○ FP represents the primary key of the fact table.
  - ○ MF {m1(Tym1), m2 (Tym2), m3 (Tym3), m4 (Tym4), ...} corresponds to the set of measures related to the fact. Each measure has its type.
- Each dimension table is composed by: DN, DK, A{ }, HD{ } with
  - ○ DN corresponds to the dimension name.
  - ○ DK corresponds to the primary key of the dimension table.
  - ○ A {a1 (Tya1), a2 (Tya2), a3 (Tya3), a4 (Tya4), ...} presents the set of attributes describing the current dimension. Each attribute has its type.
  - ○ HD {h_{1D}, h_{2D}, h_{3D}, h_{4D}, ...} is a set of ordered hierarchies. Each hierarchy has HN and P { } with
    - HN is the name of the current hierarchy
    - P{p1, p2, p3, p4, ...} is a set of ordered parameters.

From Conceptual Schema to Logical One

The purpose of this step is to move from the conceptual schemas to the logical ones. At this level, we have two types of schemas. The first ones were generated from the requirements. They present the Hospital Data Mart Conceptual Schemas (HDMCS)s and they are modeled as star. The second ones were generated from the different databases. They present Hospital Data Mart Multidimensional Schemas (HDMMS)s and they correspond to star or snowflake schemas. The generated schemas correspond to Hospital Data Mart Logical Schemas (HDMLS) and they can be presented as star or snowflake.

The validation of HDMLS is about adjusting the needs with databases so that we have the source from which we can extract data later.

In order to achieve this task:

- We compare the HDMCSs with HDMMSs to extract the closest ones: we classify the elements of the two schemas into the following categories: fact, measure, dimension, attribute or/and parameter and using the similarity matrix, we extract the closest schemas.
- We generate HDMLS by adding the necessary information from HDMMS to HDMCS. The mapping from the conceptual level to logical one is done by applying the following rules.

Rule 1: *Dimension table.*

Let Dc be the conceptual dimension table, Dl be the logical dimension table, and Dm be the multidimensional dimension table similar to Dc.

The mapping of Dc to Dl is done by keeping the name of Dm.

Example: if Dc is "PatientDim" and Dm is "Patient", the Dl in this case is "Patient".

Rule 2: *Attribute and Primary key.*

Let Ac be the attribute belonging to the conceptual dimension table, Am be the attribute belonging to the multidimensional table similar to Ac and Al be the attribute belonging to the logical dimension table.

The mapping of Ac to Al is done by keeping the name of Am and adding its corresponding type.

Example: if Ac is "FirstName" and Am is "Name" with "String" type, then Al is "Name" with "String" as type. Concerning the primary key, it is extracted from the multidimensional schema.

Rule 3: *Hierarchy.*

The conceptual schema is presented as star schema.

Let Hm be the hierarchy exiting in the multidimensional schema (if it is a snowflake schema), and Hl be the hierarchy of the logical schema having similar dimension tables.

In such case, the mapping is about copying the Hm with its parameters to the corresponding dimension to construct the Hl.

Rule 4: *Fact table.*

Let Fc be the conceptual fact table, Fm be the multidimensional fact table similar to Fc and Fl be the logical fact table. The mapping of Fc to Fl is done by respecting the name of Fm.

Example: Fc is "PharmacyOrderFact", Fm is "PharmacyOrder" the Fl is "PharmacyOrder".

Rule 5: *Measure and Primary key.*

Let Mc be the measure belonging to a specific Fc, Mm be the numeric attributes belonging to the Fm similar to Fc, and Ml be the measure that belong to Fl.

The specification of the measure requires human intervention to specify the numeric attributes and the corresponding function (SUM, MAX, AVG, etc) that should exist in the Fl.

Example: Mc is "TotalCost", Mm is "TotalCost", the Ml is SUM (Quantiy * Cost).

The primary key of the Fl is composed by the primary keys of the surrounded Dl.

Figure 16 presents the logical schema of the HDM after the mapping process. It contains the different measures and attributes with their types, and the fact name as defined by the user. The dimensions are adjusted according to databases.

Figure 16. Logical HDM schema

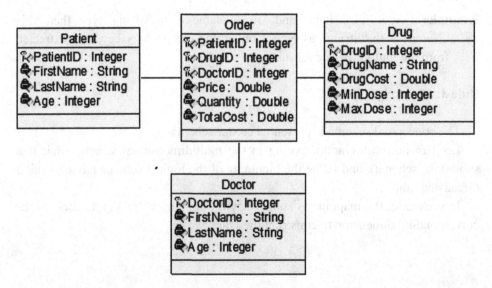

GENERATING HOSPITAL DATA WAREHOUSE SCHEMA

In order to generate the schema of the HDW, we apply the schema integration technique. Compared to that of the section "The New Schema Integration Methodology", two points are changed. The first one is related to the comparison of the elements. Indeed, we should compare, also, the types of measures and attributes. The second point is about the storage of the elements during the mapping. We need another database that takes into consideration the primary keys, the types, the hierarchies, etc.

This step is iterative. It takes two HDM logical schemas every time. At the end, it gives HDW schema. To explain this point, let us take sch1 (Figure 16) and sch2 (Figure 17) corresponding to HDM logical schemas. We apply the same steps as defined previously.

- Categorization:
  - Fact {sch1{Order}, sch2 {Order}}
  - FactKey {sch1{PatientID, DrugID, DoctorID}, sch2 {HospitalID, DrugID, DoctorID}}
  - Measure {sch1{Price, Quantity, TotalCost}, sch2{ Price, Quantity, TotalCost }}
  - Dimension {sch1 {Patient, Drug, Doctor}, sch2 {Hospital, Drug, Doctor}}
  - Attribute {sch1 {PatientID, FirstName, LastName, Age, DrugID, DrugName, DrugCost, MinDose, MaxDose, DoctorID, FirstName,

Figure 17. Logical DM schema

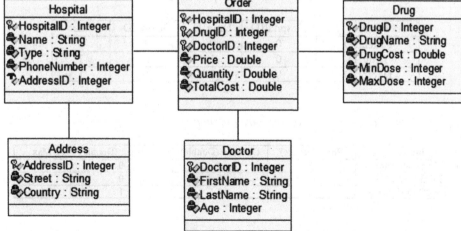

LastName, Age}, sch2 { HospitalID, Name, Type, PhoneNumber, AddressID, DrugID, DrugName, DrugCost, MinDose, MaxDose, DoctorID, FirstName, LastName, Age}}

- Construction of the similarity matrix:

Figure 18 presents the similarity matrix used to compare the two fact tables. In this case, they are similar since the value of 'Max'=1.

Figure 19 presents the similarity matrix used to compare the primary keys of the fact tables. In this case, we have the following similar pairs {DrugID, DrugID}, {DoctorID, DoctorID}.

Figure 20 presents the similarity matrix used to compare the measures. In this case, we have the following similar pairs {Price, Price}, {Quantity, Quantity} and {TotalCost, TotalCost} that they have the same type "Double". In the case of different types, we need human intervention.

Figure 21 presents the similarity matrix used to compare the dimension tables. In this case, we have the following similar pairs {Drug, Drug}, {Doctor, Doctor}.

Figure 22 presents the similarity matrix used to compare the attributes of the dimension tables "Drug/Drug". In this case, {DrugID, DrugID} with "Integer" type, {DrugName, DrugName} with "String" type, {DrugCost, DrugCost} with "Double"

Figure 18. Similarity matrix to compare the fact tables

Fact	Order	Max
Order	1	1

Figure 19. Similarity matrix to compare the fact keys

FactKey	HospitalID	DrugID	DoctorID	Max
PatientID	0	0	0	0
DrugID	0	1	0	1
DoctorID	0	0	1	1

Figure 20. Similarity matrix to compare the measures

Measure	Price (Double)	Quantity (Double)	TotalCost (Double)	Max
Price (Double)	1	0	0	1
Quantity (Double)	0	1	0	1
TotalCost (Double)	0	0	1	1

Figure 21. Similarity matrix to compare the dimension tables

Dimension	Hospital	Drug	Doctor	Max
Patient	0	0	0	0
Drug	0	1	0	1
Doctor	0	0	1	1

Figure 22. Similarity matrix to compare the attributes of the dimension tables 'Drug/Drug

Attribute of the dimension tables: Drug/Drug	DrugID (Integer)	DrugName (String)	DrugCost (Double)	MinDose (Double)	MaxDose (Double)	Max
DrugID (Integer)	1	0	0	0	0	1
DrugName (String)	0	1	0	0	0	1
DrugCost (Double)	0	0	1	0	0	1
MinDose (Double)	0	0	0	1	0	1
MaxDose (Double)	0	0	0	0	1	1

type, {MinDose, MinDose} with "Double" type and {MaxDose, MaxDose} with "Double" type are the pairs of similar attributes. In the case of different types for two similar attributes, we need human intervention.

Figure 23 presents the similarity matrix used to compare the attributes of the dimension tables "Doctor/Doctor". In this case, {DoctorID, DoctorID} with "Integer" type, {FirstName, FirstName} with "String" type, {LastName, LasName} with "String" type, and {Age, Age} with "Integer" type are the pairs of similar attributes related to the dimension "Doctor". In the case of different types, we need human intervention.

- Generation of the mapping rules: in the following, we present some of mapping rules.
  - If Similar (Order, Order) then Intersection (Order, Order) and Save (Order, Order)

Figure 23. Similarity matrix to compare the attributes of the dimension tables 'Doctor/Doctor'

Attribute of the dimension tables: Doctor/Doctor	DoctorID (Integer)	FirstName (String)	LastName (String)	Age (Integer)	Max
DoctorID (Integer)	1	0	0	0	1
FirstName (String)	0	1	0	0	1
LastName (String)	0	0	1	0	1
Age (Integer)	0	0	0	1	1

- ◦ If Similar (Price (Double), Price (Double)) then Intersection (Price (Double), Price (Double)) and Save (Price (Double), Price (Double))
- ◦ If Similar (PatientID, PatientID) then Intersection (PatientID, PatientID) and Save (PatientID, PatientID)
- ◦ If Similar (Doctor, Doctor) then Intersection (Doctor, Doctor) and Save (Doctor, Doctor)
- ◦ If Similar (FirstName, FirstName) then Intersection (FirstName, FirstName) and Save (FirstName, FirstName)
- Merging the schemas: As explained previously, it transforms the mapping rules into queries, and executes them to generate at the end the final schema of the HDW.

Compared to the previous database, we need, at this level, more details about the tables. We add a new table "FactPrimaryKey" contains the primary key of each fact table and their types. It has a primary key and a foreign key connected to the table "Fact". Concerning the table "Measure", we add the attribute "type" to specify the type of each measure. The table "Dimension" contains a new set of attributes "DimensionPrimaryKey" to specify the primary key of the dimension, "type" corresponding to the type of the primary key. This table specifies also for each dimension its level for a given hierarchy. It is described by a primary key, and a foreign key connected to the table "Schema". Finally, for the table "Attribute" gives information about the type of each attributes.

As example of queries, we can present:

- Query1 = "Insert into Fact (FactName, idSchema) values ('Order',"+ schemaId +")" ;
- Query2 = "Insert into Measure (MeasureName, MeasureType, idFact) values ('TotalCost',"+" 'Double '"+ factId +")" ;
- Query3 = "Insert into Dimension (DimensionName, Hierarchy, Level, DimensionPKName, DimensionPKType, idSchema) values ('Drug'," + null + ", '0', 'DrugID', 'Integer'" +schemaId + ") ";
- Query4 = "Insert into Attribute (AttributeName, AttributeType, idDimension) values ('DrugCost ',"+" ' Integer ' "+dimensionId +")";

With:

- schemaId: is the identifier of the new schema.
- factId: is the identifier of the new fact table.
- dimensionId: is the identifier of the new dimension table.

Once we apply the generated queries, we get the following schema (Figure 24) corresponding to the final HDW schema.

IMPLEMENTATION

To automate the schema integration, we propose the following algorithms.

Figure 25 corresponds to the main algorithm. It takes as input two schemas to give as output one schema. It is iterative. It stops when there is only one schema in the database. This algorithm starts by creating a new schema that will contain all the integrated elements. Next, it extracts the different category (fact, measure, dimension, attribute and parameter) using "Categorization" algorithm. Then, using "SchemaIntegrationFact" algorithm, it ensures the integration of the two fact tables. For each fact, it extracts the set of its corresponding measures that are integrated using "SchemaIntegrationMeasure" algorithm.

In the next step, it extracts the set of dimension tables from the two schemas, and stores them into two different lists. Using "SchemaIntegrationDimension_and_Attribute", it integrates the dimensions and their attributes. It treats also the hierarchies in the case of snowflake schemas. Finally, it deletes the two schemas that were used by applying "Delete_Schema" function that deletes the elements of each schema.

Figure 24. Hospital Data Warehouse schema

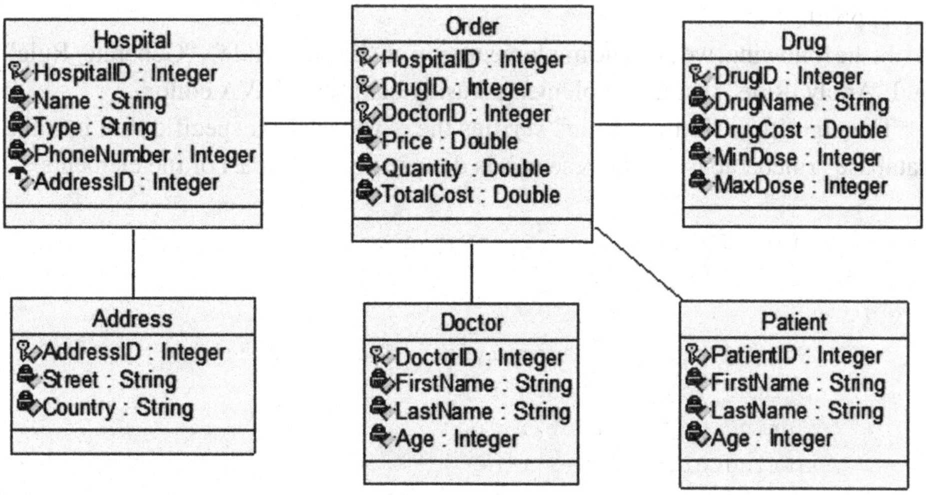

Figure 25. "SchemaIntegration" algorithm

```
1    Begin
2      Repeat
3        Categorization (sch1)
4        Categorization (sch2)
5        Create_NewSchema ( )
6        Fact1 = sch1.Fact
7        Fact2 = sch2.Fact
8        FactF = SchemaIntegrationFact (Fact2, sch1)
9        ListMeasure1 [ ] = sch1.ListMeasure (Fact1)
10       ListMeasure2 [ ] = sch2.ListMeasure (Fact2)
11       SchemaIntegrationMeasure (ListMeasure1, ListMeasure2)
12       ListDimension1 [ ] = sch1.ListDimension ( )
13       ListDimension2 [ ] = sch2.ListDimension ( )
14       SchemaIntegrationDimension_and_Attribute (ListDimension1, ListDimension2)
15       Delete_Schema ( )
16     Until (SchemaNumber = = 1)
17   End
```

Since each fact table can have many measures, we use lists that contain the measures of the fact tables. "SchemaIntegrationMeasure" algorithm (Figure 26) starts by verifying the existence of a rule corresponding to the two measures in the input. If there is one, then it applies it. If not, it calculates the degree of similarity of two measures using the formula (1). If they are similar, and have the same type, then it generates their corresponding rule, applies it and saves it. If they have different types, then we need human intervention thanks to the function Human_Generate_Rule ().

It is possible to get a set of no similar measures which are added to the chosen fact table in the previous algorithm. Concerning the rest of elements, the same steps are applied.

In the following, we give the implementation of "Extract_Rule", "Generate_Rule" and "Apply_Rule" that are implemented using eclipse as JAVA editor.

The algorithm "Extract-Rule" verifies the existence of a specific rule into the database "ruledatabase". The research is done using the names of the elements.

```
public String Extract_Rule (String elem) {
String rule = "";
try {
        String pilote = "com.mysql.jdbc.Driver";
        String login = "root";
        String mdp = "root";
        String url = new String
        ("jdbc:mysql://localhost:3307/ruledatabase");
        Class.forName(pilote);
```

Figure 26. "SchemaIntegrationMeasure" Algorithm

```
1   Begin
2     While (i < ListMeasure1.lenght)
3       While (j < ListMeasure2.lenght)
4         exist = Exist_Rule (ListMeasure1 [i], ListMeasure2[j])
5
6         If (exist) then
7           Rule = Extract_Rule (ListMeasure1 [i], ListMeasure2[j])
8           Apply_Rule (Rule, FactF)
9         Else
10            sim = DegSim (ListMeasure1 [i], ListMeasure2[j])
11            If (ListMeasure1 [i].type.equals (ListMeasure2[j].type)
12              simType = 1
13            Else
14              simType= 0
15            Fin if
16
17            If (sim == 1 && simType == 1)
18              Rule = Generate_Rule (ListMeasure1 [i], ListMeasure2[j])
19              Apply_Rule (Rule)
20              Save_Rule (Rule, meas1, meas2)
21            ElseIf (sim == 1 && simType == 0)
22              Rule = Human_Generate_Rule (ListMeasure1 [i], ListMeasure2[j])
23              Apply_Rule (Rule)
24              Save_Rule (Rule, meas1, meas2)
25            End If
26          End if
27       j++
28       i++
29     End While
30   End While
31 ListMeasNotSim [ ] = insertRest(ListMeasure1, ListMeasure2)
32 Insert (ListMeasNotSim, FactF)
33
34 End
```

```
        Connection conn = DriverManager.getConnection(url,
login, mdp);
        String requete2 = "Select * from integrationrule where
Elements = '"+elem+"';";
        Statement requete = conn.createStatement();
        ResultSet resultat = requete.executeQuery(requete2);
        while (resultat.next())
         rule = resultat.getString("Rule");}
}catch(Exception e){e.getMessage();}
return rule;}
```

Concerning the following algorithm, it generates the rule for each element. Here, we present the case for "Measure". The same

```
thing is done with the rest of elements.
public String Generate_Rule (String type, String elem, int Id-
Parent) {
String rule = "";
        if (Type.equals ("Measure"))
        rule = "Insert into Measure (MeasureName, MeasureType,
idFact) values ('"+ elem + "', '"+ type  "',"+IdParent+")";
return rule;}
The following algorithm executes the queries.
public void Apply_Rule (String rule) {
try{
        String pilote = "com.mysql.jdbc.Driver";
        String login = "root";
        String mdp = "root";
        String url = new String("jdbc:mysql://localhost:3307/
hsidatabase");
        Class.forName (pilote);
        Connection conn = DriverManager.getConnection(url,
login, mdp);
        java.sql.Statement stm = conn.createStatement();
        int resultats = stm.executeUpdate(rule);
}catch (Exception e){e.getMessage ();}}
```

CONCLUSION

The healthcare industries generate huge amount of data which makes their exploitation and their mastering a hard task. For this reason, the use of DW is considered as the best solution to store the historical data for the analysis purpose.

In this work, we proposed a new approach to generate HDW. It combines the bottom-up and hybrid. The bottom-up is necessary since the different healthcare departments do not communicate and they do not share their information and their documents. We generate, then, for each one its HDM schema then we merge them to get at the end the final HDW schema.

Concerning the HDM, they are constructed using the hybrid approach taking into consideration the users' requirements and the databases.

Concerning the collect of the needs, we proposed an assistant system (HDwADS) that facilitates the task by exploiting the previous experiences stored as traces.

As perspective, we propose extending this work by exploiting other types of data sources such as the UML databases and the XML files.

REFERENCES

Annoni, E., Ravat, F., Teste, O., & Zurfluh, G. (2006). Towards Multidimensional Requirement Design. *Proceedings of the 8th International Conference Data Warehousing and Knowledge Discovery (DaWaK)* (pp. 75-84). doi:10.1007/11823728_8

Banek, M., Tjoa, A. M., & Stolba, N. (2006). Integrating Different Grain Levels in a Medical Data Warehouse Federation. In A. M. Tjoa & J. Trujillo (Eds.), *DaWak, LNCS* (Vol. 4081, pp. 185–194). Heidelberg: Springer. doi:10.1007/11823728_18

Bennett, W., Boone, E., Parker, D., Thorpe, A., Wang, M., & White, P. T. (2009). *Data Warehousing a New Focus in Healthcare Data Management*. Retrieved from http://www.himss.org/files/HIMSSorg/content/files/EHR/DataWarehousing.pdf

Berndt, D. J., Fisher, J. W., Hevner, A. R., & Studnicki, J. (2001). Healthcare Data Warehousing and Quality Assurance. *IEEE Computer*, *34*(12), 56–65. doi:10.1109/2.970578

Berndt, D. J., Hevner, A. R., & Studnicki, J. (2003). The Catch Data Warehouse: Support for Community Health Care Decision-Making. *Decision Support Systems*, *35*(3), 367–384. doi:10.1016/S0167-9236(02)00114-8

Bizarro, P., & Madeira, H. (2002). Adding a Performance-Oriented Perspective to Data Warehouse Design. *Proceedings of 4th International Conference Data Warehousing and Knowledge Discovery* (pp. 232-244). doi:10.1007/3-540-46145-0_23

Börger, E. (1998). High Level System Design and Analysis using Abstract State Machines. In D. Hutter, W. Stephan, P. Traverso, & M. Ullmann (Eds.), Current Trends in Applied Formal Methods FM-Trends '98, LNCS (Vol. 1641, pp. 1-43). Springer-Verlag.

Chen, P. P. S. (1976). The Entity-Relationship Model-Toward a Unified View of Data. *ACM Transactions on Database Systems*, *1*(1), 9–36. doi:10.1145/320434.320440

Darmont, J. (2008). Entreposage de Données Complexes pour la Medicine d'Anticipation Personalisée. *Proceedings of the 9th International Conference on System Science in Health Care* (p. 75).

Dutta, R. (2013). Health care data warehouse system architecture for influenza (flu) diseases. Proceedings of ACER (pp. 77–89).

Einbinder, J. S., Pates, R. D., & Reynolds, R. E. (2001). Case Study: A Data Warehouse for an Academic Medical Center. *Journal of Healthcare Information Management, 15*(2), 165–175. PMID:11452578

Foundation, K. F. (2006). *Comparing Projected Growth in Health Care Expenditures and the Economy, Snapshots: Health Care Costs*. Retrieved from http://www.kff. org/insurance/snapshot/chcm050206oth2.cfm

Golfarelli, M., & Rizzi, S. (2009). *Data Warehouse Design: Modern Principles and Methodologies*. McGraw-Hill Osborne Media.

Golfarelli, M., & Rizzi, S. (2010). WAND: A CASE Tool for Data Warehouse Design. *Proceedings of 17th International Conference on Data Engineering (ICDE)* (pp. 7-9).

Gyssens, M., & Lakshmanan, L. V. S. (1997). A Foundation for Multi-dimensional Databases. *Proceedings of 23rd International Conference on Very Large Data Bases (VLDB)* (pp. 106-111).

Hüsemann, B., Lechtenbörger, J., & Vossen, G. (2000). Conceptual data warehouse design. *Proceedings International Workshop on Design and Management of Data Warehouses, Stockholm*, (pp. 3-9).

Inmon, W. H. (2005). *Building the Data Warehouse*. John Wiley & Sons Inc.

Kimball, R., & Ross, M. (2002). *The Data Warehouse Toolkit*. John Wiley & Sons.

Lee, M. L., & Ling, T. W. (1997). Resolving Constraint Conflicts in the Integration of Entity-Relationship Schemas. *Proceedings of the 16th International Conference on Conceptual Modeling,* Los Angeles, California, USA (pp. 394-407). doi:10.1007/3-540-63699-4_32

Levene, M., & Loizou, G. (2003). Why is the Snowflake Schema a Good Data Warehouse Design? *Information Systems Journal, 28*(3), 225–240. doi:10.1016/S0306-4379(02)00021-2

Malinowski, E., & Zimanyi, E. (2008). *Advanced Data Warehouse Design, From Conventional to Spatial and Temporal Applications*. Springer Verlag Berlin Heidelberg.

Mike, D. (2014). *Clinical Data Warehouse: Why You Really Need One*. Retrieved from http://www.healthcatalyst.com/clinical-data-warehouse-why-you-need-one

Moody, D. L., & Kortink, M. A. R. (2000). From Enterprise Models to Dimensional Models: a Methodology for Data Warehouse and Data Mart Design. *Proceedings of the Second International Workshop on Design and Management of Data Warehouses (DMDW)* (pp.1-12).

Mul, M. D., Alons, P., Velde, P. V. D., Konings, I., Bakker, J., & Hazelzet, J. (2012). Development of a Clinical Data Warehouse from an Intensive Care Clinical Information System. *Computer Methods and Programs in Biomedicine*, *105*(1), 22–30. doi:10.1016/j.cmpb.2010.07.002 PMID:20728956

Peralta, V., Illarze, A., & Ruggia, R. (2003). On the Applicability of Rules to Automate Data Warehouse Logical Design. *Proceedings of the 15th Conference on Advanced Information Systems Engineering* (pp. 329-340).

Sahama, T. R., & Croll, P. R. (2007). A Data Warehouse Architecture for Clinical Data Warehousing. *Proceedings of the fifth Australasian symposium on ACSW frontiers* (vol. 68, pp. 227-232).

Sen, A., & Jacob, V. S. (1998). Industrial Strength Data Warehousing. *Communications of the ACM*, *41*(9), 28–31. doi:10.1145/285070.285076

Sheta, O. E., & Eldeen, A. N. (2012). Building a Health Care Data Warehouse for Cancer Diseases. *International Journal of Database Management Systems*, *4*(5), 39–46. doi:10.5121/ijdms.2012.4503

Chapter 6
Sensorization to Promote the Well–Being of People and the Betterment of Health Organizations

Fábio Silva
Universidade do Minho, Portugal

Cesar Analide
Universidade do Minho, Portugal

ABSTRACT

Well-being is a complex notion of satisfaction towards a human being. There is no doubt that it is not essential but the greater the sense of well-being, the better are living conditions and general happiness. It can be measured and although it is not directly assessed, there are procedures that grasp its value. An example is the act of sensorization of different key related attributes. Sensorization is the ability to gather data which may be used to a plurality of objectives. The greater the number of sensorized attributed, the better evaluation on well-being can be made. But there are more benefits that can be hypothesized such as the construction of community knowledge bases and the search for abnormal relationships between well-being and the attributes sensed. A historical record of our way of life can also present clues to health organizations, both to the creation of regulations and individual diagnosis.

DOI: 10.4018/978-1-4666-9882-6.ch006

INTRODUCTION

The digital world is more than the electronic records and the internet. In there, a number of concepts exist that aim to make living easier and safer for people. For instance, the internet of things is a new paradigm in which every device is digitally connected, regardless of their function and can communicate with other devices and people over communication protocols. It applies both to fixed devices as well as portable personal devices that accompany people (Atzori, Iera, & Morabito, 2010). More examples can be enumerated by devices that are being incorporated inside the actual body, such as identification chips, smart tattoos and alike (Steele & Clarke, 2013). Along with the internet of things, smart cites development further the objective of ease of living, well-being and comfort. Smart city is a term applied to digital research and planning using computational methods and systems that results in better, easier and faster management of services and goods inside the inhabited areas. Internet of things acts in this setup as a base service which enables smart cities applications by either the collection of information directly from the environment and people or integrated fusion of data and information to the benefit of planning actions to improve the status quo. Among other concerns, health, comfort and well-being are points of concern in smart cities (Solanas et al., 2014).

If the technologies described under the concepts of smart cities and internet of things are perceived as social services, then conventional business and government agencies gain access to a new set of valuable information on both the environment and users. These trends, despite having ethical challenges of their own, present a number of opportunities for the society. Sensorization, monitoring, sharing of information are terms intimately connected to the new intelligent systems being created. They further expand the potential of the new digital world currently under construction. Applied research can be found related to health organizations and also the well-being of populations or individuals. Connected environments monitoring comfort parameters are not under active research but also regulated by governments. Air quality is an area that is actually regulated by governments, which define acceptable parameters. Concurrently, research conduct in the field of smart environments studies the impact of air composition in health, concentration tasks and psychological comfort. As expected, research directions are more specialized than government regulations and are being pushed forward by the quality of sensors and sensor networks which portrait better and better images of air composition across time and space inside environments. With this being only one example of application, there are other with equal approaches and strategies that aim to better assess and diagnose not optimised or harmful situation towards well-being and general health (Piro, Cianci, Grieco, Boggia, & Camarda, 2014).

Social well-being is considered the promotion of positive physical and psychological states in a population. Under the scope of the internet of things and smart cities, there are concerns for the perseverance of physical and psychological states and devices and procedures are described that help such tasks. The physical and psychological well-being can be coupled together for some evaluations, as one has potentially implications in the other. They can be addressed separately as well in cases where the focus is more important towards only one of the two terms.

The quest for physical well-being is addressed under smart cities by the use of indicators from personal devices such as smartwatches, sport monitors or smart bands which among other things can monitor some health parameters such as heart rate, blood oxygen levels and sport activities. Research in the body response to environment parameters is also potentiated by these personal devices that act as personal sensors (Chan, Estève, Fourniols, Escriba, & Campo, 2012). Their use to calculate more intrusive parameter such heat balance index for each individual helps perceive whether it is cold or warm in different situations. The environment condition alone is correlated to well-being and comfort status (Rana, Kusy, Jurdak, Wall, & Hu, 2013). More importantly, there are decisions that can be made using such information that may affect both physical and psychological health. Results from individuals can be aggregated into useful information about people and diagnosis of potential health hazards can result in policies to promote the adoption of better behaviours. Even more, the existence of such records is an untapped opportunity for health organizations to conduct specialized diagnosis based on the daily information of their users. Using fixed sensors over specialized areas are of interest to assess environments and their impact on heath (Atallah, Lo, & Yang, 2012). For instance, projects that monitor city or indoor air quality provide rich information about potential health risks that may impair both physical and psychological well-being. What is more, the availability of digital services allows a faster identification and actuation upon these threats. Knowledge of perilous values for health care parameters may be recognized as common sense for health institutions and their use in state of the art systems results in the prevention of potential threats. The difficulty gathering and constantly monitor such parameters leads to situations where interventions are late and the problems worse than what our common knowledge would allow. Social sustainable indicators developed to assess development of countries and populations can also be automated using sensory networks with devices directly connected with each other that can provide information that would normally require expansive survey, and field tests. In the health care community there are social indicators as well. They express concern about key health indicators that may have consequences either immediately or at later stages to public health. Some of these indicators include sound and air pollution and initiatives to monitor them already exist by the installation of sensors spread across city areas.

This chapter intends to present the untapped opportunities of the digital concepts currently under research to the well-being of people through the demonstration of research examples and applications in the state of the art review. Health organizations are mentioned due to the potential access to individual and grouped electronic records may help in a number of situations. An example can be provided in the diagnosis of potential perils that people discard due to its perceptions as something else or even when they are not perceived at all. Aggregated records provide a global picture of populations, intervention needed and where effort should be conducted in order to help public health.

BACKGROUND

Ambient Intelligence (AmI) systems aim to change how people interact with technology and the environment integrating concepts from psychology, social sciences and artificial intelligence to increase the quality of life, AmI makes this possible by anticipating and predicting future needs and desires while taking in consideration aspects like safety, economy and comfort. One concept usually linked to AmI is ubiquitous computing, a concept proposed in (Weiser, 1991) by Mark Weiser. In this environment, computational units are embedded in its surroundings functioning and hidden from view. . As figure 1 illustrates, Ambient Intelligence (AmI), covers a wide range of topics that work together to deliver the concept of AmI.

Directly connected with ambient intelligence is also how the sensing of the environment is done. In order to deliberate which actions an intelligent system may do in an environment it is necessary to obtain the information of the environment needs. Significant levels of data must be constantly and ubiquitously collected to provide the data and information needed. Towards this objective, relatively recent concepts such as the internet of thing and the idea of objects connected to each other and more importantly the internet materialize the ideas proposed (Atzori et al., 2010).

Ambient Intelligence Techniques

Monitor people well-being and increases in stress are with the problems covered by ambient intelligence and ubiquitous monitoring. As such, there are model proposals to explain and potentially predict any undesirable effects considering a series of factors believed to influence user/occupant behaviour (Acampora & Loia, 2008). Other approaches, relate environment attributes to people attributes such as heart rate which may be used to infer thermal comfort levels and detect stress induced by environment attributes and not optimised values (Liu, Lian, & Liu, 2008). In Paola

Figure 1. Ambient intelligence domain

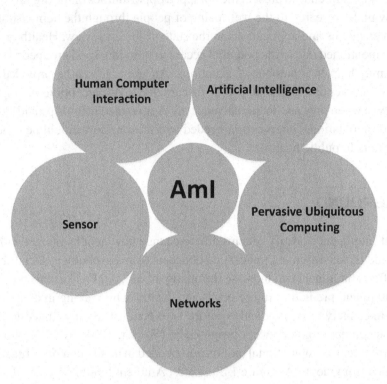

et al. (Paola, Gaglio, Re, & Ortolani, 2012), ambient intelligence is used within a sensor network testbed to derive useful from sensor spread across the environment. The data retrieved from sensors is used to derive rich information such as user attendance, perceptible temperature, user activity and preferences. All this information is learned unobtrusively by the system fusing sensor data without requiring user attention or direct user input.

The scientific research field of Ambient Intelligence provides a wide spectrum of methodologies to obtain such information in a non-intrusive manner. The types of sensors used in the environment may be divided into categories to better explain their purpose. Generally, an ambient might be divided by sensors and actuators. Sensors monitor the environment and gather data useful for cognitive and reasoning processes (Aztiria, Izaguirre, & Augusto, 2010). Actuators take action upon the environment, performing actions such as controlling the temperature, the lightning or other appliances. In terms of sensorization, environment sensors can be divided into sensor that monitor environment or sensor that monitor the user and its activities.

Learning in ambient intelligence is often made using machine learning algorithms such as time series algorithms, evolutionary algorithms and statistical inference.

These methods sanction the acquiring of past and current trends and predict future results. From information assembled from different environments, machine learning techniques may derive models of behaviour and interaction based on specialized backgrounds (e.g., users, environment, social interaction or consumption). Such techniques are applied over data extracted from data sources spread over the environment or attached to its users. The internet of things eases the problem of data availability by keeping it accurate and ideal for always on systems.

Well-being assessment is a task that requires a definition of well-being related with the available data and information. Systems to assess and monitor well-being benefit greatly from technologies provided by ambient intelligence and the internet of things. Both infrastructure and modelling techniques can be adopted from similar systems.

Well-Being Assessment

According to the Oxford Dictionary of English, well-being is the state of being comfortable, healthy, or happy. In order to assess it, the three subjects should be covered by the process conducting such evaluation. Not only that but also the context of evaluation must be considered. For instance, comfort values differ according to the task and the location context (ex. home or professional.).

In a professional environment, according the World Health Organization a healthy job is likely to be one where the pressures on employees are appropriate in relation to their abilities and resources, to the amount of control they have over their work, and to the support they receive from people who matter to them. As health is not merely the absence of disease or infirmity but a positive state of complete physical, mental and social well-being, a healthy working environment is one in which there is not only an absence of harmful conditions but an abundance of health promoting ones. Environment and physical working conditions are important organizational risk factors (Biron, Ivers, Brun, & Cooper, 2006). Previous approaches to this work focused on the physical attributes predicament such as heart rate, and comfort due to environment conditions. The work here detailed enriches the comfort evaluation with additional inputs through the use of sensor fusion and better index related with each individual such heat stress, skin wetness and temperature perception. A multilayer approach can effectively warn and monitor people discomfort inferring both the physical state of the body as well as the emotion derived from the environment.

Applied to the home and professional scenarios, though with different values, there is the thermal comfort. The once believed assumption that comfort equilibrium calculation were too complex to perform on a recurrent analysis (Fanger, 1970) are mostly proved wrong in an intelligent environment equipped with smart sensors connected to a central processing unit. Although, some of the algorithm might still be considered too complex, most formally complex mathematical can be used. From this perspective it is possible to perform scoring systems to rate the degree of comfort or discomfort a user experiences when subjected to a system. Traditional studies use ergonomic research to estimate ideal parameters that are adequate to the space, people and task performed. Considering these variables, in this study, we can analyses traditional attributes such as temperature, humidity, luminosity, relevant attributes like CO, CO2 and airborne dust. However, it is possible to increase the precision of these models, not only estimating individual assessments but also correlated assessments through dedicated indicators with sensor and data fusion techniques. As an example there are a number of indexes that can be created, namely, perfected temperature, percentage of people in discomfort and stress related with heat perception (K. Parsons, 2010) and adequate luminosity for each task. These sensors monitor the environment and its attributes looking for suboptimal attributes; however relate these attributes with user discomfort or user stress is still a relative study. There is another layer, physical human sensors that, in this case, monitor the heart rate for each individual inside smart environments. Whenever suboptimal values are detected, it will be possible to relate the physical state of each person to the environment attributes. Psychological and physiological adverse ambient conditions can produce significantly changes in a person. However authors orient this topic to a set of variables. In this particular approach sound, temperature and luminosity are studied as external factors that affect well-being and mood states. Previous authors have already researched and debated the influence of such variables in the impact of mood change in people (K. C. Parsons, 2000). In a noisy environment people have different sensitivity to sound volume, for example sensible people to sound have a predisposition to become more anxious. In hot places, when temperature increases, psychological changes may occur, such as irritability, fatigue and discomfort. Accessing this type of information from the environment allows realizing the kind of emotional reactions that may arise and classify mood states. Related studies between stress and well-being and stress recognition can also be found. In (Choi, Ahmed, & Gutierrez-Osuna, 2000) we can see a wearable system for ambulatory stress monitoring recording a number of physiological variables known to be influenced by stress. This system is not ZigBee based, it employs a radio module from TI (Texas instruments Inc.), a connection-based low-power lightweight sensor network protocol for small RF networks supporting two basic topologies: strictly peer-to-peer and a star topology. The authors use a star topology where all sensors (leaf nodes) are connected to a sensor hub (the root). In (Tauseef, 2012) author gathers values from a skin temperature sensor, a heart rate sensor and a skin conductance sensor. The signals from the sensors are input into a microcontroller where all the processing takes place and carried out though ZigBee technology. Data are stored in a computer it is stored for data analysis and feature extraction for emotion recognition.

The approach to well-being assessment covered is the mainly based on the data and information retrieved from pervasive systems and adapting the values according to task and context and location

COMFORT VALUES

Comfort is subjective directly related to a person's personality, beliefs and habits. There are however ergonomic studies that provide the necessary background to create an environment that satisfies the most common needs to keep both the people and environments healthy. The analysis here depicted entails the consideration of sample environment and personal attributes. Although not being an extensive review of possible attributes it does indicate a minimum set of possible attributes to start comfort and well-being assessments. An initial objective toward well-being monitoring is to maintain the values of comfort inside of the selected thresholds according to location, context and activity.

Environment Assessment

From the literature there are a number of attributes that can be monitored through the use of sensor platforms. There are ergonomics, medical and comfort values that can be used together with sensor data to infer useful information and knowledge about an environment. On table 1 are represented the medical and comfort values that can be used together with sensor data to infer useful information and knowledge about an environment. There are represented the medical and structural values for relative humidity, temperature, carbon monoxide and carbon monoxide, and dust within buildings for acceptable human work conditions (Silva, Olivares, Royo, Vergara, & Analide, 2013). Values outside the ranges presented are responsible for condition such as stress, mood alteration and health risks to people.

Table 1. Atmosphere attributes

Comfort Attribute	Lower Limit	Upper Limit
Humidity	20%	60%
Temperature	18 °C	25 °C
Luminosity	50 lux	107527 lux
Dust	0 $\mu g/m^3$	50 $\mu g/m^3$
Carbon Dioxide	0 ppm	35 ppm
Carbon Monoxide	0 ppm	600 ppm

Likewise, it is possible to infer a range of ideal values for attributes that while not being directly responsible for health risks, they may increase stress or influence well-being on people. The range of values presented considers an ergonomic analysis of activities and desirable conditions for people. The range of values outside this range is considered harmful towards comfort. Using data from sensor networks and sensor platforms it is possible to use sensor fusion to produce data and information with higher quality and more contextualized to the environment variables. Table 2 demonstrates the use of information about the activity of people inside a building or environment and the values for luminosity that are deemed acceptable. Energy efficiency projects could take this information to regulate artificial luminosity inside buildings while avoiding inflicting stress on people due to poor lightning. The use of different data from different sensors enables the application of sensor fusion projects empowered by sensor networks and sensor platforms that produce information contextualized to the environment and the people on it. Generally, the information analysed may also present higher quality in terms of interpretation and application. Taking into consideration the values obtained from the sensor network, it is possible to assess them using the reference values presented.

Despite providing a good start to well-being analysis, environment configuration alone does not fully represent comfort and well-being values. In order to complete such information personal attributes from the user of the environments should be taken into consideration and if possible correlated in the assessment.

Table 2. Luminosity values

Task	Lower Limit
Public Areas	20
Short Visit	50
Working areas with few visual tasks	100
Warehouses, Homes, Theatres, Archives	150
Easy Office Work	250
Normal Office, Study Library, Laboratory	500
Mechanical Workshops, Office Landscapes	750
Normal Drawing Work, Normal Detailed Work	1000
Detailed Drawing Work, Detailed Work	1500
Prolonged tasks and exacting visual tasks	2000

Personal Attributes

The analysis of environment sensor data is useful to determine whether or not an environment is set up correctly, but it is lacks how the presented conditions affect people in terms of discomfort, stress or relief. From these considerations, indexes captured in the literature can be used. In the work presented, relationships between environment conditions, physical definition of people and the tasks being performed are used to create the indexes heat stress and the percentage of people dissatisfied (PPD) based on the predicted mean vote (PMV) created by (Fanger, 1970). Likewise, temperature values can also be regulated according to the profile of people in specific environments. The knowledge about perceived temperature on human beings allows for a fine tuned control of heating appliances and reduces the stress inflicted by temperature on users. The temperature sensation might be calculated by known algorithms such as the PMV or PET algorithms, which are correlated with thermal sensation and thermal stress. In table III is possible to see the relationship between the PMV indicator and the thermal and stress sensation felt by people that has an impact on comfort. Other attribute directly related with physical index assessed by the sensor network is the heart rate. With the help of mobile wearable sensors, the value of heart rate can be saved historically, and used in comfort assessment. Tough the limits allowed for this attribute change according to the nature of the physical activity being performed, this study considers light physical activity where physical efforts are not necessary. As such reference values for sample attributes valued is presented in table3.

Other attributes can be directly assessed from the physical condition and physical of users. In this case we can enumerate attributes such as blood pressure, blood oximetry, number of steps, time walking and time running.

Similarly to the consideration made to environment attributes, well-being should include more information than just personal attributes. The reason is that personal attributes can be biased by external factors not directly correlated by environment or well-being such as diseases or emotional factors.

Table 3. Personal attributes

Physical Attribute	Optimal Lower Limit	Optimal Upper Limit
Temperature perception (PMV)	-1.5	1.5
PET	18 °C	25 °C
Heart Rate (Men)	57	75
Heart Rate (Woman)	60	78
Oximetry	90%	100%

WELL-BEING DASHBOARDS AND ASSESSMENTS

A combination of personal and environmental attributes provides a better representation of the information required to assess well-being and hypotheses about user condition, its relation to environment attributes and the activities being performed. Such information though not being medically considered as hard prove to diagnosis may be used as soft information about condition and habits of living.

With this idea in mind, taking the considerations from the knowledge base already present in the literature about the different attributes that make comfort and health analysis, it is possible to setup monitoring and deliberative system to assess, control and deliberate relevant patterns towards inefficiency in well-being. This system depends on the number of sensing devices and attributes considered to make decisions more accurate and expressive. Another concept to notice is related to the context of the analysis. Different environments have different requirements, as well as their users. It is important to adapt the notions of comfort and safety according to this view. Furthering these notions, early recognition signs that something is not the way it should be are detected by assessing situations out of the ordinary, where due to a conjunction of attributes states, patterns of future impairment situations are calculated. Taking knowledge from a knowledge base about each environment, for instance relations between sensor and event records, it is actually possible to estimate the state of well-being, both currently and in the future.

Home and Professional Environment

A home environment is a particular setup, with a very personal context. Depending on job state, a person may spend most of the time in this environment or only after work hours. Taking into consideration a typical residence with working people, it is possible to assess comfort condition and monitor and predict values of comfort.

From the installation of different sources of sensorization through the environment it is possible to measure the impact of each individual attribute in the environment. As a personal environment those should be the best suited to assess what each user deems as comfortable. However as users can have different meanings for comfort, there might exist some exceptions to this assertion. The approach undertaken is explained later, but to focus on the analysis of the home environment, the attention was turned to a set of simple attributes: temperature and luminosity according to table 4 which illustrates a summary description of the data collected.

A professional environment, though not always equal it is generally categorized by a population of individuals sharing the same environment. Each environment

Table 4. Measurements of attributes for home environment

	Mean	Standard Deviation	Max	Min
Temperature	21,76	3,70	26,35	18,03
Luminosity	318,64	441,76	2045,00	0,00
Humidity	47,57	10,82	70,01	39,91

has different requirements according to the specific tasks its users perform. For instance, as evidenced by table 2 in the section comfort values, the quantity of light necessary is dependent on the specificity of the work or area.

Figure 2 is a representation of a professional environment comprised of a single room equipped with electronic hardware and a controlled air conditioning system. During this experiment a presence control was instituted to add user presence as an attribute. The description of the summary of the data gathered is available in table 5.

The analysis of well-being is inherently different from home and professional configurations due to the fact that the context alters comfort values. Though some of the alterations remain within the acceptable range they can be used to introduce differences in the well-being analysis.

Personal Assessment

Well-being trough environment alone is an incomplete study as it disregards the effects of user interaction and user behaviour. Under normal circumstances, well-

Figure 2. Professional environment

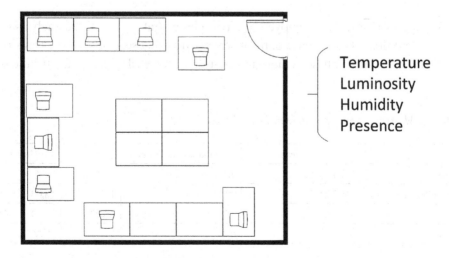

Table 5. Measurements of attributes for professional environment

	Mean	Standard Deviation	Max	Min
Temperature	19,98	1,68	24,88	17,99
Luminosity	122,53	102,49	632,00	0,00
Humidity	45,69	7,39	63,19	38,86
Number of People	2,27	1,70	10,00	0,00

being should generate values inside the satisfactory range for attributes being measured. Considering one individual alone, the existence of normal range values for environment and abnormal for the personal sensing might lead to the suspicion of something not right with the individual thus impairing well-being.

On table 6, a set of indicators gathered from sample personal sensorization hardware reveals the normal range of attribute date for a given individual. His historic data reveal how comfortable he is by assessing most common values after some period of time. As the indicator values go up or down the mean and standard deviation being considered it detects abnormal behavioural pattern and uses majority votes to decide whether it is really an uncomfortable behaviour or not.

A practical validation test can be made using records from environment and testing them against such data. It was perceived that environment conditions only directly affect personal attributes the most when they differ significantly under normal circumstances that is avoiding considerations about individual's state of mind. Environment variables ranging inside the comfort zone are less likely to produce chances in the normal values from personal sensorization.

Well-Being Assessment

Well-being assessment is employed in a two-phase strategy. First, the analysis of critical conditions through environment sensory data and secondly, the analysis of comfort. At the initial phase, a thorough analysis about each individual attribute is

Table 6. Measurements of personal attributes

	Mean	Standard Deviation	Max	Min
Steps	4177,80	7537,96	5080,00	3245,00
Blood Pressure	78,42	19,11	125,00	58,00
Oximetry	97,45	1,02	100,00	95,00
PMV	-0,79	0,86	1,20	-1,72

made to make sure that each of the sensorized values are non-risk values towards human. This evaluation is made both to environment and personal attributes. It is important to deal with information quality and validity. If the evaluation fails at this stage them uncomfortable setup is immediately generated. Even if there is only one of the attributes outside what is considered safe range, the resulting classification is deemed non satisfactory and a 0% well-being is issued as life might be endangered.

Following on to the second phase, with each user profile and environment profile, a match between activities and each attribute available is analysed. In the sample test, the temperature and luminosity of environments where chosen. Different comfort rules are created according to the dominant activities in each environment and the ideal configuration is assessed through ranges of values from medical, thermal and ergonomic studies present in configuration databases in the system. From this point, a weighted percentage is loaded from the database to allow different comfort attributes to have more or less impact in the well-being value. The final value of well-being is the weighted majority of the satisfaction comfort for each attribute. A percentage, less than 100% denotes that at least some attribute being measured is not within comfort values for a given time. Finally, a daily assessment considers the average of well-being satisfaction between measures.

Table 7 presents the relative percentages of time from the analysis of the attributes and their matching to each other. It can be seen that environment configurations are generally portrayed as good in well-being standing but the personal attributes are lacking more often. In the case of this experiment that is due to non-activity, and sedentary lifestyle. Its implications are that although the environments appear well configured, the activities of users are not being considered as good for well-being. Although with this setup, if the conditions verified are not directly correlated between both environment and personal attributes, the weighted average among all attributes decides the category of well-being.

Historical data about environment and both environment and people can be addressed making up profiles of aggregated information through the use of dashboards. These dashboards should contain valuable information for healthcare institutions and its professionals to help with patient consult for instance. More than the experience a verbal consult with a patient can produce, a virtual conversation is something

Table 7. Percentage of time in each assessment stage

	Environment Well-Being	**Personal Well-Being**	**Well-Being Assessment**
Professional environment	97%	78%	83%
Home environment	92%	82%	82%

that includes virtual data according to sensing system available. Though the system may be assessed with simulation data, it is in the real world data applied to each scenario that it usefulness can be extensively validated. For healthcare institution it is possible to navigate, through time windows and select only values of selected attributes and obtain both a measurement dashboard as well as a well-being classification. The input in the system is dependent in the number of attributes measured by the sensor network in place and the capability of its devices. The further specialized the devices and information is the further the quality of information and the validity of these analysis.

A future approach should include distribution analysis between the historical data on a given time window and the sensorized values. This envision may also help annotate different states of comfort through building and the people inside to better map how the environmental attributes of such buildings affect the well-being of people. As tried in the experimental framework to detect stressful moods (Silva et al., 2013), where a testbed was used to perceive different room states during the day and the classification of probable well-being.

FUTURE RESEARCH DIRECTIONS

In an idealistic world, all people should be able to provide all the necessary information relevant to physician's diagnosis process. Nevertheless, despite having more considerations to amount this conclusion not all the information technology can retrieve is of use. Although, most technological leaps are being taken, general access and availability is still limited to field studies and not applied.

There is however a downside to the availability of information. In high quantities, something that can only be defined by abilities of the one receiving it, it can lead to what is known as information overflow. This is state where the amount of information is greater than the capacity to review it and it can even impair good results in what refers to physician's patient diagnosis. But there is something related to the information process that should be stated. There is a different between ignoring information and not having enough information. Philosophically, when information is ignored it is not lost, is just is not considered, which can also have consequences. Even so, when information is lost so is the value it had because it will not be available anymore, and by chance if such information would be deemed important at a later stage it would not be possible to retrieve it. With these considerations, these system should evolve in two assertive directions. First the collection of data regarding environment and personal attributes, and the ability to handle such workloads of information. Secondly, the highlight of relevant information according to context.

It should be easy to find the information we are interested no matter how small it is in comparison. Like a search engine indexes and find relation between content, so should be case with historical data on these systems.

Personal and Environment Sensorization

The accuracy and relevance of these systems is dependent on the quality of the data and information gathered. There are plenty of manual devices that can track a number of health related attributes. Avoiding the loss of data and information from manual devices can be done interlinking devices to storage units as perceived by the internet of things. Not only health organizations often disregard large sums of information so do people in their daily lives. The advent of wearable devices able to perceive personal attributes such as blood pressure, blood oxygen, body temperature and galvanic skin response equates to more information being available to such systems. It should not be overlooked, that in there other attributes that are currently being developed but their integration in such platforms is definitely a requirement for the future.

Environment setup can lead to discomfort and be the root cause of some diseases. Health organization do not often possess data about this. There are a number of regulations in place such as the air quality, room temperature and humidity values. Some enterprises even go as far as monitoring it, but the data is most frequently lost after sensed. So individual and aggregated records of these attributes are lost and not available to later review. In extreme cases, where a patient develops any abnormal condition, the environmental context is only transmitted through verbal communication, which is dependent on the perception of each person. A sensing attributes could help visualize without prejudice or interpretation bias, the actual states of environment related to that person and whether or not they are relevant for the facts in question.

Community Knowledge

Large scientific projects are waking in response to the availability of data through different groups of researchers. There seems to be a unanimous consideration about the value of data to health organizations and groups alike. This interest takes different interpretations according to each groups but initiatives such as electronic exam records by some government in developed countries denotes a consideration about the refusal to loose information.

Bolder ambitions as to record everything about environments and people that technology can offer are presented in the view of large technological organizations such as Google, Microsoft, Samsung and Phillips. Their view can be summarized as gathering every information about user, user behaviour and environment through the development of intelligent devices. Moreover, it is also within their view the development of medical hardware able to perform exam and diagnosis on a continuous basis gathering the information in a large community knowledge base. With such information and through process of data mining and knowledge extraction their ambition is to tackle diagnosis on diseases in early stages as well as to identify the root causes in the relationship between sensed attributes and discomfort and common illness.

The advantages of information systems towards the evaluation, knowledge discovery and pattern identification in medical records is even recognized by healthcare institutions in general (Obenshain, 2004), (Yoo et al., 2012).

CONCLUSION

The development of our well-being is something that should not be overlooked. As with any other important matter, continuous development and improvement is desirable and an objective. Systems such as these are starting to appear through the research community and as exploratory projects within large enterprises. While not identifying themselves as health organizations, their goal is to further the investigation and promotion of well-being through the population whilst increasing the information available and building large data bases about user behaviour and environment conditions. This starts the study of communities and the impact of behaviours and environment on health and comfort through large sets of population strengthening existent knowledge with large validation test, but most importantly creating the opportunity to generate new and improved knowledge by the analysis of these records. Seemingly close behaviour in different conditions can generate different results, it can be comparable to the butterfly effect, where a small change can have great implication on the whole system towards a positive or negative result. The categorization of these conditions may help improve not only well-being but health as well. The promises and the large research body around these themes indicates that these technologies and these research considerations are valid. They are even today the object of pursuit by developed societies as a mean to improve living conditions.

REFERENCES

Acampora, G., & Loia, V. (2008). A proposal of ubiquitous fuzzy computing for Ambient Intelligence. *Inf. Sci.*, *178*(3), 631–646. doi:10.1016/j.ins.2007.08.023

Atallah, L., Lo, B., & Yang, G.-Z. (2012). Can pervasive sensing address current challenges in global healthcare? *Journal of Epidemiology and Global Health, 2*(1), 1–13. doi:10.1016/j.jegh.2011.11.005 PMID:23856393

Atzori, L., Iera, A., & Morabito, G. (2010). The Internet of Things: A survey. *Computer Networks, 54*(15), 2787–2805. doi:10.1016/j.comnet.2010.05.010

Aztiria, A., Izaguirre, A., & Augusto, J. C. (2010). Learning patterns in ambient intelligence environments: A survey. *Artificial Intelligence Review, 34*(1), 35–51. doi:10.1007/s10462-010-9160-3

Biron, C., Ivers, H., Brun, J.-P., & Cooper, C. L. (2006). Risk assessment of occupational stress: Extensions of the Clarke and Cooper approach. *Health Risk & Society, 8*(4), 417–429. doi:10.1080/13698570601008222

Chan, M., Estève, D., Fourniols, J.-Y., Escriba, C., & Campo, E. (2012). Smart wearable systems: Current status and future challenges. *Artificial Intelligence in Medicine, 56*(3), 137–156. doi:10.1016/j.artmed.2012.09.003 PMID:23122689

Choi, J., Ahmed, B., & Gutierrez-Osuna, R. (2000). Ambulatory Stress Monitoring with Minimally-Invasive Wearable Sensors. *Comput. Sci. and Eng., Texas A&M*. Retrieved from http://citeseerx.ist.psu.edu/viewdoc/download?doi=10.1.1.188.46 05&rep=rep1&type=pdf

De Paola, A., Gaglio, S., Lo Re, G., & Ortolani, M. (2012). Sensor 9 k : A testbed for designing and experimenting with WSN-based ambient intelligence applications. *Pervasive and Mobile Computing, 8*(3), 448–466. doi:10.1016/j.pmcj.2011.02.006

Fanger, P. O. (1970). *Thermal comfort: Analysis and applications in environmental engineering*. Danish Technical Press. Retrieved from http://books.google.pt/ books?id=S0FSAAAAMAAJ

Liu, W., Lian, Z., & Liu, Y. (2008). Heart rate variability at different thermal comfort levels. *European Journal of Applied Physiology, 103*(3), 361–366. doi:10.1007/ s00421-008-0718-6 PMID:18351379

Obenshain, M. (2004). Application of data mining techniques to healthcare data. *Infection Control and Hospital Epidemiology, 25*(8), 690–695. http://www.jstor. org/stable/10.1086/502460 doi:10.1086/502460 PMID:15357163

Parsons, K. (2010). *Human thermal environments: the effects of hot, moderate, and cold environments on human health, comfort and performance*. Taylor & Francis. Retrieved from http://books.google.pt/books?id=4oxA6W_Os50C

Parsons, K. C. (2000). Environmental ergonomics: A review of principles, methods and models. *Applied Ergonomics*, *31*(6), 581–594. doi:10.1016/S0003-6870(00)00044-2 PMID:11132043

Piro, G., Cianci, I., Grieco, L., Boggia, G., & Camarda, P. (2014). Information centric services in Smart Cities. *Journal of Systems and Software*, *88*, 169–188. doi:10.1016/j.jss.2013.10.029

Rana, R., Kusy, B., Jurdak, R., Wall, J., & Hu, W. (2013). Feasibility analysis of using humidex as an indoor thermal comfort predictor. *Energy and Building*, *64*, 17–25. doi:10.1016/j.enbuild.2013.04.019

Silva, F., Olivares, T., Royo, F., Vergara, M. A., & Analide, C. (2013). Experimental Study of the Stress Level at the Workplace Using an Smart Testbed of Wireless Sensor Networks and Ambient Intelligence Techniques. In J. Ferrández Vicente, J. Álvarez Sánchez, F. de la Paz López, & F. J. Toledo Moreo (Eds.), *Natural and Artificial Computation in Engineering and Medical Applications SE - 21* (Vol. 7931, pp. 200–209). Springer Berlin Heidelberg; doi:10.1007/978-3-642-38622-0_21

Solanas, A., Patsakis, C., Conti, M., Vlachos, I., Ramos, V., Falcone, F., & Martinez-Balleste, A. et al. (2014). Smart health: A context-aware health paradigm within smart cities. *IEEE Communications Magazine*, *52*(8), 74–81. doi:10.1109/MCOM.2014.6871673

Steele, R., & Clarke, A. (2013). The Internet of Things and Next-generation Public Health Information Systems. *Communications and Network*, *05*(03), 4–9. doi:10.4236/cn.2013.53B1002

Tauseef, M. (2012). *Human Emotion Recognition Using Smart Sensors*. Massey University.

Weiser, M. (1991). The Computer for the Twenty-First Century. *Scientific American*, *264*(3), 94–103. doi:10.1038/scientificamerican0991-94 PMID:1675486

Yoo, I., Alafaireet, P., Marinov, M., Pena-Hernandez, K., Gopidi, R., Chang, J.-F., & Hua, L. (2012). Data mining in healthcare and biomedicine: A survey of the literature. *Journal of Medical Systems*, *36*(4), 2431–2448. doi:10.1007/s10916-011-9710-5 PMID:21537851

KEY TERMS AND DEFINITIONS

Ambient Intelligence: It is use to refer electronic environments that are sensitive and responsive to the presence of people, without the perception of people.

Attribute: A quality or feature of interest that is a part of someone or something that can be measured and used in studies.

Comfort Values: Range of values in specific units measuring attributes that can be related to environments and activities where the user is not supposed to feel the need to change alter.

Community Knowledge: Knowledge hold by a community and observable through their beliefs, actions and decisions.

Data-Mining: The use of computational algorithms and mathematical procedures to discover patterns of similar data to be used for activities such as classification prediction and forecast, knowledge discovery and clustering.

Healthcare: It considers the provision of medical care to individuals that is part of an organised plan by governments, agencies, institutions and practitioners.

Internet of Things: The connection of uniquely identifiable devices and embedded objects through internet communication protocols where they can share and receive information.

Smart-Cities: It considers cities with intelligent infrastructure, supported by public and private internet services designed to promote sustainability, sustainable development and well-being of its population.

Testbed: It is a term that refers to a physical or intangible platform for experimentation of projects, which allows for rigorous and replicable tests. This permits the verification of scientific theories, computational tools, new technologies and procedures under controllable settings.

Well-Being: Mental and physical state where the needs are satisfied. It generally connected with comfort, mental and physical health.

Chapter 7

Optimizing the Use and Adoption of Healthcare Information Systems:
A Systematic Review

Wilfred Bonney
University of Dundee, UK

ABSTRACT

Advancements in Information and Communication Technology (ICT) have led to the development of various forms of electronic records to support general practitioners and healthcare providers in capturing, storing, and retrieving routinely collected medical records and/or clinical information for optimal primary care and translational research. These advancements have resulted in the emergence of interoperable Healthcare Information Systems (HIS) such as Electronic Health Records (EHRs), Electronic Medical Records (EMRs) and Personal Health Records (PHRs). However, even as these systems continue to evolve, the research community is interested in understanding how the use and adoption of HIS can be optimized to support effective and efficient healthcare delivery and translational research. In this chapter, a systematic literature review methodology was used not only to explore the key benefits and technical challenges of HIS, but also to discuss the optimization approaches to maximizing the use and adoption of HIS in healthcare delivery.

DOI: 10.4018/978-1-4666-9882-6.ch007

INTRODUCTION

Advancements in Information and Communication Technology (ICT) have led to the development of various forms of electronic records to support general practitioners and healthcare providers in capturing, storing, and retrieving routinely collected medical records and/or clinical information for optimal primary care and translational research. These advancements have resulted in the emergence of interoperable Healthcare Information Systems (HIS) such as Electronic Health Records (EHRs), Electronic Medical Record (EMRs) and Personal Health Records (PHRs). However, even as these systems continue to evolve, the research community is still interested in understanding:

- What constitutes Health or Healthcare Information Systems?
- What are the key benefits, challenges, and obstacles of using Health or Healthcare Information Systems?
- What optimization techniques and approaches can be used to maximize the use and adoption of Health or Healthcare Information Systems in healthcare delivery?

HIS are powerful ICT-based processes, tools and applications that support effective and efficient healthcare delivery and translational research (Rodrigues, 2010). HIS have the potential to not only support seamless exchange of clinical information, but also improve both service efficiency and effectiveness for both inpatient and outpatient services (Harrison & McDowell, 2008). Hence, the need for optimizing HIS is of great essence in the healthcare industry.

The objective of this paper was to use a systematic literature review methodology not only to explore the key benefits and technical challenges of HIS, but also to discuss the optimization approaches to maximizing the use and adoption of HIS in healthcare delivery. The first part of the paper describes the systematic review methodology. In the second part, the focus is on the overview of HIS and their associated key benefits and challenges in the healthcare domain. The third part focuses on the optimization techniques and approaches to maximizing the use and adoption of HIS to support effective and efficient healthcare delivery and translational research.

METHOD

A systematic literature review, based on peered reviewed articles from 2000 to 2014, was used not only to explore the key benefits and technical challenges of HIS, but also to discuss the optimization approaches to maximizing the use and adoption of HIS in healthcare delivery. The methodology involved a systematic review of relevant peered reviewed publications, found and accessed with the help of ProQuest (with multiple databases option) and EBSCOhost databases. Additional sources were retrieved using the SAGE Journals Online, ScienceDirect, PubMed, Google Scholar, and ACM digital libraries. The targeted search terms consisted of the combination of keywords and/or phrases including: (a) healthcare information systems; (b) health care information systems; (c) health information systems; (d) health AND/OR healthcare AND/OR health care AND information systems; (e) healthcare information systems AND benefits; (f) healthcare information systems AND challenges; (g) healthcare information systems AND optimization techniques; (h) information systems AND evaluative methods; and (i) information technology AND evaluative methods.

Overall, 198 abstracts were screened and 40 of them were reviewed in full. Findings from the reviewed articles were synthesized, paraphrased and categorized under three broad themes: *Overview of Healthcare Information Systems; Key Benefits and Challenges of Healthcare Information Systems;* and *Optimization Approaches to Healthcare Information Systems*. Studies were included in the analysis if they reported not only on key benefits and technical challenges of HIS, but also discussed the optimization approaches to maximizing the use and adoption of HIS in healthcare delivery. The inclusion criteria also required that the selected full-text articles were (a) published in English language; (b) published in the date range between 2000 and 2014; and (c) electronically available in full-text. All identified studies that did not meet the requirements for the inclusion criteria were excluded from the systematic review. The PRISMA (Preferred Reporting Items for Systematic reviews and Meta-Analysis) flow diagram (Moher, Liberati, Tetzlaff, & Altman, 2009) for the systematic review is shown in Figure 1.

RESULTS

Overview of Healthcare Information Systems

The term *Healthcare Information Systems, Health Care Information Systems* or *Health Information Systems* (HIS) is commonly used to encompass several healthcare information technologies such as Electronic Health Records (EHRs), Electronic Medical Records (EMRs), Personal Health Record (PHRs), Telemedicine, Laboratory Information System (LIS), Radiology Information System (RIS), and Clinical Decision Support Systems (CDSS) (Fadlalla & Wickramasinghe, 2004; Harrison & McDowell, 2008; LeRouge, Mantzana, & Wilson, 2007; Haux, 2006; Rada, 2008; Saleem, Jones, Van Tran, & Moses, 2006). Hospital Information System is not HIS,

Figure 1. PRISMA flow diagram for the systematic review

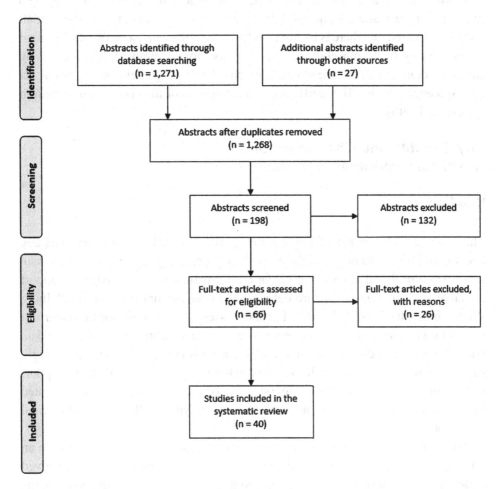

but an instance of HIS (Haux, 2006). HIS comprise of several different systems and/ or applications that support the clinical and administrative processes of healthcare delivery (Locatelli et. al, 2012; Rada, 2008). HIS may be defined as a congruence of complex systems for processing clinical and administrative data, information and knowledge in healthcare environments (Haux, 2006). Essentially, HIS "integrate data collection, processing, reporting, and use of the information necessary for improving health service effectiveness and efficiency through better management at all levels of health services" (Lippeveld, Sauerborn, & Bodart, 2000, p. 2).

Health Information Technology (HIT) has contributed immensely to the success of HIS development and deployment. According to LeRouge et al. (2007), HIT is "no longer perceived as just a supporting tool, but has become a strategic necessity for developing an integrated healthcare IT infrastructure that can improve services and reduce medical errors" (p. 669). This perception of HIT has contributed to the increasing use and adoption of HIS in many hospitals and clinics. Jamal et al. (2009) also noted that there is enough evidence to suggest that a "properly designed information system can become an important tool for preventing medical errors by enforcing clinician adherence to evidence-based clinical guidelines" (p. 34). Rada (2008) recognized that HIS partly apply the concepts of management information systems to healthcare.

Key Benefits and Challenges of Healthcare Information Systems

Key Benefits

There are several benefits of implementing HIS in healthcare delivery. The key benefits of HIS are to help healthcare providers create, generate, and disseminate germane clinical and administrative data, information and knowledge to support effective and efficient healthcare delivery and translational research (Fadlalla & Wickramasinghe, 2004; Saleem et al., 2006). Essentially, HIS provide the underpinning vital knowledge for patient-centered care by generating and converting data into information for clinical decision-making at a point of care. HIS are increasingly gaining popularity in the healthcare domain because of their capability to support legacy software systems and/or components to operate seamlessly in an integrated healthcare environment (Cavanaugh, Garland, & Hayes, 2000; Haux, 2006; Jamal et al., 2009).

HIS also continue to assume critical role in providing quality patient care in an effective and efficient manner (Saleem et al., 2006). Opening with the perceived under-utilization of HIT, Adler-Milstein and Bates (2010) indicated that many of the healthcare problems associated with paper charts and human errors can be prevented with the use of information technologies. Adler-Milstein and Bates (2010) argued that HIS are "increasingly being considered a natural tool for aiding providers, as computers can easily store up-to-date information on domains like medications and their contraindications" (p. 120). These properties of HIS coupled with their ability to support personalized medicine and evidence-based practice resonate very well amongst healthcare providers and healthcare IT professionals.

Key Challenges

There are various challenges and obstacles facing the expansion and use of HIS in healthcare delivery (LeRouge et al., 2007). The key challenges of HIS are attributed to the healthcare environment in which the systems operate. As a case in point, Fadlalla and Wickramasinghe (2004) associated healthcare delivery to a "highly fragmented delivery system that lacks even rudimentary clinical information capabilities resulting in inadequate information flows and poorly designed care processes characterized by unnecessary duplication of services, long waiting times, and delays" (p. 65). These poorly designed clinical workflow processes affect and/or constrain successful implementation of HIS.

Failures in healthcare IT systems development and deployment are not generally reported in the literature because they do not speak well for the organizations involved in the deployment of the information systems. Avison, Gregor, and Wilson (2006) attributed failures in IT systems to three factors: "complexity of application system software; poor IT governance; and relatively inexperienced and/or powerless IT staff lacking clout among corporate decision makers" (p. 92). Healthcare IT professionals often underestimate the complexity of routine clinical and managerial workflow processes in the healthcare environment (LittleJohns, Ludwick & Doucette, 2009). Specifically, healthcare IT professionals fail to take into consideration the social and professional cultures of healthcare organizations (Little Johns, p. 862). These processes and organizational cultures are crucial when it comes to the use and adoption of HIS in the healthcare domain.

Part of the clinicians' resistance to the adoption of EHRs and EMRs is attributed to the complexity of application systems and poor IT governance structure. In most cases, the information systems are developed by IT professionals that are not knowledgeable enough about the information flow and use in the healthcare settings. This often leads to the development of information systems that complicate and slow down the routine workflow of clinicians. For example, Gibb and Haar (2009) recognized the significance role of IT in the healthcare industry by noting that greater IT interface challenges negatively influences e-business activity conducted by general practitioners. This might explain why the use of EHRs and EMRs in hospitals still remain less attractive to clinicians and healthcare providers at large.

In another study, Reti, Feldman, and Safran (2009) found that lack of properly defined governance structure limits the broad use of PHRs. In order to facilitate the communication between clinicians and patients, Reti et al. (2009) proposed a governance structure that recognizes clinicians and patients as key stakeholders of PHRs and include them as members. It is in this regard that Avison et al. (2006) asserted that IT project success can be achieved only by applying proper and prudent management controls to the development and deployment of information systems. Diamond and Shirky (2008) made similar assessment by defending the notion that technology and policy are inseparable and that clear policy statements are needed to guide the design of technology.

Optimization Approaches to Healthcare Information Systems

This component of the research discusses ways to optimize HIS so as to maximize their use and adoption in the healthcare domain. The optimization approaches involved four broad themes: *Interoperable Health Data Standards; Component-oriented Approach; Social Actor Theory*; and *Evaluative Methods*.

Interoperable Health Data Standards

The use of interoperable health data standards in HIS has enormous potential to accelerate their use and adoption within the healthcare industry. Hammond et al. (2014) unequivocally acknowledged the importance of interoperable standards by asserting that health data standards are required when excessive diversity creates inefficiencies or impedes effectiveness. Interoperable standards play a crucial role in enhancing security and improving interoperability of HIS (Gritzalis, 1998).

Interoperable standards afford the capability to standardize patient records and management procedures across the continuum of disparate healthcare providers. In a study conducted to compare and contrast the different facets of interoperability being considered in the development of HIS, Halley, Sensmeier, and Brokel (2009) found that interoperable health data standards need to be maintained in order to support the information-sharing needs across care settings, providers, patients, and population healthcare environments. According to Halley et al. (2009), it is "only through the interoperable exchange of health information that expected decreases in costs will be realized, such as eliminating duplicate tests, improving administrative efficiencies, increasing access to patient clinical results, and providing information to decrease repetitive input" (p. 310). These findings from Halley et al. (2009) call for the deployment of the HIS in an interoperability environment where interoperable standards are used explicitly and efficiently.

The interoperability environment could involve the use of data exchange or messaging standards (e.g. Health Level Seven (HL7) Version 2 & 3 Messaging Standard and Digital Imaging and Communications in Medicine (DICOM)); and classification and terminology standards such as Read Codes, International Classification of Diseases: Tenth Revision (ICD-10), Logical Observation Identifiers Names and Codes (LOINC), and Systemized Nomenclature of Medicine - Clinical Terms (SNOMED CT). Terminology and classification standards promise to provide the common medical language necessary for EHRs, EMRs, PHRs, quality clinical data recording and reporting, safety, clinical trials, biosurveillance, and reimbursement (Campbell & Giannangelo, 2007). Watkins et al. (2009) recognized the importance of the interoperability environment by asserting that healthcare organizations operate in dynamic environment and the standardization of healthcare data within the context of clinical workflow is essential in providing the foundation for future translational research and the increasingly vital quality and regulatory reporting. Watkins et al. (2009) also noted that the accurate and consistent representation of clinical data and ultimately interoperability, are necessary to serve patient-centered care, where healthcare information exists with many providers.

Component-Oriented Approach

The component-oriented approach is a software development methodology that could be adopted to optimize HIS. Mei et al (2003) considered the component-oriented approach as an effective and efficient way to improve the productivity and quality of software development as well as in building distributed systems. More importantly, the component-oriented approach to software development has emerged as an important means to (a) control the complexity of software systems; (b) improve software quality; and (c) support software development and software reuse (Mei et al. 2006). The component-oriented approach emphasizes component-based system development and security risk analysis that builds on existing infrastructure framework supported by additional requirement specifications (Brændeland & Stølen, 2006).

Application of component-oriented software development to HIS development not only results in more reusable software components, but also enables the production of reusable artifacts in a systematic fashion (Park et al., 2004; Pinto et al., 2002). The essence of the component-oriented approach to software development is to facilitate reusability, rapid development, cost effectiveness, and dynamic service, thereby, leading to cost reduction, improved reliability and a faster development of software components (Berbener et al., 2005; Park et al., 2004). As part of organizational change, Berg (2001) cautioned that the implementation of HIS should not be run as a mere technical project, but rather be managed as a process of organizational development, in which IT is drawn upon as a strategic asset to transform healthcare organizational goals, structures and routine workflows.

Service-oriented architecture (SOA) is also a good fit for the component-oriented approach. Supplementing the component-oriented approach with service-oriented architecture will provide a rich environment in which secure exchange of health information can be established to support efficient use and adoption of HIS. Secure exchange of clinical information is very crucial in optimizing wider adoption of HIS (Agrawal, Grandison, Johnson, & Kiernan, 2007; Kahn, Aulakh, & Bosworth, 2009). For example, protecting the confidentiality, security, and data integrity of personalized health information contained in HIS is of prime concern to many patients and healthcare providers. According to Agrawal et al. (2007), secure exchange of clinical information is important in promoting evidence-based practice, medical research, assisting decision support, and increasing knowledge available for patient care. Using the component-oriented approach will enlighten healthcare providers to identify and document the security risks and gaps at the component level of HIS development.

Social Actor Theory

Organizational cultures, roles and social identities remain some of the key challenges in successfully implementing HIS in the healthcare domain. Social informaticians consider the social actor theory as a solution to leverage, mitigate and handle issues of organizational cultures, roles, and social identities (Strong et al., 2009). The social actor theory was first introduced by Lamb and Kling (2003). Rowlands (2006) characterized the social actor theory by asserting that "people's individual autonomy (their agency) and their behaviors are shaped by the social norms, institutional forces, and the social and physical structures that surround them" (p. 1540). This characterization is very useful in optimizing the development of HIS.

The social actor theory could be applied to the development of EHRs, EMRs and PHRs. Conceptualizing healthcare professionals as social actors will require examining their affiliations, environment, interactions and identity (Lamb and Kling, 2003) to understand social structures and processes that might need to be considered before deploying HIS in the healthcare domain. This is crucial because different healthcare professionals have different social identities, and they are often not compatible with the social identity of IT users (Strong et al., 2009). Hence, any implemented HIS will require that the system is engineered in a way that fits the workflow of the healthcare professionals. In other words, the system should be enabling, not constraining.

One approach to optimizing HIS is identifying healthcare actors during the development phase. According to Mantzana, Themistocleous, Irani, and Morabito (2007), the healthcare actors involved in the adoption of HIS can be "any human and/or organisation that accepts, provides, supports or controls healthcare services" (p. 33). Mantzana et al. (2007) emphasized the importance of healthcare actors by asserting that an earlier identification of the actors will enable decision and policy-makers to better understand actors' views and roles and hence, enable more informed decisions regarding the adoption of information systems in the healthcare environment. The social actor theory promotes users' participation in systems design and will enable healthcare IT professionals to develop information systems that will support the workflow of different healthcare professionals, thereby, improving the quality and efficiency of healthcare delivery. For example, Van Akkeren and Rowlands (2007) used the social actor theory to study how mandated HIS adoption was perceived by different healthcare professionals.

Evaluative Methods

Evaluative methods such as *IT Portfolio Management* and *Value Chain Analysis* could be used to assess the impact of already implemented HIS so as to identify gaps and ways to optimize them.

IT Portfolio Management

Information Technology Portfolio Management (ITPM) may be defined as a strategic way of managing IT as a "portfolio of assets similar to a financial portfolio and striving to improve the performance of the portfolio by balancing risk and return" (Jeffery & Leliveld, 2004, p. 41). More importantly, successful implementation of ITPM will benefit organizations in assessing investment in information technology usage (Jeffery & Leliveld, 2004; Ward & Peppard, 2002). For example, Jeffery and Leliveld (2004) introduced the ITPM maturity model as a new tool that can be used to assess what constitutes best-practice ITPM. The model segments a company's ITPM into stages to support efficient evaluation of IT usage.

ITPM implementation is often not an easy undertaking, as there are implementation hurdles such as poor execution and deep-rooted divide between business and IT (Jeffery & Leliveld, 2004; Ward & Peppard, 2002). It is in this regard that Helferich, Schmid, and Herzwurm (2006) noted that establishing an effective integration and communication between business and IT is a challenge to most organizations because it requires a change of existing workflow processes and can lead to a clash of cultures. To overcome these hurdles, Jeffery and Leliveld (2004) identified four best practices for successfully deploying ITPM in an organization: "staged implementation strategy, creating a process for upgrading ITPM, ensuring that staff members are trained, and involving business-side people from the beginning" (p. 47). Luftman (2003), on the other hand, proposed six categories for assessing IT/business alignment: communications, competency/value measurements, governance, partnership, technology scope, and skills maturity. HIS could be evaluated using the six categories, proposed by Luftman (2003), for evaluating the effectiveness of the current application portfolio in an organization. The overall alignment score, obtained from the alignment assessment, will help healthcare providers and stakeholders in determining the success level of implemented HIS in a given organization.

Value Chain Analysis

Value chain analysis is another evaluative method that could be used to help healthcare IT professionals and healthcare providers to identify strategic planning techniques to enhancing HIS development and deployment. Value chain analysis not only provides a key to discovering the business-to-business customers' strategic needs, but it also uncover the strategically relevant activities through which an organization conducts its business (Bhatt & Emdad, 2001; Crain & Abraham, 2008; Zokaei & Simons, 2006). Zokaei and Simons (2006) defined value chain analysis as "a structured method of analyzing the effects of all the core activities on cost and/or differentiation of the value chain" (p. 147). Specifically, value chain analysis is a method of analyzing the value chain for competitive advantage.

The value chains are used to "delineate the value-added stages from raw material to end-user as a product is manufactured and distributed, with each stage representing an industry" (Crain & Abraham, 2008, p. 29). Drawing upon the work of Porter (1985), Bhatt and Emdad (2001) noted that the initial conceptualization of the value chain was primarily targeted toward manufacturing firms. However, in the present digital age, a majority of organizations are conducting their business in an electronic environment, in which information systems become the main medium through which business transactions are exchanged (Bhatt & Emdad, 2001). Bhatt and Emdad (2001), therefore, categorized value chains into two types: physical value chain and virtual value chain. Whereas the physical value chain activities are concerned with fulfilling customer orders and assembling final products and services; the virtual value chain activities are concerned with providing information access to customers, suppliers, and/or manufacturers (Bhatt & Emdad, 2001). In a similar study, Rayport and Sviokla (1995) characterized virtual value chain as a way of gathering, organizing, selecting, synthesizing, and distributing information.

In the e-Health environment, the application of the value chain analysis will mostly involve the use of virtual value chain, as strategic business activities in the virtual value chain are performed with and around information. Bhatt and Emdad (2001) recommended on the need for businesses to integrate virtual value chain with physical value chain so as to realize the full potential of their products and services. Value chain analysis has been used in the healthcare environment to support business activities. For example, Gamble, Savage, and Icenogle (2004) used value chain analysis to examine structural and executional cost for deploying two telemedicine applications (i.e. teleradiography and telerehabilitation) in rural health program. Gamble et al. (2004) were motivated by the fact that current value chains for some clinical applications are structured in a manner that requires subsidies to cover costs. Findings from Gamble et al.'s (2004) study suggested that the value chains of telemedicine applications offer considerable cost savings relative to traditional delivery models.

DISCUSSION AND CONCLUSION

This chapter has discussed and explored the key benefits, technical barriers, challenges, and optimization approaches to maximizing the use and adoption of HIS in healthcare delivery. HIS are becoming a critical component in the healthcare industry and continue to play a pivotal role in helping healthcare providers create, generate, and disseminate germane clinical and administrative data, information and knowledge to support effective and efficient healthcare delivery and translational research. The research has the potential to benefit healthcare providers, policy-makers, and stakeholders in determining the optimization techniques for improving the use and adoption of HIS so as to support effective and efficient healthcare delivery and translational research. There is an expectation that future development of HIS will increase in scope and complexity while providing significant opportunities for data quality assessment and improvement.

Accelerating wider use and adoption of HIS is an expensive and complex undertaking in the healthcare industry. Protecting the confidentiality, security, and data integrity of personalized health information contained in HIS is of prime concern to many patients and healthcare providers. Healthcare providers and stakeholders are not willing to invest in information systems that do not provide adequate protection for personalized health data. However, using the component-oriented approach will enlighten healthcare providers to identify and document the security risks and gaps at the component level of HIS development.

Engaging and involving the government in the development and deployment of the HIS is necessary to increase their use and adoption in medical practice. This is because government involvement will not only help accelerate and promote healthcare IT implementation, but it will also provide opportunities for fully interoperable HIS that would improve the use and adoption of evidence-based medicine in both medical practice and translational research. Future research should focus on identifying techniques in involving the government as part of the stakeholders (i.e. social actor) in the development of HIS. Beyond the need for accessing the impact and optimization techniques of HIS in medical practice, it is also important to measure patient outcomes and develop a standardized reporting procedure to support translational research.

REFERENCES

Adler-Milstein, J., & Bates, D. W. (2010). Paperless healthcare: Progress and challenges of an IT-enabled healthcare system. *Business Horizons*, *53*(2), 119–130. doi:10.1016/j.bushor.2009.10.004

Agrawal, R., Grandison, T., Johnson, C., & Kiernan, J. (2007). Enabling the 21st century health care information technology revolution. *Communications of the ACM*, *50*(2), 34–42. doi:10.1145/1216016.1216018

Avison, D., Gregor, S., & Wilson, D. (2006). Managerial IT unconsciousness. *Communications of the ACM*, *49*(7), 89–93. doi:10.1145/1139922.1139923

Berbner, R., Grollius, T., Repp, N., Heckmann, O., Ortner, E., & Steinmetz, R. (2005). *An approach for the management of Service-oriented Architecture (SoA) based Application Systems* (pp. 208–221). EMISA.

Berg, M. (2001). Implementing information systems in health care organizations: Myths and challenges. *International Journal of Medical Informatics*, *64*(2-3), 143–156. doi:10.1016/S1386-5056(01)00200-3 PMID:11734382

Bhatt, G. D., & Emdad, A. F. (2001). An analysis of the virtual value chain in electronic commerce. *Logistics Information Management*, *14*(1/2), 78–85. doi:10.1108/09576050110362465

Brændeland, G., & Stølen, K. (2006). Using model-based security analysis in component-oriented system development. Paper presented at the *QoP '06: Proceedings of the 2nd ACM Workshop on Quality of Protection*, Alexandria, Virginia, USA (pp. 11-18). doi:10.1145/1179494.1179498

Campbell, K. E., & Giannangelo, K. (2007). Language barrier: Getting past the classifications and terminologies roadblock. *Journal of American Health Information Management Association*, *78*(2), 44–46, 48. PMID:17366992

Cavanaugh, B., Garland, H., & Hayes, B. (2000). Upgrading legacy systems for the integrating the healthcare enterprise (IHE) initiative. *Journal of Digital Imaging*, *13*(S1), 180–182. doi:10.1007/BF03167655 PMID:10847393

Crain, D. W., & Abraham, S. (2008). Using value-chain analysis to discover customers' strategic needs. *Strategy and Leadership*, *36*(4), 29–39. doi:10.1108/10878570810888759

Diamond, C., & Shirky, C. (2008). Health information technology: A few years of magical thinking? *Health Affairs*, *27*(5), W383. doi:10.1377/hlthaff.27.5.w383 PMID:18713827

Fadlalla, A., & Wickramasinghe, N. (2004). An integrative framework for HIPAA-compliant I*IQ healthcare information system. *International Journal of Health Care Quality Assurance*, *17*(2/3), 65–74. doi:10.1108/09526860410526673 PMID:15301262

Gamble, J. E., Savage, G. T., & Icenogle, M. L. (2004). Value-chain analysis of a rural health program: Toward understanding the cost benefit of telemedicine applications. *Hospital Topics*, *82*(1), 10–17. PMID:15490956

Gibb, J., & Haar, J. (2009). e-business connections in the health sector: IT challenges and the effects of practice size. *Journal of Management & Organization*, *15*(4), 500–513. doi:10.5172/jmo.15.4.500

Gritzalis, D. A. (1998). Enhancing security and improving interoperability in healthcare information systems. *Informatics for Health & Social Care*, *23*(4), 309–323. doi:10.3109/14639239809025367 PMID:9922951

Halley, E., Sensmeier, J., & Brokel, J. (2009). Nurses exchanging information: Understanding electronic health record standards and interoperability. *Urologic Nursing*, *29*(5), 305–313. PMID:19863037

Hammond, W. E., Jaffe, C., Cimino, J. J., & Huff, S. M. (2014). Standards in Biomedical Informatics. In E. H. Shortliffe & J. J. Cimino (Eds.), *Biomedical Informatics: Computer Applications in Health Care and Biomedicine* (4th ed., pp. 211–253). New York: Springer-Verlag; doi:10.1007/978-1-4471-4474-8_7

Harrison, J. P., & McDowell, G. M. (2008). The role of laboratory information systems in healthcare quality improvement. *International Journal of Health Care Quality Assurance*, *21*(7), 679–691. doi:10.1108/09526860810910159 PMID:19055276

Haux, R. (2006). Health information systems–past, present, future. *International Journal of Medical Informatics*, *75*(3-4), 268–281. doi:10.1016/j.ijmedinf.2005.08.002 PMID:16169771

Heeks, R. (2006). Health information systems: Failure, success and improvisation. *International Journal of Medical Informatics*, *75*(2), 125–137. doi:10.1016/j.ijmedinf.2005.07.024 PMID:16112893

Helferich, A., Schmid, K., & Herzwurm, G. (2006). Product management for software product lines: An unsolved problem? *Communications of the ACM*, *49*(12), 66–67. doi:10.1145/1183236.1183268

Jamal, A., McKenzie, K., & Clark, M. (2009). The impact of health information technology on the quality of medical and health care: A systematic review. *Health Information Management Journal*, *38*(3), 26–37. PMID:19875852

Jeffery, M., & Leliveld, I. (2004). Best practices in IT portfolio management. *MIT Sloan Management Review*, *45*(3), 41–49.

Kahn, J., Aulakh, V., & Bosworth, A. (2009). What it takes: Characteristics of the ideal personal health record. *Health Affairs, 28*(2), 369–376. doi:10.1377/hlthaff.28.2.369 PMID:19275992

LeRouge, C., Mantzana, V., & Wilson, E. (2007). Healthcare information systems research, revelations and visions. *European Journal of Information Systems, 16*(6), 669–671. doi:10.1057/palgrave.ejis.3000712

Lippeveld, T., Sauerborn, R., & Bodart, C. (2000). *Design and implementation of health information systems*. Geneva: World Health Organization.

Littlejohns, P., Wyatt, J. C., & Garvican, L. (2003). Evaluating computerised health information systems: Hard lessons still to be learnt. *BMJ (Clinical Research Ed.), 326*(7394), 860–863. doi:10.1136/bmj.326.7394.860 PMID:12702622

Locatelli, P., Restifo, N., Gastaldi, L., & Corso, M. (2012). Health care information systems: Architectural models and governance. *Innovative information systems modelling techniques* (Ch. 4, pp. 73-98). Intech.

Ludwick, D. A., & Doucette, J. (2009). Adopting electronic medical records in primary care: Lessons learned from health information systems implementation experience in seven countries. *International Journal of Medical Informatics, 78*(1), 22–31. doi:10.1016/j.ijmedinf.2008.06.005 PMID:18644745

Luftman, J. (2003). Assessing IT/business alignment. *Information Systems Management, 20*(4), 9–15. doi:10.1201/1078/43647.20.4.20030901/77287.2

Mantzana, V., Themistocleous, M., Irani, Z., & Morabito, V. (2007). Identifying healthcare actors involved in the adoption of information systems. *European Journal of Information Systems, 16*(1), 91–102. doi:10.1057/palgrave.ejis.3000660

Mei, H., Chen, F., Feng, Y. D., & Yang, J. (2003). ABC: An architecture based, component oriented approach to software development. *Journal of Software, 14*(4), 721–732.

Mei, H., & Shen, J. R. (2006). Progress of research on software architecture. *Ruan Jian Xue Bao* [Journal of Software], *17*(6), 1257–1275.

Moher, D., Liberati, A., Tetzlaff, J., & Altman, D. G.The PRISMA Group. (2009). *Preferred Reporting Items for Systematic Reviews and Meta-Analyses: The PRISMA Statement. PLoS Medicine, 6*(6), e1000097. doi:10.1371/journal.pmed.1000097 PMID:19621072

Park, H., Suh, W., & Lee, H. (2004). A role-driven component-oriented methodology for developing collaborative commerce systems. *Information and Software Technology, 46*(12), 819–837. doi:10.1016/j.infsof.2004.02.002

Pinto, M., Fuentes, L., Fayad, M. E., & Troya, J. M. (2002). Separation of coordination in a dynamic aspect oriented framework. *Proceedings of the 1st international conference on Aspect-oriented software development* (pp. 134-140). New York, NY: ACM. doi:10.1145/508386.508403

Porter, M. E. (1985). *Competitive advantage: Creating and sustaining superior performance*. New York, NY: Free Press.

Rada, R. (2008). *Information Systems and Healthcare Enterprises*. Hershey, PA: IGI Publishing. doi:10.4018/978-1-59904-651-8

Rayport, J., & Sviokla, J. (1995). Exploiting the virtual value chain. *Harvard Business Review, 73*(6), 75–85.

Reti, S. R., Feldman, H. J., & Safran, C. (2009). Governance for personal health records. *Journal of the American Medical Informatics Association, 16*(1), 14–17. doi:10.1197/jamia.M2854 PMID:18952939

Rodrigues, J. J. P. C. (2010). Preface. In J. J. P. C. Rodrigues (Ed.), *Health Information Systems: Concepts, Methodologies, Tools, and Applications* (pp. i–vi). Hershey, PA: Medical Information Science Reference. doi:10.4018/978-1-60566-988-5

Rowlands, B. H. (2006). The user as social actor: A focus on systems development methodology enactment. *Paper presented at the SAC '06: Proceedings of the 2006 ACM Symposium on Applied Computing*, Dijon, France (pp. 1540-1545). doi:10.1145/1141277.1141634

Saleem, N., Jones, D. R., Van Tran, H., & Moses, B. (2006). Forming design teams to develop healthcare information systems. *Hospital Topics, 84*(1), 22–30. doi:10.3200/HTPS.84.1.22-31 PMID:16573013

Strong, D. M., Volkoff, O., Johnson, S. A., Bar-On, I., & Pelletier, L. (2009). Electronic health records and the changing roles of health care professionals: A social informatics perspective. *Proceedings of AMCIS 2009 Paper 560*. Retrieved from http://aisel.aisnet.org/amcis2009/560

Van Akkeren, J., & Rowlands, B. (2007). An epidemic of pain in an Australian radiology practice. *European Journal of Information Systems, 16*(6), 695–711. doi:10.1057/palgrave.ejis.3000715

Ward, J., & Peppard, J. (2002). *Strategic planning for information systems* (3rd ed.). New York, NY: Wiley.

Watkins, T. J., Haskell, R. E., Lundberg, C. B., Brokel, J. M., Wilson, M. L., & Hardiker, N. (2009). Terminology use in electronic health records: Basic principles. *Urologic Nursing, 29*(5), 321–326. PMID:19863039

Zokaei, A. K., & Simons, D. W. (2006). Value chain analysis in consumer focus improvement. *International Journal of Logistics Management, 17*(2), 141–162. doi:10.1108/09574090610689934

Chapter 8
Evaluation of the Length of Hospital Stay through Artificial Neural Networks Based Systems

Vasco Abelha
University of Minho, Portugal

Fernando Marins
University of Minho, Portugal

Henrique Vicente
University of Evora, Portugal

ABSTRACT

The mentality of savings and eliminating any kind of outgoing costs is undermining our society and our way of living. Cutting funds from Education to Health is at best delaying the inevitable "Crash" that is foreshadowed. Regarding Health, a major concern, can be described as jeopardize the health of Patients – Reduce of the Length of Hospital. As we all know, Human Health is very sensitive and prune to drastic changes in short spaces of time. Factors like age, sex, their ambient context – house conditions, daily lives – should all be important when deciding how long a specific patient should remain safe in a hospital. In no way, ought this be decided by the economic politics. Logic Programming was used for knowledge representation and reasoning, letting the modeling of the universe of discourse in terms of defective data, information and knowledge. Artificial Neural Networks and Genetic Algorithms were used in order to evaluate and predict how long should a patient remain in the hospital in order to minimize the collateral damage of our government approaches, not forgetting the use of Degree of Confidence to demonstrate how feasible the assessment is.

DOI: 10.4018/978-1-4666-9882-6.ch008

1. INTRODUCTION

Over the past few years, the dogma of reducing costs has grown rapidly. We are currently facing a worldwide economic crisis that is affecting every sector of our society. This leads to erroneous behaviors and actions by our leaders, when trying to delay and repeal the possibility of a foreshadowed economic crash. And how do they try to bypass the crash? Reduction of all costs. Sections such as Education, Health, Social Security, etcetera, are being forced to cut down the costs, to counterbalance the lack of funding by the government. In education, schools are closing down, teachers are fired or compelled to lecture more students and to work for more hours, culminating in a diminution of performance in the art of teaching and learning. The same can be applied to Health.

Nowadays, closing health facilities and laying off medical staff are some of the headlines of our lives, both doctors and patients are suffering the consequences of our leader's convictions in reducing costs. None is getting the respect they deserve. Health practitioners are, as well as teachers, enforced to practice extra hours, to reduce the duration of medical evaluations and, last but not the least, to prioritize the health of the institution above the patient health, which ends up in minimizing the length of the patient's stay at the hospital.

Ethically, this view is unacceptable. Objectively, this is happening. In no circumstances, should a medical patient be seen as a number, as a monetary cost. The Hospital must be regarded only as a tool, a place to treat maladies, illness. A Patient's fate must not be decided by arithmetic, but by his health condition, his context, his past and present. These are the only decisive aspects to determine the duration of a sick person in the medical facility. And what is this context?

In the medical universe, the context can be referred as the life story of a patient. In order to make any type of medical judgment, a health professional has to consult all the information on the patient. This information comes from two sources:

- Patient
- Hospital

From the patient, we can obtain age, sex, comorbidities - physiological / morphological features - as well as data related to their daily lives. It is important to note that this information is subjective and may also not correspond to the truth, since we can never confirm the honesty of the patient. The ill-founded can induce the health professional in error through lies or due to memory problems.

The data relative to the Hospital includes all kinds of medical history of the patient: examinations, consultations, cultures and medical journals. It can be said that this information is objective and concrete, as these are obtained through medical procedures and exact methods.

We can see, based on the literature, that these information sources fit perfectly in the medical universe, specifically, SOAP note - (an acronym for subjective, objective, assessment, and plan) is a method of documentation employed by health care providers to write out notes in a patient's chart.

The aspects, previously enumerated, are more than necessary, as presented in a wide-range of literature or among experts, to do a risk assessment– Determine, with a certain Degree of Confidence, if a patient should stay in health care or not. Of course not all aspects have the same importance (Fry, 1993; Pritchard, 1981; World Health Organization [WHO], 1978). The most prominent aspects can be linked to Patient History, Comorbidity and Daily Context. To shed some light, the latter refers to the patient daily lives. If they have no conditions to be "set out in the open" – home hygienic conditions, no guidance - they ought to stay in the hospital, because, if not, they will most likely deteriorate their health and be routed once again to the hospital in a near future and even increase their cost to the hospital.

"It is better to do it right the first time and not having the past come back to bite". Nevertheless and in spite of these politics, this is exactly what happens most of the times. Patients tend to decrease their already short time span of admission in the hospital. The rest of aspects are easy to infer their relevance and why they should as well be taken into consideration. Such variables as *current treatments, exams and daily hospital diaries* have a correlation between them. Most of the time they share information or complement each other.

Thus and in order to easily apply and explain the concepts soon to be described. The aspects needed to determine the length of stay in a hospital were clustered in 4 groups displayed in *Figure 1*. All the data relative to the patient such as age, sex, and comorbidity are linked to the Biological Factors. Patient History refers to the detailed patient medical history. The information here comes from the sufferer, himself, or any past records that the health system has regarding his previous admissions. Ambient Factors is simply the context embracing the patient. Anything that surrounds him is, as well, important for determining the length of stay. Hospital Factor simply summarizes every exam, diagnosis he did at the hospital.

After a briefly description of the relevance and meaning of the values, one setback that arises is the incomplete information, noise and uncertainty. Sometimes we may not be completely certain of such information or we may not even have access to that specific data. Our investigation aims to speculate and estimate the necessary length of stay in a hospital of a certain patient, while reducing any mishap in their health. This is achieved by the use of logical programming based approach to knowledge representation and reasoning, complemented with a computational framework based on Artificial Neural Networks.

Figure 1. Variables relevant on the length of stay

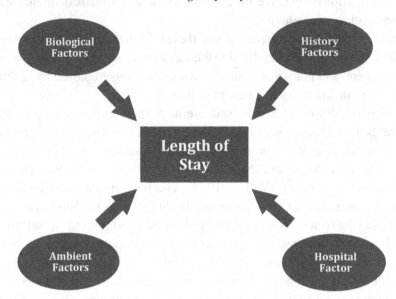

2. KNOWLEDGE REPRESENTATION AND REASONING

Many approaches for knowledge representation and reasoning have been proposed using the *Logic Programming* (*LP*) paradigm, namely in the area of Model Theory (Pereira, 2009; Neves, Machado, Analide, Abelha, & Brito, 2007; Neves, 1984) and Proof Theory (Halpern, 2005; Kovalerchuck & Resconi, 2010). We follow the proof theoretical approach and an extension to the *LP* language, to knowledge representation and reasoning. An *Extended Logic Program* – acronym E.L.P – is a finite set of clauses in the form:

$$p \leftarrow p_1, \ldots, p_n, not\ q_1, \ldots, q_m \tag{1}$$

$$?(p_1, \ldots, p_n, not\ q_1, \ldots, q_m)\ (n, m \geq 0) \tag{2}$$

where *?* is a domain atom denoting falsity, the p_j, q_j, and p are classical ground literals, i.e., either positive atoms or atoms preceded by the classical negation sign ¬ (Kovalerchuck & Resconi, 2010). Under this representation formalism, every program is associated with a set of abducibles (Pereira & Anh, 2009; Neves, Machado, Analide, Abelha, & Brito, 2007; Neves, 1984) given here in the form of exceptions to the extensions of the predicates that make the program. Once again, LP emerged as an attractive formalism for knowledge representation and reasoning tasks, introducing an efficient search mechanism for problem solving.

Due to the growing need to offer user support in decision making processes some studies have been presented (Lucas, 2011; Machado, Abelha, Novais, João Neves, & José Neves, 2010), related to the qualitative models and qualitative reasoning in Database Theory and in Artificial Intelligence research. With respect to the problem of knowledge representation and reasoning in Logic Programming (LP), a measure of the *Quality-of-Information* (*QoI*) of such programs has been object of some work with promising results (Liu & Sun, 2007; Caldeira et al., 2010). The *QoI* with respect to the extension of a predicate *i* will be given by a truth-value in the interval [0,1], i.e., if the information is *known* (*positive*) or *false* (*negative*) the *QoI* for the extension of *predicate*$_i$ is 1. For situations where the information is unknown, the *QoI* is given by:

$$QoI_i = \lim_{n \to \infty} \frac{1}{n} = 0 \left(N \gg 0 \right) \tag{3}$$

where *N* denotes the cardinality of the set of terms or clauses of the extension of *predicate*$_i$ that stand for the incompleteness under consideration. For situations where the extension of *predicate*$_i$ is unknown but can be taken from a set of values, the *QoI* is given by:

$$QoI_i = \frac{1}{Card} \tag{4}$$

where *Card* denotes the cardinality of the *abducibles* set for *i*, if the *abducibles* set is disjoint. If the *abducibles* set is not disjoint, the *QoI* is given by:

$$QoI_i = \frac{1}{C_1^{Card} + \ldots + C_{Card}^{Card}} \tag{5}$$

where C_{Card}^{Card} is a card-combination subset, with *Card* elements. The next element of the model to be considered is the relative importance that a predicate assigns to each of its attributes under observation, i.e., w_i^k, which stands for the relevance of attribute *k* in the extension of *predicate*$_i$. It is also assumed that the weights of all the attribute predicates are normalized, i.e.:

$$\sum_{1 \le k \le n} w_i^k = 1, \forall_i \tag{6}$$

where ∀ denotes the universal quantifier. It is now possible to define a predicate's scoring function $V_i(x)$ so that, for a value $x = (x_1, \cdots, x_n)$, defined in terms of the attributes of $predicate_i$, one may have:

$$V_i(x) = \sum_{1 \leq k \leq n} w_i^k \times \frac{QoI_i(x)}{n} \tag{7}$$

It is now possible to engender all the possible scenarios of the universe of discourse, according to the information given in the logic programs that endorse the information depicted in Figure 3, i.e., in terms of the extensions of the predicates *Biological Factors, Historical Factors, Hospital Factors and Ambient Factors*.

It is now feasible to rewrite the extensions of the predicates referred to above, in terms of a set of possible scenarios according to productions of the type:

$$predicate_i\left(X_1, \ldots, X_n\right) :: QoI \tag{8}$$

Figure 3. A summary of the Relational Database model

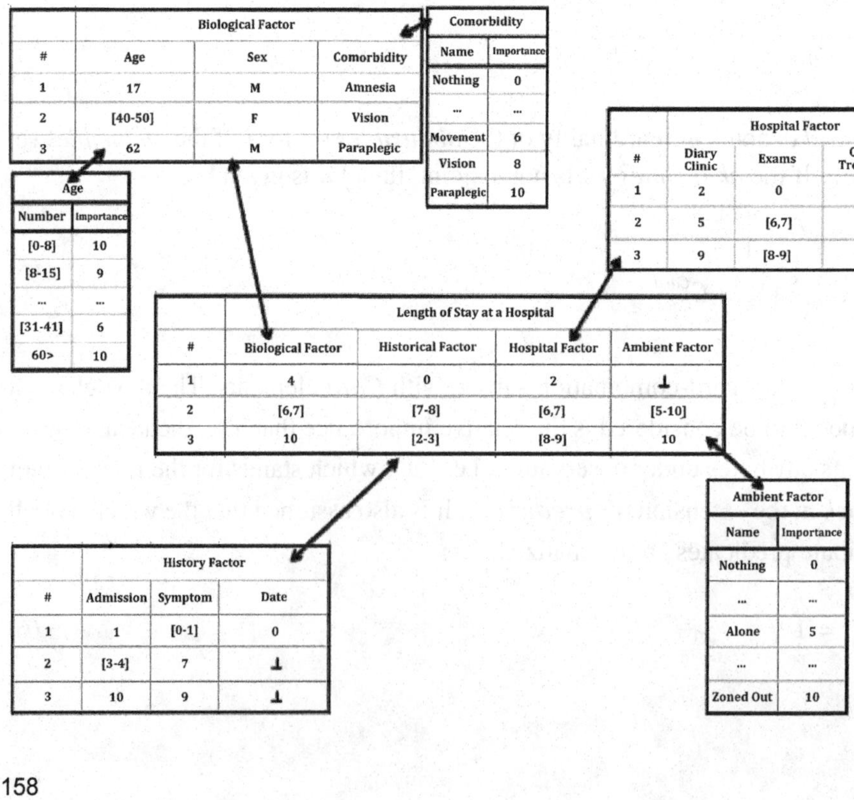

and evaluate the *Degree of Confidence* (*DoC*) given by $DoC = V_i\left(x_1, \cdots, x_n\right)/n$, which denotes one's confidence in a particular term of the extension o f $predicate_i$. To be more general, let us suppose that the Universe of Discourse is described by the extension of the predicates:

$$a_1\left(\ldots\right), a_2\left(\ldots\right), \ldots, a_n\left(\ldots\right) \text{ where } \left(n \geq 0\right) \tag{9}$$

Therefore, for a given *scenario_i*, one may have (where $\perp$ denotes an argument value of the type unknown; the values of the others arguments stand for themselves):

$$\begin{cases} \neg a_1\left(x_1, y_1, k_1, z_1\right) \leftarrow not\ a_1\left(x_1, y_1, k_1, z_1\right) \\ \quad a_1\left(27, [10,12], 15,\right) :: 0.5 \\ \quad \underbrace{[25,30][10,12][3,25][0,5]}_{\text{atribute's domains for } x_1, y_1, k_1, z_1} \\ \neg a_2\left(x_2, y_2, k_2, z_2\right) \leftarrow not\ a_2\left(x_2, y_2, k_2, z_2\right) \\ \quad a_2\left([33,42], 10, [10,12], \perp\right) :: 0.48 \\ \quad \underbrace{[20,50][8,10][6,14][20,50]}_{\text{atribute's domains for } x_2, y_2, k_2, z_2} \end{cases}$$

⬇ *1st interaction: transition to continuous intervals*

$$\begin{cases} \neg a_1\left(x_1, y_1, k_1, z_1\right) \leftarrow not\ a_1\left(x_1, y_1, k_1, z_1\right) \\ \quad a_1\left([27,27], [10,12], [15,15], [0,5]\right) :: 0.5 \\ \quad \underbrace{[25,30][10,12][3,25][0,5]}_{\text{atribute's domains for } x_1, y_1, k_1, z_1} \\ \neg a_2\left(x_2, y_2, k_2, z_2\right) \leftarrow not\ a_2\left(x_2, y_2, k_2, z_2\right) \\ \quad a_2\left([33,42], 10, [10,12], [20,50]\right) :: 0.48 \\ \quad \underbrace{[20,50][8,10][6,14][20,50]}_{\text{atribute's domains for } x_2, y_2, k_2, z_2} \end{cases}$$

⋮

$$2nd\ interaction:\ normalization\ \frac{Y - Y_{min}}{Y_{max} - Y_{min}}$$

$$\begin{cases} \neg a_1\left(x_1, y_1, k_1, z_1\right) \leftarrow not\ a_1\left(x_1, y_1, k_1, z_1\right) \\ a_1\left(\left[\dfrac{27-25}{30-25}, \dfrac{27-25}{30-25}\right], \left[\dfrac{10-10}{12-10}, \dfrac{12-10}{12-10}\right], \left[\dfrac{15-3}{25-3}, \dfrac{15-3}{25-3}\right], \left[\dfrac{0-0}{5-0}, \dfrac{5-0}{5-0}\right]\right) \equiv \\ \quad a_1\left([0.4, 0.4], [0, 1], [0.545, 0.545], [0, 1]\right) :: 0.5 \\ \quad \underbrace{[0,1][0,1][0,1][0,1]}_{\text{atribute's domains for } x_1, y_1, k_1, z_1} \\ \neg a_2\left(x_2, y_2, k_2, z_2\right) \leftarrow not\ a_2\left(x_2, y_2, k_2, z_2\right) \\ a_2\left(\left[\dfrac{33-20}{50-20}, \dfrac{42-20}{50-20}\right], \left[\dfrac{10-8}{10-8}, \dfrac{10-10}{10-8}\right], \left[\dfrac{10-6}{14-6}, \dfrac{12-6}{14-6}\right], \left[\dfrac{20-20}{50-20}, \dfrac{50-20}{50-20}\right]\right) \equiv \\ \quad a_2\left([0.433, 0.733], [1, 0], [0.5, 0.75], [0, 1]\right) :: 0.48 \\ \quad \underbrace{[0,1][0,1][0,1][0,1]}_{\text{atribute's domains for } x_2, y_2, k_2, z_2} \end{cases}$$

$$\vdots$$

The *Degree of Confidence (DoC)* is evaluated using the equation $DoC = \sqrt{1 - \Delta l^2}$, as it is illustrated in Figure 2. Here Δl stands for the length of the arguments' intervals, once normalized.

Below, one has the expected representation of the universe of discourse, where all the predicates' arguments are nominal. They speak for one´s confidence that the unknown values of the arguments fit into the correspondent intervals referred to above.

Figure 2. Degree of Confidence evaluation

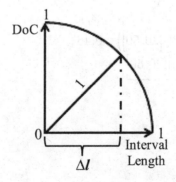

$$
\left[
\begin{array}{l}
\neg a_{1_{DoC}}\left(x_1, y_1, k_1, z_1\right) \leftarrow not\ a_{1_{DoC}}\left(x_1, y_1, k_1, z_1\right) \\
\qquad a_{1_{DoC}}\left(1, 0, 1, 0\right) :: 0.5 \\
\qquad \underbrace{\left[0.4, 0.4\right]\left[0, 1\right]\left[0.545, 0.545\right]\left[0, 1\right]}_{\text{atribute's domains for } x_1, y_1, k_1, z_1} \\
\qquad\qquad \underbrace{\left[0, 1\right]\left[0, 1\right]\left[0, 1\right]\left[0, 1\right]}_{\text{atribute's domains for } x_1, y_1, k_1, z_1} \\
\neg a_{2_{DoC}}\left(x_2, y_2, k_2, z_2\right) \leftarrow not\ a_{2_{DoC}}\left(x_2, y_2, k_2, z_2\right) \\
\qquad a_{2_{DoC}}\left(0.95, 0, 0.97, 0\right) :: 0.48 \\
\qquad \underbrace{\left[0.433, 0.733\right]\left[1, 0\right]\left[0.5, 0.75\right]\left[0, 1\right]}_{\text{atribute's domains for } x_2, y_2, k_2, z_2} \\
\qquad\qquad \underbrace{\left[0, 1\right]\left[0, 1\right]\left[0, 1\right]\left[0, 1\right]}_{\text{atribute's domains for } x_2, y_2, k_2, z_2} \\
\qquad\qquad\qquad \vdots
\end{array}
\right.
$$

3. A CASE STUDY

Therefore, and in order to exemplify the applicability of our model, we will look at the relational database model, since it provides a basic framework that fits into our expectations (Vicente et al., 2012), and is understood as the genesis of the LP approach to knowledge representation and reasoning.

Consider, for instance, and speaking hypothetically, where a relational database is given in terms of extends of the relations or predicates depicted in Figure 3, which stands for a situation where one has to interpret the various information and data about a Patient. Adding to this, there is the hypothesis of surfacing some incomplete data. For instance, in relation *Ambient Factors* the presence/absence of underlying problems for Case 1 is unknown, while in Case 2, it varies from 5 to 7. The Length of Stay Database (Figure 3) is populated according to the various results of the different columns:

- Biological Factors;
- Historical Factors;
- Hospital Factors;
- Ambient Factor.

These are all the necessary variables to estimate the importance/risk of a patient remaining in Hospital Care, as well as their boundaries.

It should be reminded and noted that every single value is classified from level 0 to 10. The higher the level goes the more important it is. As seen in the Figure 3 every set has the equivalent result. Nevertheless, we must remark and not forget that these values, present on Figure 3 are merely example to aid on the explanation of the algorithm. These will and can be later calibrated by the medical staff for their needs.

Through this we can deduct and describe the extension of the length predicate as:

$$length: Bio \text{ Factor, Hist. Factor, Hosp. Factor, Amb. Factor } \rightarrow \{0,1\}$$

where 0 (zero) and 1 (one) denote, respectively the aspect of *non need or need* of keeping them in health care. It is now possible to give the extension of the predicate length, in the form:

$$\{$$
$$\neg length\left(Bio, Hist, Hosp, Amb\right) \leftarrow not\ length(Bio, Hist, Hosp, Amb)$$

$$length(\ \underbrace{4,0,2,\perp}_{\substack{\text{attribute's values} \\ [0,10][0,10][0,10][0,10] \\ \text{attribute's domains}}}\ ) :: 1$$

$$length(\underbrace{[6,7],[7,8],\perp,[5,10]}_{\substack{\text{attribute's values} \\ [0,10][0,10][0,10][0,10] \\ \text{attribute's domains}}}) :: 1$$
$$\}$$

In this program, the first clause denotes the closure of predicate *length*. The next clauses correspond to the four terms taken from the extension of the *length* relation. For example, the second clause corresponds to a female patient "2": a age uncertain, somewhere between 40 to 50 years with problems in her vision – blind.

Analyzing Table Age with Comorbidity (both are filtered), we realize the values from 0-10 to her respective age can be between [6,7]. Assuming her age is between 40 and 50, it can belong to *level 6 [31,41] or level 5 [41,51] – interval should be [5,6].* Comorbidity of vision corresponds to level 8. So doing an average of the respective values to her biological factors will give us a variable between [6,7]. We keep doing these kinds of operations for all the aspects that aren't unknown. If they are unknown we just assume the level can go from 1 to 10. To eliminate any doubt, Case 1, refers to a patient that should no longer remain in Health Care, while Case 2 is the opposite and ought to remain held for further examination and care. For further enlightenment, it is essential to explain that – in the Table History Factor – *Admission, Symptom* and *Date* is relative to the severity of his past status. Date is the number of times he has been in the hospital. The latter – admission and symptom – is referent to his health condition and how it evolved during the admission and posterior time on the medical facility.

Moving on, the next step is to transform all values into continuous intervals and then normalize the predicate to obtain the *Degree of Confidence* of the length predicate.

$$\{$$
$$\neg length\big(Bio, Hist, Hosp, Amb\big) \leftarrow not\ length(Bio, Hist, Hosp, Amb)$$

$$length\big(\ \underbrace{[0.4,0.4],[0,0],[0.2,0.2],[0,1]}_{\substack{\text{attribute's values ranges once normalized} \\ [0,1][0,1][0,1][0,1] \\ \text{attribute's domains}}}\ \big) :: 1$$

$$length\big(\ \underbrace{[0.6,0.7],[0.7,0.8],[0.1,0.1],[0.5,1]}_{\substack{\text{attribute's values ranges once normalized} \\ [0,1][0,1][0,1][0,1] \\ \text{attribute's domains}}}\ \big) :: 1$$

$$\}$$

The logic program referred to above, is now presented in the form:

{

$$\neg length(Bio, Hist, Hosp, Amb) \leftarrow not\ length(Bio, Hist, Hosp, Amb)$$

$$length_{DoC}\left(\underbrace{1,1,1,0}_{\text{attribute's confidence values}} \right) :: 1$$

$$\underbrace{[0.4, 0.4], [0,0], [0.2, 0.2], [0,1]}_{\text{attribute's values ranges}}$$

$$\underbrace{[0,1][0,1][0,1][0,1]}_{\text{attribute's domains}}$$

$$length_{DoC}\left(\underbrace{0.99, 0.99, 1, 0}_{\text{attribute's confidence values}} \right) :: 1$$

$$\underbrace{[0.6, 0.7], [0.7, 0.8], [0.1, 0.1], [0,1]}_{\text{attribute's values ranges}}$$

$$\underbrace{[0,1][0,1][0,1][0,1]}_{\text{attribute's domains}}$$

}

where its terms make the training and test sets of the Artificial Neural Network given in Figure 4.

4. ARTIFICIAL NEURAL NETWORKS

Neves et al. (2010, 2012, 2013) demonstrated how Artificial Neural Networks (ANNs) could be successfully used to model data and capture complex relation-ships between inputs and outputs. ANNs simulate the structure of the human brain being populated by multiple layers of neurons. As an example, let us consider the case where one may have a situation in which a prolonged stay is needed, which is given in the form:

{

$length\ attributes : (Bio, Hist, Hosp, Amb)$

Figure 4. A possible Artificial Neural Network Topology

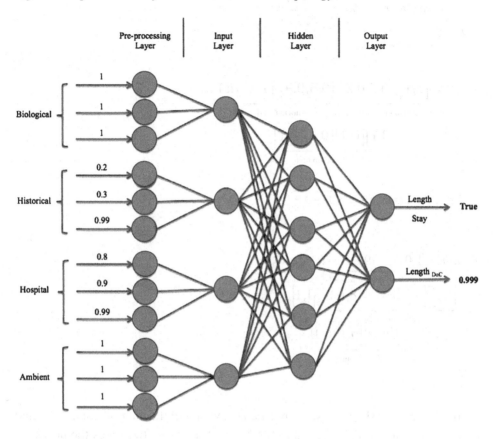

$$length \left(\underbrace{10,[2,3],[8,9],10}_{\text{attribute's values}} \right) :: 1$$

$$\underbrace{[0,10][0,10][0,10][0,10]}_{\text{attribute's domains}}$$

⬇ *1st interaction: transition to continuous intervals*

$$length \left(\underbrace{[10,10],[2,3],[8,9],[10,10]}_{\text{attribute's values ranges}} \right) :: 1$$

$$\underbrace{[0,10][0,10][0,10][0,10]}_{\text{attribute's domains}}$$

$\Downarrow$ *2nd interaction: normalization* $\dfrac{Y - Y_{min}}{Y_{max} - Y_{min}}$

$$length\left(\underbrace{[1,1],[0.2,0.3],[0.8,0.9],[1,1]}_{\text{attribute's values ranges once normalized}} \right) :: 1$$

$$\underbrace{[0,1][0,1][0,1][0,1]}_{\text{attribute's domains}}$$

$\Downarrow$ *DoC calculation:* $DoC = \sqrt{1 - \Delta l^2}$

$$length\left(\underbrace{1, 0.99, 0.99, 1}_{\text{attribute's confidence values}} \right) :: 1$$

$$\underbrace{[1,1],[0.2,0.3],[0.8,0.9],[1,1]}_{\text{attribute's values ranges}}$$

$$\underbrace{[0,1][0,1][0,1][0,1]}_{\text{attribute's domains}}$$

}

In Figure 4 it is shown how the normalized values of the interval boundaries and their *DoC* values work as inputs to the ANN. The output translates the necessity of increasing the length of stay on a Hospital of a patient, and *DoC* the confidence that one has on such a happening.

5. CONCLUSION AND FUTURE WORK

To understand if the increase of the length of hospital stay is mandatory for the well being of the patient is a hard and complex task, which needs to consider many different conditions with intricate relations among them. These characteristics put this problem into the area of problems that may be tackled by AI based methodologies and techniques to problem solving. Despite that, little to no work has been done in that direction. This work presents the founding of a computational framework that uses powerful knowledge representation and reasoning techniques to set the structure of the information and the associate inference mechanisms. This representation is above everything else, very versatile and capable of covering every possible instance by considering incomplete, contradictory, and even unknown data. The main contribution of this work is to be understood in terms of the evaluation of the *DoC*, and the possibility to address the issue of incomplete information. Indeed, the new paradigm of knowledge representation and reasoning enables the use of the normalized values of the interval boundaries and their *DoC* values, as inputs to the ANN. The output translates the necessity of keeping a patient in a hospital order to improve their health and the degree of confidence that one has on such a happening. Future work may recommend that the same problem must be approached using other computational frameworks like Case Based Reasoning or Particle Swarm, just to name a few.

REFERENCES

Caldeira, A. T., Martins, M. R., Cabrita, M. J., Ambrósio, C., Arteiro, J., Neves, J., & Vicente, H. (2010). *Aroma Compounds Prevision using Artificial Neural Networks Influence of Newly Indigenous Saccharomyces SPP in White Wine Produced with Vitis Vinifera Cv Siria.*

Ferreira Maia Neves, J. C. (1984, January). A logic interpreter to handle time and negation in logic databases. *Proceedings of the 1984 annual conference of the ACM on The fifth generation challenge* (pp. 50-54). ACM. doi:10.1145/800171.809603

Fry, J. (1993). *General practice: the facts.* Radcliffe Medical Press.

Gelfond, M., & Lifschitz, V. (1988, August). *The stable model semantics for logic programming* (Vol. 88, pp. 1070–1080). ICLP/SLP.

Halpern, J. Y. (2003). *Reasoning about uncertainty* (Vol. 21). Cambridge: MIT press.

Kakas, A. C., Kowalski, R. A., & Toni, F. (1998). The role of abduction in logic programming. Handbook of logic in artificial intelligence and logic programming, 5, 235-324.

Kovalerchuk, B., & Resconi, G. (2010, July). Agent-based uncertainty logic network. *Proceedings of the 2010 IEEE International Conference on Fuzzy Systems (FUZZ)* (pp. 1-8). IEEE. doi:10.1109/FUZZY.2010.5584836

Liu, Y., & Sun, M. (2007, November). Fuzzy optimization BP neural network model for pavement performance assessment. *Proceedings of the IEEE International Conference on Grey Systems and Intelligent Services GSIS '07* (pp. 1031-1034). IEEE.

Lucas, P. (2004). *Quality checking of medical guidelines through logical abduction* (pp. 309–321). Springer London. doi:10.1007/978-0-85729-412-8_23

Machado, J., Abelha, A., Novais, P., Neves, J., & Neves, J. (2010). Quality of service in healthcare units. *International Journal of Computer Aided Engineering and Technology*, 2(4), 436–449. doi:10.1504/IJCAET.2010.035396

Neves, J., Machado, J., Analide, C., Abelha, A., & Brito, L. (2007). The halt condition in genetic programming. In *Progress in Artificial Intelligence* (pp. 160–169). Springer Berlin Heidelberg. doi:10.1007/978-3-540-77002-2_14

Pereira, L. M. (2009). Evolution prospection. In *New Advances in Intelligent Decision Technologies* (pp. 51–63). Springer Berlin Heidelberg. doi:10.1007/978-3-642-00909-9_6

Pritchard, P. M. (1981). *Manual of primary health care: its nature and organization*. Oxford University Press.

Vicente, H., Dias, S., Fernandes, A., Abelha, A., Machado, J., & Neves, J. (2012). Prediction of the quality of public water supply using artificial neural networks. *Journal of Water Supply: Research & Technology - Aqua*, 61(7), 446–459. doi:10.2166/aqua.2012.014

Vicente, H., Roseiro, J. C., Arteiro, J. M., Neves, J., & Caldeira, A. T. (2013). Prediction of bioactive compound activity against wood contaminant fungi using artificial neural networks. *Canadian Journal of Forest Research*, 43(11), 985–992. doi:10.1139/cjfr-2013-0142

World Health Organization, & Unicef. (1978). Primary health care: a joint report.

Chapter 9
An Approach for the Semantic Interoperability of SNOMED:
Improving Quality of Health Records

Magda Amorim
Universidade do Minho, Portugal

Filipe Miranda
Universidade do Minho, Portugal

ABSTRACT

The semantic and syntactic interoperability introduces the capability of two machines to communicate and understand each other improving then the quality of Electronic Health Records. In this work, is presented an independent application of the medical record, using a web service (with protocol TCP/IP) capable of provide human interaction with interfaces in different devices (web, android app., browser). SNOMED CT is a comprehensive and scientifically validated health care terminology resulting in an organized computer processable collection of medical terms. This can be mapped into other systems of codes like ICD also used in our application. A data base (SNOMED codes and relations) was created capable of answer to all sort of queries from the users using the browser or the mobile application. The first hospital unit to enjoy this system was the pathological anatomy unit of the CHAA hospital. Here after receiving a "piece" and a task, the responsible performs all kind of procedures with the purpose of performing a report (diagnosis for example). With

DOI: 10.4018/978-1-4666-9882-6.ch009

the implementation of SNOMED CT, to produce reports a physician could search for the name of the "piece" or the code and immediately upload in that patient HER the diagnosis. The usage of this codes leads to report uniformed that could be read and understood around the world. Another important feature of the application is the incorporation within the AIDA, AIDA-PCE and AIDA-BI. Experiments with real user show a successful software implementation judging by the utilization rate and medical personal acceptance. The mobile application should suffer an upgrade allowing the patient usage for example.

INTRODUCTION

Health information Systems (HIS) refer to any system that captures, stores and manages or transmits information related to the health of individuals or the activities of organizations within the health sector. Since the 60's this systems suffered an intense transformation alongside the technological evolution. According with the World Health Organization (WHO) (World Health Organization, 2008):

The health information systems provides the underpinnings for decision-making and has four key functions: data generation, compilation, analysis and synthesis, and communication and use. The health information systems collects data from the health sector and other relevant sectors, analyses the data and ensures their overall quality relevance and timeliness, and converts data into information for health-related decision-making.

While some people think the purpose of this systems is only for monitoring and evaluate, the reality is much different. It's true they are essential in booth that fields but also they server broader ends, providing alerts for capability, supporting patient and healthcare facility management, enabling planning, supporting global reporting and underpinning communication of health challenges to diverse users (World Health Organization, 2008).

A strong HIS is the backbone of a strong health system getting the right information into the right hands at the right time, enabling policymakers, managers, and individual service providers to make informed choices about everything from patient care to national budgets (Duarte, et al., 2010). They represent a hospital subsystem of socio-technological development that covers information processing, resources, flows and people (Duarte, et al., 2010; The International Health Terminology Standards Development Organisation, 2012))

The Electronic Health Record (EHR) is a digital version of patient´s clinical sheet working like a real time centered record making information available almost instantly to authorized users (The International Health Terminology Standards Development Organisation, 2012).

An electronic health record systems goes beyond the standard medical history and patient history. This systems can contain patient's medical history, diagnoses, medications, treatments plans. Allows the access to evidence-based tools that can be used to infer decisions about patient's care (The International Health Terminology Standards Development Organisation, 2012). Perhaps the key feature of an EHR is possibility of share health information in a digital format across more than one health organization.

The use of techniques that allow expanding the structured and uniformed data throughout the EHR has been increasing, resorting in mechanisms that seek to facilitate the data collection and analysis (Chute, Cohn, & Campbell, 1998). The user of standard terms and concepts in medical records is one of most important tools in this field. This data standardization involves the underlying terminologies like classifications and nomenclatures.

Furthermore, the standardization of health records ensures a better communication between health professionals and the interoperability between systems, allowing the automation of the hospital records. The standards are divided in clinical information representation standards, communication standards and image standards. Its use ensures that the EHR is understood by any health professional anywhere, also allowing the machines to interpret symptoms and assist physicians in diagnosis and treatment (Duarte, et al., 2010; Duarte, Portela, Abelha, Machado, & Santos, 2011).

The major challenge in eHealth is the semantic interoperability of electronic health records (EHR) systems (European Community, 2009; Matinez-Costa, Menárguez-Tortosa, & Fernández-Breis, 2011).

This paper introduces a project which aims to implement SNOMED CT in a real context and expose the benefits of that introduction. Providing semantic interoperability between EHR systems, using an independent application from the platform of medical record using web services technologies to achieve that integration. Firstly introduced in Anatomical Pathological unit in a Portuguese major hospital allows the physician to code or decode is findings during the medical procedure.

More than advertise the process of implementation or the languages and tools used for the development of the application the present work aims to explain the impact generated by the use of this software. The concept of standardization of the records and the use of international codes for diagnosis and procedures is a huge improvement in this field.

SEMANTIC INTEROPERABILITY

Semantic interoperability is the ability of computer systems to exchange data and interpret that shared data (HIMSS, n. d.). This foundation enables machine computable logic, inference, and knowledge discovery and data federation between information systems (HIMSS, n. d.). This is central concept in the sharing of clinical information. When the subject A produces a medical report, the subject B (who requested de procedure) needs to understand the meaning of the result. The best way to accomplish data is using international codes and available libraries.

Interoperability is defined by the Healthcare Information and Management Systems Society (HIMSS) as an extent to which systems and devices can exchange and interpret the shared data. Two systems become interoperable, if they are able to exchange data and subsequently present it in a way that can be understood by a user (HIMSS, n. d.).

The definitions produced above are essentially the semantic interoperability (systems capable of exchange data) using languages like SQL or XML. On other hand the semantic interoperability refers the ability of automatically interpret information exchanged meaningfully and accurately (Walker, et al., 2005).

Looking now for the ability of different HIS to work together, the technical/ semantically interoperability essentially refers to the integration between applications, pretended when defining the architecture for Electronic Health Record (EHR). The Service Oriented Architecture (SOA) is the latest development in the integration of applications. This architecture enables the definition and creation of transversal processes supported by applications of different types (Walker, et al., 2005).

The critical issue for the health information exchange and interoperability is the adoption of electronic communication platform that allows the integrated parts to transmit receive and store data (Walker, et al., 2005; Eichelberg, Aden, Riesmeier, Dogac, & Laleci, 2005; Medicity, n. d.).

The automatic transference of patent's information between locations reduces the delivery time and reduces the number of tests and procedures. The automatic detection of warnings reduces the occurrence of medical errors (Medicity, n. d.; Stroetmann, et al., 2009).

The ability of health organizations, in different responsibility levels, to communicate and operate is called EHR interoperability. For this is essential the information share and communication between EHRs themselves, or with different HIS (Santos, 2008; Commission recommendation of 2 July 2008 on cross-border interoperability of electronic health record systems, 2008).

The web applications are essential to accomplish the exchange of information and to access that information. The implemented software presents a search tool for

SNOMED CT codes and a way to classify the diagnostic correctly. At the end is to move forward from a free text situation into one where all is coded and understood all around the world.

The next section aims to explain the material involved in all process. So the SNOMED CT database is explained in detail, as well as the AIDA and AIDA-PCE that will integrate and provide the information across different platforms (web and mobile application).

SNOMED CT

The only way two systems to communicate and understand each other is to speak a common language. The Systematized Nomenclature of Medicine Clinical Terms simply or SNOMED, is a comprehensive and scientifically-validated healthcare terminology resulting in an organized computer processable collection of medical terms. The primary purpose is the encoding of meanings used in health information to support the effective clinical recording of data with the intent to improve patient care (International Health Terminology Standards Development Organization, 2014).

SNOMED results from the joint venture between the National Health Service (NHS) in England and the College of American Pathologists (CAP). Formed in 1999 by the convergence of SNOMED RT and the United Kingdom's Clinical Terms Version 3 (formerly known as the Read Codes). In 2007, the SNOMED CT intellectual property rights were transferred from the CAP to the SNOMED SDO® in the formal creation of the IHTSDO (The International Health Terminology Standards Development Organization, 2014; Spackman, Campbell, Côte, & D., 1997).

The comprehensive coverage of this collection includes clinical findings, symptoms, anatomical locations, diagnosis, procedures and even specific medical tools. Its use provides interoperable encoded data that enhance the implementation of evidence-based practice, facilitates decision support rules and contributes to improve the quality of care provided to patients (Martney, et al., 2012; Schulz, Suntisrivaraporn, Baader, & Boeker, 2009).

Another important feature is the possibility to cross-map to other international standards and classifications improving the quality of the HER and patients care. The next section addresses the SNOMED CT structure.

Snomed Structure

The core components types in SNOMED CT are concepts, descriptions and re-lationships. The last version includes more than 311,000 active concepts and the associated descriptions surpass the one million with unique meanings (International Health Terminology Standards Development Organization, 2014).

The logical model specifies a structured representation of the concepts (used to represent clinical meanings), the descriptions used to refer to these, and the relationships between the concepts. The figure 1 illustrates the stated above.

A concept is clinical meaning, referenced with a unique, numeric and machine-readable identifier, unambiguous with no human interpretable meaning.

A set of descriptions (human readable form) is linked to each concept composed by a Fully Specified Name (FSN) and a Synonym. The first one is a unique and unambiguous description of the concept meaning. It's important to retain that the FSN is no intended to appear in medical records, only used to disambiguate the distinct meaning of each different concept. The second one represent a term that can be used to display or select a concept. Several synonyms could be related to one concept allowing the user to select the best one for that situation (preferred term) (The International Health Terminology Standards Development Organisation, 2012).

The relationships represent an association between two concepts. These are used to define the meaning of a concept so it can be processed by a computer. The connection between two concepts is made by a third one called attribute (International Health Terminology Standards Development Organization, 2014). Almost all SNOMED CT concepts are the source of at least one "is a" relationship, except the root concept which is the most general concept. The use of this relation can be seen in the figure 1. Other examples are the "finding site", which shows the disease

Figure 1. Logical model of SNOMED CT

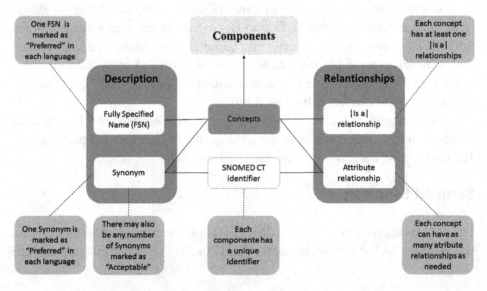

localization (topography); and "morphology", which describes the morphology that characterizes a particular disease. Following the links created by relationships we can have a hierarchy, or a textual representation, which defines the concept as is required by the service that uses this nomenclature (Eichelberg, Aden, Riesmeier, Dogac, & Laleci, 2005).

SNOMED CT includes over 50 attributes capable of define some of the existing categories in the conceptual mode. After specifying the top level concepts is possible to arrange a considerable number of other concepts in a subtype hierarchy.

Some examples of this top level concepts are "clinical finding," "procedure," "situation with explicit content," "organism," "pharmaceutical," "physical object," "organism," etc.

The domain is the hierarchy to which a specific attribute can be applied, for example:

- The domain attribute |associated morphology| is the |clinical finding| hierarchy. Therefore, a |procedure| cannot have a |associated morphology|. However, a |procedure| can have a |procedure morphology|

The set of SNOMED CT concepts that are allowed as the value of a specified attribute is named the "range" of the attribute. The combination of these attributes to the hierarchies causes a clinical data retrieval more useful and relevant (Lee, Cornet, Lau, & Keizer, 2012).

Beyond this, the SNOMED structure allows consistent retrieval of clinical information for a wide range of purposes, including decision support, audit, epidemiology, research, service management, billing and statutory reporting.

At the end SNOMED is a basis in which healthcare organizations can develop effective data analysis for support of decision and project the best treatment available. SNOMED and other code systems can be the central piece to fully enjoy the benefits of HER, improving communication and increasing the availability of relevant information.

Mapping SNOMED to ICD

The International Classification of Diseases (ICD) is the standard diagnostic tool for epidemiology, health management and clinical purposes. This includes the analysis of the general population health situation monitoring incidence and prevalence of diseases and other health problems (Health, 2014). In addition enables the storage and retrieval of diagnostic information for clinical, epidemiological and quality purposes.

Clinical information gathered with SNOMED CT may include data that is relevant to reports, statistical purposes, etc. that need to be encoded using a specific code system or statistical classification such as ICD-10. Mapping allows relevant information to be used for those purposes, minimizing the additional manual data entry.

Maps are associations between particular codes, concepts or terms in a system A and the similar codes, concepts or terms in the code system B. When a set of maps is defined the process is called mapping. The maps are developed with a specific purpose, so there may be different maps between the same pair of code systems in accordance with different purposes.

The main propose of the SNOMED CT to ICD-10 map ("The map") is to support semi-automated generation of ICD10-CM codes from clinical data encoded in SNOMED-CT for reimbursement and statistical purposes (Health, 2014).

The "Map" may be used in two distinct scenarios. Firstly, a real-time use by the healthcare provider, the map embedded in the problem list application of the EHR. The problem list is updated with the SNOMED code and then occurs the mapping into ICD-10 codes (The International Health Terminology Standards Development Organization, n. d.).

On the second way, the Map is used within an application suggesting a candidate ICD-10-CM codes to professionals based on stored SNOMED CT encoded problem list. Textual advice may be present to facilitate the process .The map will be periodically update to increase SNOMED CT coverage (U.S. National Library of Medicine, n. d.).

IHTSDO has a formal working arrangement with the WHO to develop and assure maps with rule-based approach and linkages between SNOMED and WHO Classifications, more precisely the ICD-10. The first maps were released in 2013, but the goal is to complete the international maps to ICD-10 in 2014

AIDA

Agency for Integration, Diffusion and Archive of Medical Information (AIDA) is a platform that consists in a Multi-Agent System (MAS) that tries to overcome the difficulty of reunite all clinical systems, as well as support the medical and administrative complexity of different Hospital information sources (Duarte, et al., 2010). AIDA was created by a group of researchers from Minho University (Artificial Intelligence Group), and is currently installed at some major Portuguese hospitals. It is an electronic platform that provides employees with intelligence featuring a pro-active behavior in its main functions: communication between heterogeneous systems, storage management and hospital information; response to requests in time;

sending and receiving information from hospital sources like laboratories, medical reports, images, prescriptions, and others. AIDA has an easy access for her users, allowing the management of clinical information anywhere in the hospital. The platform enables the sending of messages via phone or e-mail. At the same time, establishes connection with all Systems of medical information: EHR; Administrative Information System (AIS); Medical Information System (MIS); and Nursing Information System (NIS) (Duarte, Portela, Abelha, Machado, & Santos, 2011). Figure 2 shows the central role of AIDA.

AIDAS's covers all task needed to execute a medical examination and ate the same time agents ensure that information is shared with other hospital subsystems. Therefore, clinical professionals can also access all information through their specifics systems of record. The information will still be available in other platforms like MIS, NIS or AIS (Duarte, et al., 2013) but the importance of AIDA is reunite and provide patient health record at one place.

AIDA-PCE

The AIDA-PCE is an EHR implemented in the "Centro Hospitalar do Porto" developed by the same creators of AIDA platform. The AIDA-PCE follows a problem-oriented organization suggested by Lawrence Weed in the 60's. In this type of organization, clinical information (annotations, therapeutic, diagnostic) should be recorded in a

Figure 2. The central role of AIDA [6]

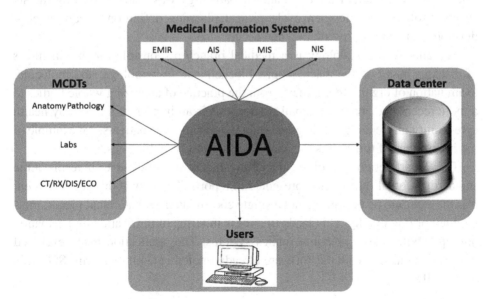

tree structure creating an organized list of issues. In this cadre each problem derives from the main branch (Pereira, et al., 2012) and is classified as active or inactive. This first type are those where the disease is still active or even when intervention is required immediately. On the other hand, inactive problems require no urgent action. These EHR problems assets are monitored and recorded daily using a SOAP (Subjective, Objective, Assessment and Planning) framework. Thus, each record contains the patient's symptoms, a doctor's observation, an analysis of diagnosis and a treatment plan that the patient is subject to (Duarte, et al., 2010; Pereira, et al., 2012).

In order to implement AIDA-PCE a set of requirements must be considered in order to benefitting the staff job and patient health. This systems has many features in common with PCP, overcoming this in response time, speed and security.

The structure of this EHR allows seamless integration with existing HIS by promoting the ubiquity of records between different specialties and services. It's possible to generate documents and customized reports for specific purposes with information standardized and uniform (Duarte, et al., 2010; Pereira, et al., 2012).

This section explained the methods and the systems used to implement this application. The next section explains where the application was implemented and how was implemented.

IMPLEMENTATION

The application implemented at anatomy pathology was made respecting the six stages of software development cycle: project, planning, definition of requirements, development and test, installation and acceptance.

The anatomical pathology is a medical branch responsible for the diagnosis of diseases based on the macroscopic, biochemical, immunologic and molecular examination of organs and tissues. From the practice of analyzing whole bodies to a more recent one analyzing small tissues, this is an important unit of any health care facility influencing the diagnosis and treatment of the patients. An example of the importance of this unit is the analysis of tissues from biopsies.

The Department of pathological anatomy had some deficiencies in terms of the standardization of information presented in reports. The only codification existent was the exams to be performed not a single code related to anatomical pieces, morphology or topography. This leads to a mess in terms of unification and semantic interoperability with other informatics systems. The application here developed will work alongside with the software already implemented in that unit (SONHO, SAM, AIDA).

Following the steps for development of this type of works, the software should accomplish some basic objectives and requirements. This one's define the main functions of our application, and are specified in Table 1.

All the above functions require SNOMED CT information stored in a way that can be easily accessed and updated. To support the search and retrieval of information the best tool is a creation of a solid data base. This is implemented beneath all web applications. The SNOMED CT data base uses the SQL language for queries purposes, must be able to handle a lot of information and constant updates. Following a relational model (tables and relations) it's an ideal fit for SNOMED CT structure (concepts, hierarchies, relations between concepts). The notation of primary key and foreign key relates all tables and a time stamp indicates if some concept is still used or not.

The SOA technology allows the integration of applications from different sources and languages using the principle of request/reply for communicating between client and server.

The Web service, accessible throw internet connection, has a central role on the platform architecture for the semantic interoperability, making the service available across multiple web applications. This is exemplified in figure 3 where all the request made throw URL are understood and answered in XML format by the server after SQL queries in the SNOMED CT database.

The web page (browser) and android application are the interface for the clients in our service where various pages are accessed as results of the implementation of Web Services. Their main goal is analyze the impact, resulting when semantic interoperability is introduced in reports at the unit. A user friendly design and simplicity are extremely important for a general acceptance.

The SNOMED BROWSER was created using ASP.NET and AJAX ensuring the practicality and fluidity of the page. His basic functions are the classification

Table 1. Application requirements

Objective	Requirements
Classification of anatomical concepts	Searching in SNOMED database for the anatomical concepts included in (topography, morphology, etiology) and classify the severity associated with morphology, when applicable;
Concepts research	Providing possibility to obtain information about any SNOMED concept;
Diagnosis supporting	Using the relationships between SNOMED concepts to obtain a diagnostic suggestion according to topography and morphology previously introduced.

Figure 3. Model of application built

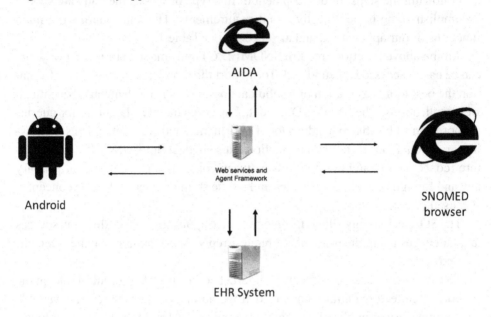

of medical terms and diagnosis, suggested according to location, etiology and morphology of the sample following the standards of CHAA. Following the SNOMED CT structure is possible to insert more information about sample location namely with relationships above stated "part of" and "laterally".

The mobile application developed with Android Development Tools enables the search of information from the SNOMED CT database for medical terms and defined codes, as well the location, morphology, etc. The design is as simple as possible allowing persons without formation use it.

In the end the basic functionalities of the service implemented are:

- Search for SNOMED CT concepts;
- Classify anatomical terms, diagnosis including location and sample morphology;
- Access to clinical history in chronological order;
- Support the diagnosis of Anatomical Pathological procedures;

This section explained the basic features of application and served to explain the complexity of all process as well as the advantages in implement this kind of software.

Interface Interaction

The classification of a diagnosis or medical term is suggested according with location, etiology and morphology of the sample. Using this search options the medical error is reduced and is possible to analyze in real time the possible connection of a morphology with some diagnosis. The inverse is also possible, some SNOMED CT code is presented and the software presents a list of possible locations and morphologies.

The classification process begins with the introduction of sample site. The physician selects by anatomical location or by SNOMED code. More information can be added through relationships "part of" and "laterality" with the local previously chosen. The second step of this process should indicate the morphology detected in the sample, such as the location. Also here there is a support to the user after the introduction of the name or the respective code. At the end of the process it is returned a list of all concepts that, by following relationships concerning the topography and morphology, represents a disease that encompasses the information initially introduced. Besides the usual process classification process, it is also possible to check which are the diseases associated only with a particular location or morphology. The reverse is also possible, so indicating the names or SNOMED codes of disease it's possible to check the locations and morphologies. The mobile application is much simple and interactive only with the search function.

In sum the software responses the numeric SNOMED CT or possible connection for that code simplifying the live of health care professionals and avoiding potential mistakes in the diagnosis of a sample.

The Semantic Web Agent's Implementation

The agents are another approach to integrate SNOMED CT in health care facilities. Although, there is no common accepted definition for the term Agent, it's possible to define as a computer system able of two basics capabilities: the first one related to autonomous action and the capability of deciding for themselves what they need to do in order to satisfy their design objectives. The second one related with the interaction between agents exchanging data and engaging in social activities such as coordination, cooperation and negotiation (Semantic Web, n. d.).

In sum the Semantic Web Agent activities can be describe as (Kumar, 2012):

- Receiving tasks and preferences from the service requester;
- Seeking information from the Web sources;
- Communicating with other agents;
- Comparing information about user requirements and preferences;

- Giving answer to the service requester or user;
  The technologies used by Semantic Web Agent are (Kumar, 2012):
- Ontologies used to assist in Web searches, using metadata for identifying and extracting information from Web sources. That way, agents can also interpret retrieved information and communicate with other agents;
- Agent specific communication language used for communicating with other agents;
- One of the most important activities of agents are the Negotiation, this process in which a group of agents reach to a mutually acceptable agreement on some matter;
  A multiple agent systems (MAS) it's a group of intelligent agents interacting with each other, having specific tasks.

This systems present an enormous potential to assure the interoperability on the SIS mainly by compacting the whole system.

The use of this technology in the application, allows the automation of the integration processes of search results of SNOMED concepts made by users. They may be integrated into clinical administrative platforms such as SAM /SAPE and SONHO, used by the National System of health (NHS) to EHR. However, these systems are used only ICD codes, the mapping is crucial to ICD10 already addressed (Araújo, Faria, & Cruz, 2007).

The application was installed and after that tested by the service director verifying if fulfilled the initial requisites.

RESULTS AND DISCUSSION

The application was successfully implemented at the CHAA with direct connections to AIDA and AIDA-PCE. This step is important once the diagnosis is ready the result is automatically upload to the PCE allowing other units to access that information. This is a huge improvement in the interoperability and the diffusion of information across different platforms.

This numeric code resulting from the medical query into our application is introduced in the patient health record alongside the normal report in free text. The doctor responsible for that patient with access to AIDA has direct to this information this and could initiate immediately the treatment. While the access to the report was possible with AIDA-PCE the existence of a code specific for that patient medical condition is knew. Automatic alert systems could be created. The AIDA could analyze the code and in case of cancer alert the patient with mail or SMS. This is the best feature of our work.

After 3 months of use and based on inquiries made directly into database the results were positive. The following table shows the number of reports published with the SNOMED classification and the total of Reports published by each doctor of pathological anatomy. The percentage of utilization is very high which shows the good acceptance of this application by clinical professionals.

The implementation of AIDA allowed the automatisms for some important tasks. For example, after its installation, the AIDA platform now sends an email to the oncology service for each published report with one specific SNOMED code. This new AIDA feature is very important because it accelerates the process of patient treatment in case of some identified diagnoses, which can be vital for patient health. Other example of these automatisms is the importing of diagnosis for the alerts of medical record. A patient that has an examination result on pathological anatomy with report of the SNOMED, his results will be available on the medical record platform and all of the physician can have access to that report and their all diagnoses. Furthermore, after this implementation, physicians began making statistics by diagnosis more effectively.

More results were obtained through interviews with staff of the Department of pathological anatomy. They all agree that this application has improved the quality of information, benefiting the service provided to the patient. For the administrative staff this implementation made the workflow easier whereas for the physician the most important improvements were to help prevent errors; to speed up the bureaucracy processing of the patient treatment; to avoid lost diagnoses and allow for statistics by diagnosis.

An important facet of this work is the possibility of integrate this system within the AIDA-BI a platform developed by the same group as AIDA. With the information gathered it's possible to develop a data warehouse and reunite some indicator with business inelegance tools.

The mobile application can be improved in feature work mainly the integration of new features and access to more information anywhere at any time.

Table 2. Number of published reports

	Column A (*t*)	**Column B** (*t*)	**Column B** (*t*)
Total reports	1301	1671	519
Reports with SNOMED	1300	1667	517
Percentage	99,9%	99,8%	99,6%

CONCLUSION

The importance of the EHR is unquestionable allowing the centering and standardization of all clinical information. The problem with this centralization is the duplication of information or some technical problem that prevents the access to information. Apart from that reunite all the SIS under the same roof is lengthy process and the best way to accomplish that is throw the interoperability.

The SNOMED CT is organized in concepts, descriptions and relations becoming the best tool for the RCE respecting reports and diagnosis.

Various approaches for implementing and facilitate the interaction between machine and user are already implemented in several health units. Recent advances in technologies and a growing field of mobile applications makes the information available almost anywhere.

During this project was implemented and installed a system for classifying medical examination results in a real hospital environment. Although extreme importance for the hole process the implementation step was left aside. Only with a simple explanation of the tolls and the resources available in each situation. More important than implementation is the concept of gather same application patient basic information, all the patient medical history and in case of that patient medical reports. The main goal of the application is the classification of pathological anatomy reports made through AIDA. The page has the function to classify certain diagnosis suggested according to the location and morphology of the sample.

This reports written in a way that can be read anywhere and understood. The usage of international codes like SNOMED and ICD is the key point of this work. Alongside this codification the AIDA platform is extremely important allowing the integration of this information with the electronic health record.

The business intelligence introduction (AIDA-BI) is a tremendous step forward is handling and measurement of clinical information. The introduction of BI platforms helps specialists and the management staff to understand in numbers or charts the different problems in hands.

The system usability and acceptance will continue throughout meetings and questionnaires and intermediate reports will be under construction.

REFERENCES

Araújo, S., Faria, J., & Cruz, J. (2007). *Propostas de Melhoria da Segurança dos Sistemas de Informação Clínica em Portugal*. Portugal: Faculdade da Universidade do Porto.

Chute, C. G., Cohn, S. P., & Campbell, J. R. (1998). A framework for comprehensive health terminology systems in the United States: Development guidelines, criteria for selection, and policy implications. *Journal of the American Medical Informatics Association*, 5(6), 503–510. doi:10.1136/jamia.1998.0050503 PMID:9824798

Commission recommendation of 2 July 2008 on cross-border interoperability of electronic health record systems. (2008). Off. J. Eur. Union.

Duarte, J., Pontes, G., Salazar, M., Santos, M., Abelha, A., & Machado, J. (2013). Stand-alone electronic health record. *Proceedings of the 2013 IEEE International Conference on Industrial Engineering and Engineering Management IEEEM2013*, Bangkok, Thailand.

Duarte, J., Portela, C. F., Abelha, A., Machado, J., & Santos, M. F. (2011). Electronic health record in dermatology service. M. M. Cruz-Cunha, J. Varajão, P. Powell, & R. Martinho, (Eds.), Communications in Computer and Information Science, 221 (pp. 156-164).

Duarte, J., Salazar, M., Quintas, C., Neves, J., Santos, M., Neves, J., . . . Machado, J. (2010). Data quality evaluation of electronic health records in the hospital admission process. *Proceedings of the 2010 IEEE/ACIS 9th International Conference on Computer and Information Science ICIS* (pp. 201-206).

Eichelberg, M., Aden, T., Riesmeier, J., Dogac, A., & Laleci, G. B. (2005, December). A survey and analysis of electronic healthcare record standards. *ACM Computing Surveys*, 37(4), 277–315. doi:10.1145/1118890.1118891

European Community. (2009). Semantic interoperability for better health and safer healthcare. *Deployment and research roadmap for Europe*.

World Health Organization. (2014). *International Classifications of Diseases*.

HIMSS. (n. d.). *Transforming healthcare through IT*. Retrieved from http://www.himss.org/library/interoperability-standards/what-is

International Health Terminology Standards Development Organization. (2014). *International Health Terminology Standards Development Organization*. Retrieved from http://www.ihtsdo.org/snomed-ct/snomed-ct0/

Kumar, S. (2012). *Semantic Web Agents-Based Semantic Web Service Composition*. doi:10.1007/978-1-4614-4663-7

Lee, D., Cornet, R., Lau, F., & Keizer, N. (2012). A survey of SNOMED CT implementations. *Journal of Biomedical Informatics, 46(1), 87-96.* PMID:23041717

Martney, S. A., Warren, J. J., Evans, J. L., Kim, T. Y., Coenen, A., & Auld, V. A. (2012, August). Development of the nursing problem list subset of SNOMED. *Journal of Biomedical Informatics*, *45*(4), 683–688. doi:10.1016/j.jbi.2011.12.003 PMID:22202620

Matinez-Costa, C., Menárguez-Tortosa, M., & Fernández-Breis, J. (2011). Clinical data interoperability based on archetype transformation. *Journal of Biomedical Informatics*, *44*(5), 869–880. doi:10.1016/j.jbi.2011.05.006 PMID:21645637

Medicity. (n. d.). *Medicity: Semantic Interoperability in HIE's*. Retrieved from www.medicity.com

Pereira, R., Duarte, J., Salazar, M., Santos, M., Abelha, A., & Machado, J. (2012). Usability of an electronic health record. *Proceedings of the 4th IEEE International Conference on Industrial Engineering and Engineering Management*. Hong Kong.

Santos, P. (2008, October). *Content Addressable Multimedia Database Server for Medicine: Registro Eletrónico de Saúde "PANORAMIX"* [Content Addressable Multimedia Database Server for Medicine: Registro Eletrónico de Saúde "PANORAMIX"] [Master's Thesis]. Instituto Superior Técnico.

Schulz, S., Suntisrivaraporn, B., Baader, F., & Boeker, M. (2009). SNOMED reaching its adolescence: Ontologists and logicians health check. *International Journal of Medical Informatics*, *78*(Suppl. 1), S86–S94.

Semantic Web. (n. d.). *Semantic Web*. Retrieved from http://semanticweb.org/wiki/Main_Page

Spackman, K. A., Campbell, K. E., & Côte, R. A. (1997). SNOMED RT: A reference terminology for health care. Proceedings of the AMIA annual Fall symposium (pp. 640–644). PMID:9357704

Stroetmann, N., Kalra, D., Lewalle, P., Rector, A., Rodrigues, M., & Stroetmann, A. (2009). *Semantic Interoperability for better health and safer healthcare*. Deployment and Research for Europe.

The International Health Terminology Standards Development Organisation. (2012, July 31). *The International Health Terminology Standards Development Organisation: SNOMED CT Technical Implementation Guide*. Retrieved from http://ihtsdo.org/fileadmin/userupload/doc/download/docTechnicalImplementationGuideCurrent-en-USINT20120731.pdf

The International Health Terminology Standards Development Organization. (2014, July). SNOMED Clinical Terms User Guide.

The International Health Terminology Standards Development Organization. (n. d.). *SNOMED-CT-Supporting Meaningful User.*

U.S. National Library of Medicine. (n. d.). *NIH.* Retrieved from http://www.nlm. nih.gov/research/umls/mapping projects/snomedcttoicd10cm.html

Walker, J., Pan, E., Johnston, D., Adler-Milstein, J., Bates, D. W., & Middleton, B. (2005). The Value of Health Care Information Exchange and Interoperability. *Health Affairs.* doi:10.1377/hlthaff.w5.10 PMID:15659453

Health Information Systems, Toolkit on monitoring health systems strengthening. (2008). *World Health Organization.* Retrieved from http://www.who.int/healthinfo/ statistics/toolkit_hss/EN_PDF_Toolkit_HSS_InformationSystems.pdf

Chapter 10
Nosocomial Infection Prediction Using Data Mining Technologies

Eva Silva
Universidade do Minho, Portugal

Ricardo Faria
Universidade do Minho, Portugal

Luciana Cardoso
Universidade do Minho, Portugal

Manuel Santos
Universidade do Minho, Portugal

ABSTRACT

The existence of nosocomial infection prediction systems in healthcare environments can contribute to improve the quality of the healthcare institution. Also, can reduce the costs with the treatment of those patients. The analysis of the information available allows to efficiently prevent these infections and to build knowledge that can help to identify the eventual occurrence of nosocomial infections. Good models induced by the DM classification techniques SVM, DT and NB, were achieved (sensitivities higher than 91.90%). Therefore, this system is able to predict these infections consequently, reduce the nosocomial infection incidence. The platform developed presents important information, as well as supports healthcare professionals in their decisions, namely in planning infection prevention measures. So, the system acts as a CDSS capable of reducing nosocomial infections and the associated costs, improving the healthcare and, increasing patient's safety and well-being.

DOI: 10.4018/978-1-4666-9882-6.ch010

INTRODUCTION

A nosocomial infection is one that occurs during the first 48 hours after the patient's hospitalization, during three days after his/her discharge or during the 30 days that follow a surgery. Also, this infection must not have been present or in incubation at the moment of the patient's admission (Clean Care is Safer Care Team, 2011; Inweregbu, Dave & Pittard, 2005; Rigor, Machado, Abelha, Neves & Alberto, 2008). These infections also include healthcare institution's occupational infections (Clean Care is Safer Care Team, 2011).

A patient with a nosocomial infection stays more time hospitalized resulting in an additional financial burden for the healthcare institution (Inweregbu et al., 2005; Rigor et al., 2008). Moreover, nosocomial infections have a great impact on patient's morbidity and mortality. Especially in intensive care units where the occurrence of nosocomial infections is significantly higher. This happens because of the compromised immune systems of the patients in these units, as well as the invasive procedures and treatments performed there (Inweregbu et al., 2005; Rigor et al., 2008). These reasons make the control and prevention of nosocomial infections crucial for healthcare institutions.

So, the occurrence of these infections can be used to evaluate the quality of the care delivered in the healthcare units and the effectiveness of the infection control and/or prevention plans implemented.

Besides that, according to Inweregbu et al. (2005), it is proved that about one third of nosocomial infections can be prevented by implementing appropriate infection control measures.

There are several factors that contribute to the occurrence of a nosocomial infection, for instance the patient's immune status, his/her age, the hospitalization duration, the use of antibiotics, the diagnostic and treatment methods used, etc. (Rigor et al., 2008). Besides that, great amounts of microorganisms exist in healthcare units, therefore, even a small flaw in the infection prevention programs can easily contribute to the occurrence of an infection.

Thus, it is very important to prevent nosocomial infections. This prevention can be accomplished by performing predictions using data that is capable to characterize the patient health status, as well as his/her hospitalization period and the procedures performed during that period. Data mining (DM) technologies can be used to create predictive models about data. Said that, it is possible to make predictions by applying these models to the new data.

The present work arises from the need to prevent the occurrence of nosocomial infections. It is also related to the healthcare professional's need to take fast, reasoned and accurate decisions to improve the efficiency as well as the productivity of the healthcare organization and the quality of the delivered care.

Through nosocomial infection prediction this work is capable to help healthcare professionals in the study of these infection and in the infection related decision-making process.

Therefore, the main goal is to study the applicability of DM techniques to perform clinical predictions related to the occurrence of nosocomial infections in the Medicine Units of CHP (*Centro Hospitalar do Porto*). To achieve this goal, the design of classification DM models is needed. The best model achieved with this process must be applied to the new data and be integrated to a BI (Business Intelligence) platform that was previously developed to study the nosocomial infection incidence (Silva, Cardoso, Marins, Abelha & Machado, 2014). This part of the platform will be used to indicate the probability of a patient doesn't belong to a risk group of acquiring a nosocomial infection, based on the presence of certain risk factors.

The BI system developed is composed by a DM module and a BI platform. This system can perform as a CDSS (Clinical Decision Support System) because of the information presented by the BI platform. Said that, this work can be used to support decision-making. For that, is necessary to study the nosocomial infection incidence and the infection occurrence prediction.

This platform presents the results of the predictions accomplished allowing healthcare professionals to identify possible occurrences of nosocomial infections. Therefore, it is possible for them to plan and implement specific infection prevention measure. With this being said, it is possible to prevent the occurrence of infections improving the patient's safety and well-being (increasing the quality of the healthcare).

Besides the introduction, this article includes six more sections. The first is related to the background and provides an overview of the BI technology and the main benefits in healthcare sector. Also, the main concepts of Knowledge Discovery in Databases (KDD) and DM are explored there. The second section refers to the implementation of DM in healthcare. The third section presents the DM study for nosocomial infection prediction performed in this work and its main results. The fourth section presents the BI platform to predict the occurrence of infections and the main results obtained. The fifth section suggests some future work measures and the last section presents the main conclusions of the work.

BACKGROUND

Business Intelligence

The term BI refers to a set of concepts and methods used to improve the decision-making process in an organization by using computerized systems (Foshay & Kuziemsky, 2014; Power, 2008).

A BI system is a data-driven Decision Support System (DSS) that includes several tools and methodologies. These tools are capable to integrate, analyze and make available the data about the activities and processes that happen inside an organization. From these data, BI systems extract and present useful information for the decision-making process (Bonney, 2013; Power, 2008; Prevedello, Andriole, Hanson, Kelly, & Khorasani, 2010).

A BI system integrates huge amounts of data from different data sources and converts them into a unified format. Then, the data is loaded into a Data Warehouse (DW). This technology also provides the analytical tools for the analysis and for explore that data. A typical BI system is composed of tools to implement the Extract Transform Load (ETL) process, a DW (Data Werehouse) and analytical software such as On-line Analytical Processing (OLAP) tools, querying tools, reporting tools and DM tools (Bonney, 2013).

The BI technology main goal is to promote more informed and faster decisions that can accomplish better results. Therefore, this technology improves the quality and the quickness to obtain the information to consider in the decision-making process (Mettler & Vimarlund, 2009). Thus, these systems provide relevant information to help the decision-making process. This way, they are a competitive advantage for the organizations that implements them.

In the healthcare sector BI systems are an efficient and adequate method to integrate and explore huge amounts of data collected. Therefore, it is possible to use these data for decision support. The information extracted from the data by the BI systems may be very useful to identify, characterize and monitor the activities and processes that happen inside of the healthcare environment. Thus, it is possible to identify problems and improvement opportunities. So, BI may improve the quality and safety of the care delivered by the healthcare institutions. In addition, contributes to the adoption of evidence-based practice, helping managers and healthcare professionals to make more accurate decisions by accessing to relevant information about the activities and processes that occur inside the organization (Bonney, 2013; Foshay & Kuziemsky, 2014).

Knowledge Discovery in Databases and Data Mining

DM refers to the process of finding unknown patterns in huge amounts of complex data and use that information to build predictive models that are capable of help decision-making (Koh & Tan, 2005).

According to Fayyad, Piatetsky-Shapiro, & Smyth (1996), DM is just one stage of the KDD process. The KDD process refers to the discovery of useful knowledge on data. In other hand, DM refers only to the analysis of data and application of algorithms to induce models about data or extract patterns from them.

There are four more steps of the KDD process: data selection, data pre-processing, data transformation and the interpretation and evaluation of the DM stage results. These steps are essential to ensure the extraction of useful knowledge from data (Fayyad et al., 1996).

Data selection consists of choosing the useful data to solve the problem. The pre-processing stage is responsible for cleaning the data in order to make them consistent. The transformation stage manipulates it, in order to make them suitable for the DM algorithms. Finally, the last step, is the interpretation and evaluation of the mined patterns, as well as applying them in the decision-making process (Azevedo & Santos, 2008; Fayyad et al., 1996).

The quality of the DM stage results is strictly related with the quality of the data used in the DM stage. Therefore, the quality of the extracted knowledge depends on the quality of the data used and that is a crucial factor to take good decisions (Koh, & Tan, 2005).

There are several DM techniques to make tasks such as classification, clustering, linear regression, association, etc. (Fayyad et al., 1996). The most used DM techniques are decision trees, genetic algorithms, artificial neuronal networks and nearest neighbors (Chaudhuri, Dayal, & Narasayya, 2011; Fayyad et al., 1996; Paramasivam, Yee, Dhillon, & Sidhu, 2014). The algorithms to apply depend on the DM goal and there is not a universal and an ideal DM technique because each technique is more suitable for certain problems than the others (Fayyad et al., 1996).

A DM tool is capable to perform a deeper and more detailed analysis than OLAP tools or querying (Chaudhuri et al., 2011). While OLAP tools or querying require human interaction to discover relationships between data, DM technology is capable to automatically find these relationships.

DATA MINING IN HEALTHCARE

In the healthcare sector, DM is becoming more popular and essential. Healthcare institutions must improve the quality of the healthcare while reducing costs (Hardin & Chhieng, 2007). Moreover, huge amounts of data are collected every day by the healthcare institutions and their complexity and volume makes them hard to analyze. DM technology is capable of transform these data into useful information for decision-making. (Koh & Tan, 2005). Therefore, it is well suited to provide decision support in healthcare (Hardin & Chhieng, 2007).

DM is also capable of make predictions that can be useful in the medical and biomedical context. The main goal of these predictions is to lower the level of subjectivity in the clinical decision-making process and improve the daily workflow of the healthcare institution. The predictive models produce excellent knowledge to support the healthcare professionals work (Paramasivam et al., 2014).

It can be used in several contexts to solve several problems. It can be used by healthcare insurers to help to detect fraud and abuse. It can be used to help administrative decisions. And can be used to identify best practices and effective treatments (Koh & Tan, 2005).

Today DM is used in a large number of applications that have included both DM and CDSS and it attracts considerable attention. Healthcare organizations want DM to improve physician practices, resource utilization as well as disease management (Hardin & Chhieng, 2007).

DATA MINING FOR NOSOCOMIAL INFECTION PREDICTION

DM technology can be applied to healthcare to build predictive models to perform predictions in real environments using real clinical data.

It is important to know when nasocomial infections can occur and that can be performed through the application of DM techniques to predict the probability of the occurrence of an infection in the presence of certain variables. Therefore, this DM study intends to develop DM models that are capable to classify if a patient is in risk of acquire nosocomial infection. This process is done using risk factors that describe his/her clinical condition. These models allow to explore the relationship between the occurrence of infections and the characteristics and risk factors present in the patients hospitalized.

This DM module is part of a BI system and the best results achieved by the study are integrated in a BI platform.

Cross Industry Standard Process for Data Mining Methodology

There are several methodologies to implement the KDD process but the most used is the Cross Industry Standard Process for Data Mining (CRISP-DM). The DM study presented in this work was performed using this methodology and the stages of this methodology will be presented next.

It is important to emphasize that the sequence of the CRISP-DM stages is not rigid because it is frequently necessary to return to previous steps. The result of one stage determines the action to implement in the next stage. Besides that, the KDD process is cyclical and does not finish with the last stage, because the knowledge obtained during this process can trigger new business questions, frequently more focused, that force the cycle to restart again (Chapman et al., 2000).

Business Understanding

As mentioned, the main goal of this DM study is to predict the occurrence of nosocomial infections in the presence of certain risk factors. Moreover, the DM goal is the prediction through classification of patients. For that is necessary to use a DM technique to classify variables. Classification consists on the prediction of a target variable that has different classes and maps elements of a dataset in those predefined classes (Fayyad et al., 1996; Koh & Tan, 2005).

At this stage, the problem to solve was formulated as the question "What is the probability of a patient not belonging to a group risk for the occurrence of nosocomial infections when intrinsic risk factors or extrinsic risk factors are present in his/her clinical condition?".

Data Understanding

Considering the question formulated, the data capable to contain a relationship between the variables to study and the variable associated with the nosocomial infection were selected. In this study a dataset composed of CHP nosocomial infection forms data collected between September 30 2013 and December 31 2013 was considered. Besides that, the study considers only data from the Medicine Units of this healthcare institution (specialties Medicine A, Medicine B and Medicine C).

Not all of the attributes collected with the nosocomial infection forms had enough quality or relevance to be used in the DM process. For that reason, a careful selection of attributes was performed in order to choose the representative variables for the study. The following variables that model the problem were chosen:

- Nosocomial Infection: variable that dictates the result of the diagnosis simulated by the DM techniques and has two possible values, "Yes" or "No";
- Age, Gender, Clinical Specialty, Hospitalization Days: variables that characterize the patient and his/her hospitalization;
- Risk Factors: variable that represents the presence or the absence of any intrinsic risk factor, such as alcoholism, diabetes, coma, malnutrition, etc.;
- Urinary Catheter, Peripheral Catheter, Central Catheter, Nasogastric Intubation and Nasotracheal Intubation: variables that represent the presence or absence of the different invasive device, i.e. extrinsic risk factors, used during the patient's hospitalization period.

Data Preparation

After selecting the data and variables, it was necessary to perform the data pre-processing, a stage that allows to build a dataset with the important data. This stage of the CRISP-DM process reduces the search space because it eliminates all the null values and noise present in the data. The columns or lines without interest, are eliminated, leaving the dataset only with the records of interest.

After this stage, the dataset was formed by 283 records from which only 26 are associated with the occurrence of a nosocomial infection.

At this stage data and variables were also aggregated in class in order to model the problem in a more accurate way. The following classes were created:

- **Age Class:** Aggregation of the patient's age in ranges that correspond to different age groups;
- **Intubation:** Aggregation of all the invasive devices related to intubation in a single class (nasogastric intubation and nasotracheal intubation);
- **Catheterization:** Aggregation of all the invasive devices related to catheterization in a single class (Urinary Catheter, Peripheral Catheter and Central Catheter).

Moreover, oversampling was applied to the dataset in order to replicate the data associated with the occurrence of a nosocomial infection. Thus it was possible, to obtain a number of records associated with the occurrence of a nosocomial infection, that is approximated to the number of records associated with the non-occurrence of an infection. This technique consists on the minority class data replication in order to increase its weight. This is necessary because the classifiers tend to produce more classification errors in the presence of minority classes (Barua, Islam, & Kazuyuki, 2013). In the case of this work, this technique was applied because of the difference between the number of forms associated with the occurrence of a nosocomial infection and because of the number of forms associated with the non-occurrence of an infection was very significant. Thus, the meaning of the nosocomial infection occurrences could get lost because of its lower occurrence rate in the population to study. After the oversampling, the dataset had 517 records.

With this stage of the CRISP-DM three datasets were created: a dataset without replicated data (Approach A), a dataset with replicated data (Approach B) and a dataset with replicated data and the variable age aggregated into classes (Approach C).

Modelling

In this study Support Vector Machines (SVM), Decision Trees (DT) and Naïve Bayes (NB) were the classification techniques used to perform DM. These techniques were used to automatically induce the classification models with Oracle Data Miner [i], a SQL Developer extension that allows to build, evaluate and apply DM models. These techniques were selected considering their efficiency and the interpretability of the models they generate.

SVM is a powerful algorithm that is based on the statistical learning theory and find the best decision plans that split data into different sets, can be used to model complex problems and has a great capacity of generalization of the model to new data (Oracle, 2008; Paramasivam et al., 2014).

DT are based on conditional probabilities and they recursively divide the dataset in discrete subcategories in order to maximize the distance between classes, producing good results and models in a very fast way (Oracle, 2008; Paramasivam et al., 2014).

NB is also based on conditional probabilities, makes predictions considering the Bayes Theorem and it is very fast and scalable (Oracle, 2008).

Considering the different chosen variables, several scenarios were considered to build the models:

- **Absence of Risk Factors (Scenario 1):** All of the variables were used in the model except the variable Risk Factors, i.e., the variables Age or Age Class, Sex, Hospitalization Days, Clinical Specialty, Intubation, Catheterization and the target variable Nosocomial Infection were used;
- **Absence of Intubation (Scenario 2):** All of the variables were used in the model except the variable Intubation, i.e., the variables Age or Age Class, Sex, Hospitalization Days, Clinical Specialty, Risk Factors, Catheterization and the target variable Nosocomial Infection were used;
- **Absence of Catheterization (Scenario 3):** All of the variables were used in the model except the variable Catheterization, i.e., the variables Age or Age Class, Sex, Hospitalization Days, Clinical Specialty, Risk Factors, Intubation and the target variable Nosocomial Infection were used;
- **All the Variables (Scenario 4):** All of the variables were used in the model, i.e., the variables Age or Age Class, Sex, Hospitalization Days, Clinical Specialty, Risk Factors, Intubation, Catheterization and the target variable Nosocomial Infection were used.

These four scenarios were modeled according to the three different datasets previously created (Approach A, Approach B and Approach C). The DM techniques were then applied to all combinations of scenarios and approaches (Situations), in order to create new knowledge and the best model. So, the four scenarios were modeled by the three DM classification techniques, the three approaches and a target variable. At the end, 36 DM models were obtained.

The models generated can be used to analyze the relationship between the variables considered and their impact in the occurrence of a nosocomial infection. These models can be represented by the following expression:

$$M_n \equiv <A_f, S_i, TDM_y>$$

According this expression, the Predictive Model n (M_n) belongs to the DM Approach f (A_f) and is composed by the Situation i (S_i) and the DM Technique y (TDM_y).

For instance, for the Approach A:

A_f {Classification}

TDM_y {SVM, DT, NB}

S_i {Scenario 1 and Approach A, …, Scenario 4 and Approach A},

for Approach B:

A_f {Classification}

TDM_y {SVM, DT, NB}

S_i {Scenario 1 and Approach B, …, Scenario 4 and Approach B}

and for Approach C:

A_f {Classification}

TDM_y {SVM, DT, NB}

S_i {Scenario 1 and Approach C, …, Scenario 4 and Approach C}

At this stage the data were split in test data (30%) and train data (the remaining 70%).

Evaluation

As a result of the DM process several models are obtained. These models must be evaluated in order to check their quality and, therefore, chose the one that allows to obtain the best results.

The most used technique to evaluate the models is the Confusion Matrix, a matrix that measures the correction of the predictions (Oracle, 2008). This matrix as four types of results: True Positives (TP), False Positives (FP), True Negatives (TN) and False Negatives (FN). A TP is a positive case correctly classified. A FP is a case incorrectly classified as positive. A TN is a case correctly classified as negative. Finally, a FN result is a case incorrectly classified as negative.

With the estimation of each of these results it is possible to apply a set of statistical measures to evaluate the quality of the results, being the most used sensibility, specificity and acuity (Kohavi & Provost, 1998).

- **Sensibility:** The capacity of the model detecting the occurrence of an event when present and it measures the proportion between the number of TP results and all the positive results, i.e...
- **Specificity:** The capacity of the model classify correctly the non-occurrence of an event and it is the ratio between the number of TN results and all the negative values, i.e...
- **Acuity:** The agreement between the correctly detected values and the real values and it is the proportion between all the true results and all the cases, i.e...

The quality of the models obtained with this work was evaluated with these statistical measures. In the case of this work, it is necessary to predict the non-occurrence of a nosocomial infection.

Some of these models allowed to achieve the best overall four results for each one of the DM techniques used (Table 1). The best models were selected considering the values of sensitivity because it is important to identify all the non-occurrences of infection. Knowing the non-occurrences of infection, it is possible to consider all the other predictions as risk groups capable of acquiring a nosocomial infection.

Deployment

After the evaluation of the models, the knowledge obtained can be used by healthcare professionals to predict the occurrence of an infection in the presence of the studied risk factors. The combination of variables that have a higher probability to result in the occurrence of an infection can also be identified. Then, the nosocomial

Table 1. Top 4 models for each DM technique (Adapted from (Silva et al., 2014))

Support Vector Machine			
	Specificity	Sensitivity	Acuity
Scenario 1 and Approach B	0.763	0.919	0.838
Scenario 2 and Approach B	0.741	0.942	0.831
Scenario 1 and Approach C	0.731	0.793	0.766
Scenario 3 and Approach C	0.675	0.845	0.754
Decision Tree			
	Specificity	Sensitivity	Acuity
Scenario 1 and Approach C	0.855	0.798	0.818
Scenario 4 and Approach C	0.673	0.982	0.786
Scenario 4 and Approach B	0.673	0.982	0.786
Scenario 2 and Approach B	0.67	1	0.786
Naïve Bayes			
	Specificity	Sensitivity	Acuity
Scenario 1 and Approach B	0.733	0.941	0.825
Scenario 2 and Approach B	0.733	0.941	0.825
Scenario 4 and Approach B	0.733	0.941	0.825
Scenario 4 and Approach C	0.733	0.941	0.825

infection control and prevention measures can be planned and justified. Therefore, the best model achieved by the DM techniques was integrated on a BI platform in order to implement a CDSS capable to predict the occurrence of a nosocomial infection in new patients through old data. The BI platform will be presented after the presentation and discussion of the achieved results.

Discussion

The ideal behavior of a classification model is to have sensibility values higher than 90%. In the case of this study, the models with higher sensibility percentages are capable to detect correctly the non-occurrence of the target variable and good values of sensitivity (values higher than 91.90%) were achieved. Therefore, the overall results are acceptable and the models are capable to predict, with a high degree of certainty, the non-occurrence of an infection.

The best combination of scenario and approach for all the DM techniques was situation Scenario 2 and Approach B, because it has the highest value of sensibility for all the techniques used. It also has high values of acuity.

The sensibility achieved was 100% when modelled with DT. Therefore, this model is capable to predict the non-occurrence of nosocomial infections with great certainty. For that reason, from all the combinations of situations and techniques, this is the model that best predicts the non-occurrence of an infection. All the cases that are not classified as not having infection are expected to be the risk groups capable of acquiring an infection. In this case, specificity and acuity values of 78.60% and 67% were achieved.

The Table 2 presents, for each of the DM algorithms applied to the situation Scenario 2 and Approach B, the number of incorrectly and correctly classified cases. It also presents the percentage of correctly classified cases for each of the algorithms.

According to the results presented in Table 2, the more efficient algorithm applied to situation Scenario 2 Approach B was SVM because it allowed to achieve the highest percentage of correct answers (83.12%). In spite of having the highest value of sensibility with DT, this situation also has the smallest value of sensibility. Thus, its value of acuity is not very high.

In general, the values of specificity were also acceptable and varied between 67% and 85.50%. So the models are capable of predicting the occurrence of a nosocomial infection even though that classification introduces a certain error.

The acuity varied between 75.40% and 83.80%, so there is an overall agreement between the values correctly detected and the real values.

It can be verified that, overall, the sensibility values were higher than the specificity values which means that the models obtained are better to predict the non-occurrence of a nosocomial infection than to predict the cases where the infection is present.

This paper demonstrated that through the application of DM classification techniques to real clinical data it is possible to obtain classification models. This models can be applied to predict if a patient will acquire or not a nosocomial infection. The models are satisfactory and can support the decision-making of healthcare professionals. These models allow the application of the appropriate preventive measures, necessary to ensure the risk patient's safety and well-being.

Table 2. Number of incorrectly and correctly classified cases and percentage of correctly classified cases for situation Scenario 2 and Approach B

	Incorrect	Correct	% of Correct
Support Vector Machine	26	128	83.12
Decision Tree	33	121	78.57
Naïve Bayes	27	127	82.47

BUSINESS INTELLIGENCE PLATFORM FOR NOSOCOMIAL INFECTION PREDICTION

The best model obtained (Scenario 2 and Approach B for DT algorithm) was integrated on a BI platform. The BI platform is a web application created with Pentaho Community Edition. This is an open source BI tool that allows several BI tasks, such as the creation of reports and dashboards. Also, allows the implementation of DM and OLAP and other features, to help its users to visualize and analyze data. In this work only the main component of Pentaho Community Edition, the Business Analytics Platform, was used.

Using Oracle Data Miner, the best model was applied to 2013 nosocomial infection data in order to calculate the probability of the non-occurrence of a nosocomial infection. The result of the prediction was a table with the predicted value, the probability of the result being "No" and a set of attributes that characterize the patient. This table were used to build the predictive models (Age, Sex, Clinical Specialty, Hospitalization Days, Risk Factors, Intubation, Catheterization).

Later, a dashboard to present the probability of a selected patient to acquire a nosocomial infection was created using Community Dashboard Editor (CDE), a module of Pentaho's Business Analytics Platform. CDE allows and simplifies the development of powerful, interactive and visually attractive dashboards, making information interpretation easier for the user.

This dashboard allows the users to choose the episode (a code given to the patient when he/she is hospitalized in CHP) to predict using a combo box.

The result of the prediction is present in the dashboard on a dial chart (Figure 1), in which 100% corresponds to the non-occurrence of an infection and the other values represent risk groups capable of having an infection. Therefore, the lower the predicted value, higher the risk of acquiring an infection.

In the case of Figure 1, the patient associated with the episode 12033354 has 80% of probability of not acquiring a nosocomial infection.

The values of the variables considered in the construction of the models (Specialty, Age, Sex, Hospitalization Days, Risk Factors, Catheterization, Intubation) for the episode selected are also presented in the dashboard.

According to Figure 2, the episode 12033354 is associated with a 76-year-old female patient that was hospitalized for 56 days, presented risk factors and was submitted to catheterization but not to intubation.

This dashboard allows clinical professionals to identify the patients that belong groups in risk of acquiring a nosocomial infection. Therefore, they can notice the patients that should be more accompanied and apply the necessary preventive measures. Thus, it is possible to reduce the costs related to the occurrence of a nosocomial infection and ensure patient's well-being and safety.

Figure 1. Example of a prediction made by the BI platform

Episode
12033354

Prediction Result

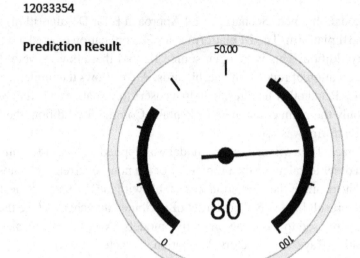

Figure 2. Example of the patient's characteristics presented by the BI platform

Patient's Characteristics

Specialty ⌄	Age ⌄	Gender ⌄	Hospitalization Days ⌄	Risk Factors ⌄	Catheterization ⌄	Intubation ⌄
Medicine A	76	Feminine	56	With Risk Factors	Yes	No

This allows the dashboard to work as a CDSS capable to predict the non-occurrence of a nosocomial infection in new patients through clinical data. Moreover, can help healthcare professionals in their decision-making because it identifies the patients that belong to groups of risk. With this information, healthcare professionals can monitor these patients with more attention. Therefore, they can plan and implement the necessary measures to prevent and control these infections.

FUTURE RESEARCH DIRECTIONS

The repetition of the DM study with other data and DM techniques as well as the incorporation of other variables in the predictive model would be also interesting tasks.

The best model achieved must also be applied to present data in order to make real time nosocomial infection predictions in new hospitalized patients.

It is also important to evaluate the usability and functionality of the platform to find improvement opportunities that are related with the performance of the system or related with important features to its users.

CONCLUSION

The prevention of nosocomial infections is crucial because these infections can put at risk the security and well-being of patients and healthcare professionals. Moreover, the diagnoses and treatment originates in additional costs for healthcare institutions.

DM technology can be applied to clinical data in order to predict the occurrence of infections. Through the use of real data extracted from nosocomial infection forms recorded in CHP, the DM module of this work demonstrated that it is possible to obtain classification DM models. This models are capable to predict if a patient with certain risk factors will or not acquire a nosocomial infection.

In this DM study CRISP-DM methodology was followed and three classification algorithms were used: SVM, DT and NB. It is possible to conclude that these techniques associated with real clinical data allow to predict nosocomial infection cases (Silva et al., 2014). Good models to predict the non-occurrence of infection were achieved (sensibilities higher than 91.90%). The integration of the best model obtained in the BI platform is of great worth because it allows the classification of patients. Therefore, the induction of DM predictive models for nosocomial infection can be seen as a great contribution to the development of CDSS to this sector.

The best predictive model was only applied to data from 2013, but in the future the system can be expanded to predict present cases of infection. This will allow to predict nosocomial infections in new patients in real time. Moreover, being nosocomial infections an important problem in the healthcare environment, it is important to emphasize that the best model achieved with this study can be applied to other specialties of CHP.

The BI platform gives more autonomy and flexibility to healthcare professional, allowing them to analyze data and interpret information extracted in a quicker and simpler way. Healthcare professionals can apply the information presented in the platform to plan specific and customized infection prevention measures according to the real needs of each patient. So, the platform helps these professional performing their jobs. Besides that, open source BI tools allow the creation of new knowledge through information presentation without any additional costs for healthcare organizations.

The BI system presented in this chapter is capable to present relevant and useful information for nosocomial infection related decision-making, allowing to predict them. In other hand, it is capable of acting as a CDSS for healthcare professionals. Therefore, it can help to reduce nosocomial infection rate and associated costs.

The work presented in this chapter is of great importance for society because the developed BI platform allows the prevention and reduction of nosocomial infections through the promotion of an evidence-based clinical practice. More, it decreases the risk of complications to patients and improving their safety and well-being. It is important to note that, being nosocomial infections an extremely important problem in healthcare institutions, the methodology presented in this chapter can be adapted to generate predictive models other institutions.

REFERENCES

Azevedo, A., & Santos, M. F. (2008). KDD, SEMMA and CRISP-DM: A parallel overview. *Proceedings of the IADIS European Conference on Data Mining* Amesterdam, Netherlands (pp. 182-185).

Barua, S., Islam, M. M., & Murase, K. (2013). ProWSyn: Proximity weighted synthetic oversampling technique for imbalanced data set learning. In J. Pei, V. S. Tseng, L. Cao, H. Motoda, & G. Xu (Eds.), *Advances in Knowledge Discovery and Data Mining* (pp. 317–328). Berlin: Springer Berlin Heidelberg. doi:10.1007/978-3-642-37456-2_27

Bonney, W. (2013). Applicability of business intelligence in electronic health record. *Procedia: Social and Behavioral Sciences, 73*(0), 257–262. doi:10.1016/j.sbspro.2013.02.050

Chapman, P., Clinton, J., Kerber, R., Khabaza, T., Reinartz, T., Shearer, C., & Wirth, R. (2000). *CRISP-DM 1.0 Step-by-step data mining guide*. SPSS. Retrieved from ftp://ftp.software.ibm.com/software/analytics/spss/support/Modeler/Documentation/14/UserManual/CRISP-DM.pdf

Chaudhuri, S., Dayal, U., & Narasayya, V. (2011). An overview of business intelligence technology. *Communications of the ACM, 54*(8), 88. doi:10.1145/1978542.1978562

Clean Care is Safer Care Team (2011). *Report on the burden of endemic health care-associated infection worldwide: Clean care is safer care*. Geneva: World Health Organization. Retrieved from http://apps.who.int/iris/bitstream/10665/80135/1/9789241501507_eng.pdf?ua=1

Fayyad, U., Piatetsky-Shapiro, G., & Smyth, P. (1996). From data mining to knowledge discovery in databases. *AI Magazine, 17*(3), 37–54. doi:10.1609/aimag.v17i3.1230

Foshay, N., & Kuziemsky, C. (2014). Towards an implementation framework for business intelligence in healthcare. *International Journal of Information Management, 34*(1), 20–27. doi:10.1016/j.ijinfomgt.2013.09.003"ttp://

Hardin, J. M., & Chhieng, D. C. (2007). Data mining and clinical decision support systems. In E. S. Berner (Ed.), *Clinical Decision Support Systems* (pp. 44–63). New York, USA: Springer; doi:10.1007/978-0-387-38319-4_3

Inweregbu, K., Dave, J., & Pittard, A. (2005). Nosocomial infections. *Continuing Education in Anaesthesia. Critical Care & Pain, 5*(1), 14–17. doi:10.1093/bjaceaccp/mki006

Koh, H. C., & Tan, G. (2005). Data mining applications in healthcare. *Journal of Healthcare Information Management, 19*(2), 64–72. PMID:15869215

Kohavi, R., & Provost, F. (1998). Glossary of terms. *Machine Learning - Special Issue on Applications of Machine Learning and the Knowledge Discovery Process, 30*(2-3), 271-274

Mettler, T., & Vimarlund, V. (2009). Understanding business intelligence in the context of health care. *Health Informatics Journal, 15*(3), 254–264. doi:10.1177/1460458209337446 PMID:19713399

Oracle (2008). Oracle data mining concepts. Retrieved from http://docs.oracle.com/cd/B28359_01/datamine.111/b28129/toc.htm

Paramasivam, V., Yee, T. S., Dhillon, S. K., & Sidhu, A. S. (2014). A methodological review of data mining techniques in predictive medicine: An application in hemodynamic prediction for abdominal aortic aneurysm disease. *Biocybernetics and Biomedical Engineering, 34*(3), 139–145. doi:10.1016/j.bbe.2014.03.003

Power, D. J. (2008). Understanding data-driven decision support systems. *Information Systems Management, 25*(8), 149–154. doi:10.1080/10580530801941124

Prevedello, L. M., Andriole, K. P., Hanson, R., Kelly, P., & Khorasani, R. (2010). Business intelligence tools for radiology: Creating a prototype model using open-source tools. *Journal of Digital Imaging, 23*(2), 133–141. doi:10.1007/s10278-008-9167-3 PMID:19011943

Rigor, H., Machado, J., Abelha, A., Neves, J., & Alberto, C. (2008). A web-based system to reduce the nosocomial infection impact in healthcare units. *Proceedings of the WEBIST 2008 - International Conference on Web Information Systems,* Madeira, Portugal.

Silva, E., Alpuim, A., Cardoso, L., Marins, F., Quintas, C., Portela, C. F., & Abelha, A. et al. (2014). Business intelligence and nosocomial infection decision making. In A. Azevedo & M. Santos (Eds.), *Integration of Data Mining in Business Intelligence Systems* (pp. 193–215). Hershey, PA: IGI Global; doi:10.4018/978-1-4666-6477-7. ch010

Silva, E., Cardoso, L., Marins, F., Abelha, A., & Machado, J. (n). *Business intelligence platform for nosocomial infection incidence.*

ADDITIONAL READING

Gonçalves, J., Portela, F., Santos, M. F., Silva, Á., Machado, J., Abelha, A., & Rua, F. (2014). *Real-time predictive analytics for sepsis level and therapeutic plans in intensive care medicine. IJHISI - International Journal of Healthcare Information Systems and Informatics.* Springer.

Loshin, D. (2012). *Business intelligence: The savvy manager's guide* (2nd ed.). San Francisco, CA: Morgan Kaufman Publishers Inc.

Nagy, P. G., Warnock, M. J., Daly, M., Toland, C., Meenan, C. D., & Mezrich, R. S. (2009). Informatics in radiology automated web-based graphical dashboard for radiology operational. *Radiographics, 29*(7), 1897–1906. doi:10.1148/rg.297095701 PMID:19734469

Prevedello, L. M., Andriole, K. P., & Khorasani, R. (2008). Business intelligence tools and performance improvement in your practice. *Journal of the American College of Radiology, 5*(12), 1210–1211. doi:10.1016/j.jacr.2008.08.018 PMID:19027686

Santos, M. Y., & Ramos, I. (2006). *Business Intelligence: Tecnologias da informação na gestão de conhecimento.* Lisbon, Portugal: FCA - Editora de Informática.

Spruit, M., Vroon, R., & Batenburg, R. (2014). Towards healthcare business intelligence in long-term care. *Computers in Human Behavior, 30*(0), 698–707. doi:10.1016/j.chb.2013.07.038

KEY TERMS AND DEFINITIONS

Business Intelligence: Group of technologies and methods that treat and analyse data, in order to present relevant and strategic information to crate knowledge capable to help the decision-making process of an organization.

Clinical Decision Support System: Software system created to assist the decision-making process of the healthcare professionals.

CRISP-DM: A very popular methodology used to implement the KDD process.

Data Mining: Technology that allows to discover interesting, previously unknown and relevant patterns in large datasets.

Knowledge Discovery in Databases: Process that allows to turn data into useful knowledge.

Nosocomial Infection: Infection acquired in the hospital during the period of 48 hours after hospital admission, 3 days after discharge or 30 days after an operation, and that was not present or in incubation in the moment of admission.

Open Source: Software whose source code is available for use and/or modification and can be freely used and shared by any of its users.

Chapter 11
Monitoring Time Consumption in Complementary Diagnostic and Therapeutic Procedure Requests

Ana Alpuim
University of Minho, Portugal

Sónia Pereira
University of Minho, Portugal

Marisa Esteves
University of Minho, Portugal

Manuel Santos
University of Minho, Portugal

ABSTRACT

Over the years, information technologies and computer applications have been widespread amongst all fields, including healthcare. The main goal of these organizations is focused on providing quality health services to their patients, ensuring the provision of quality services. Therefore, decisions have to be made quickly and effectively. Thus, the increased use of information technologies in healthcare has been helping the decision-making process, improving the quality of their services. For an example, the insertion of Business Intelligence (BI) tools in healthcare environments has been recently used to improve healthcare delivery. It is based on the analysis of data in order to provide useful information. BI tools assist managers and health professionals through decision-making, since they allow the manipulation and analysis of data in order to extract knowledge. This work aims to study and analyze the time that physicians take to prescribe medical exams in Centro

DOI: 10.4018/978-1-4666-9882-6.ch011

Hospitalar do Porto (CHP), though BI tools. The main concern is to identify the physicians who take more time than average to prescribe complementary means of diagnosis and treatment, making it possible to identify and understand the reason why it occurs. To discover these outliners, a BI platform was developed using the Pentaho Community. This platform presents means to represent information through tables and graphs that facilitate the analysis of information and the knowledge extraction. This information will be useful to represent knowledge concerning not only the prescription system (auditing it) but also its users. The platform evaluates the time prescription, by specialty and physician, which can afterwards be applied in the decision-making process. This platform enables the identification of measures to unravel the time differences that some physicians exhibit, in order to, subsequently, improve the whole process of electronic medical prescription.

INTRODUCTION

The Electronic Health Record (EHR) is a Health Information System (HIS) that collects all the information of a patient from various information systems, including his medical history. The EHR covers several hospital departments and units, enabling an analysis of the clinical process. It should be noted that it is oriented to the patient and not the service unit or even the diseases to which they are subject, i.e., it stands with the firm intention of benefiting the patients (Duarte et al., 2011; Hasman, 1998).

The EHR is nothing more than a set of standardized documents used for the registration of medical procedures rendered to a given patient in a given hospital unit by health professionals. Essentially, it is a set of information compiled by health professionals, which corresponds to the full data record of a given patient, including all the existing information about him. Hereupon, it tracks the general state of the individual and allows the preparation of the same clinical history, chronologically, and it also enables remote and simultaneous access to any clinical process (Duarte et al., 2011; Hasman, 1998).

This HIS is seen as a set of registration annotations and use of clinical information for better delivery of healthcare services to the patient. This being the task of practically everyone who works in the hospital, they all contribute to a better delivery of services. The EHR integrates information from various sources, from other HIS or other applications based on Information and Communication Technologies (ICT) in all its aspects, in order to replace the part, improve and speed up the assistance to the patient to accelerate certain processes, prevent medical errors, and also ease the work of all health professionals (Duarte et al., 2011; Hasman, 1998).

Besides registration, consultation and research set of clinical information, resulting from the provision of healthcare to a given patient, the EHR system also allows the prescription of medicines and Complementary Diagnostic and Therapeutic Procedures (CDTP), called the Electronic Medical Prescription (EMP). The EMP is a procedure performed by the ICT through an application, the SAM – *Sistema de Apoio ao Médico* – (Support Medical System)[1].

The EMP reduces some existing problems by improving the legibility, which does not exist in handwritten requests – data security and confidentiality of data relating to patients – since access will be assuredly restricted. It also helps with revenue management and diagnostic tests (Ammenwerth et al., 2008).

The EHR integrates the data with other information systems via the internet: collects, processes and updates data; supports research and can return the information to patients in various ways. Finally, it also allows to obtain different types of reports with a variety of font types and sizes, and still images which simplifies and assists the perception of the diagnosis by health professionals (Duarte et al., 2011).

On the other hand, the change from a manual to an electronic record affects the established communication practices by changing the content and patterns of communication between departments. Communication via computers can increase the speed of communication between professionals but, in some cases, can also cause misunderstandings and consequently some flaws, by passing the manual records to digital format (Chiasson et al., 2007; Heeks, 2006).

SAM has a large potential for improvement and, despite some limitations, the use of electronic prescribing is clearly advantageous compared to manual prescription. This system has numerous potential, one of which being the registration times that health professionals spend for prescribing CDTP.

Every prescription is recorded at least once, at the time of the request, but may be recorded several times, regarding the tasks of each request. Each one of those tasks matches a required form, when prescribing a CDTP. The time of the request corresponds to a total time starting from the moment the professional registers the order of a CDTP, ending when the process is complete. In the meantime, when prescribing a CDTP, the physician is required to complete one or more forms, which vary depending on the test request. Particular examination may not even have an associated form. The task time refers to the period it takes the physician to answer all the questions of the form(s) and click OK. The request time is always higher, because it includes the times of the tasks.

Analyzing these times becomes an essential task for improving the EMP process. Thus, an evaluation and analysis of these times is necessary. By analyzing the times recorded in databases, it is possible to separate them, either by the prescribing physician of the CDTP as well as the various specialties. To solve this problem, a platform within CHP was developed. CHP is a large healthcare organization in northern Portugal, and their data are the source for the platform developed. This platform allows us to identify the professionals who take longer than the average time on CDTP prescription process, which is a time that is essential during the day-to-day queries. This platform was developed by using the Pentaho Community software, which is an open source BI tool.

BACKGROUND

Medical Record

The user's medical record (MR) is a rich source of data, often carried out by nurses for clinical research, acting as a repository of information of a user (Gregory & Radovinsky, 2012). It is often used as a primary source of data for epidemiological analysis purposes and it is also considered standard in any study to identify demographic, clinical data variables, specific aspects related to treatment and mortality schemes (Cassidy et al., 2002; Murray et al., 2003). Data collection through the MR involves the review of their specific sources. These include nursing, consultation notes, admission and high reports, laboratory tests, surgical reports, and other clinical and administrative documentation, which, however, is not easily done if the registration is manual. A good strategy before starting data collection is necessary (Eder et al., 2005; Gearing et al., 2006; Pan et al., 2005). The tool used in the EHR for data collection should be systematically organized and should be easy to use (Gregory & Radovinsky, 2012). The MR has always been recognized as a rich source of information for conducting clinical research, decision-making and identification of diagnosis. Nonetheless, researchers should include the development and testing of the tools used for the collection (Gregory & Radovinsky, 2012).

The data collected from the EHR is essential to establish a health history on users, in order to investigate the prediction of disease. It is estimated that every year numerous lives are lost due to poorly coordinated medical information (Chiasson et al., 2007). The advantages of using data obtained from the EHR through a retrospective analysis of the records include the ability to access large amounts of data at a relatively low cost (Gregory & Radovinsky, 2012).

Over the years, a variety of systems were developed and implemented in an attempt to improve the delivery of healthcare. These systems include EHR that replaces paper records storage and search of information. Every day that passes, healthcare is becoming increasingly complex (Waegemann, 2003). With the many advances in the ICT in the last 20 years, particularly in health, many ways have been discussed in EHR but, further, developed and implemented. Nowadays, many people involved in healthcare are expecting to move to a paperless environment. This is an important step but, at the moment, it has only been achieved with success in some institutions (Waegemann, 2003).

The ICT offer many advantages over manual records on paper for storage and searching of data of users. Although it has been possible, but not fully implemented, it is expected that in the future, all records will be stored and viewed on a computer and mobile devices (Tavakoli et al., 2011).

In the past few years, many organizations have underestimated the strategic importance of information and its associated technologies, which results in a lack of potential planning the ICT. In many cases, organizations have failed to realize the strategic benefits of the ICT because they have been considering them as a mere replacement of manual and administrative functions and not as a powerful strategic resource as it should be (Saleem et al., 2009).

The data collection can be done in a document or through an electronic register. Both types of data collection instruments have some advantages and limitations. Generally, in the department of medical records, a paper document is often more cost effective and easier to use to collect data (Allison et al., 2000). However, using a paper document requires that data has to be then introduced into an electronic database in order to analyze the knowledge through computers (Gregory & Radovinsky, 2012). For this purpose, the researchers usually send copies of MR on paper to the data center where data managers belong in the database. This routine paper has many drawbacks that results in the insertion of erroneous data in the database leading to a longer duration of the clinical trial, especially for a larger amount of data, since more data the longer it takes to insert them in an electronic register (Kawado et al., 2003; Paul et al., 2005). Even under the best circumstances, the data entry process is fraught with the possibility of error occurrence, and the analysis and the results of data studies will be influenced. Nonetheless, the collection of data directly from an electronic DB, reduces the possibility of errors in the input thereof, which may result in a more reliable collection and consequently a better analysis and decision-making is more reasoned (Worster & Haines, 2004). Furthermore, for large investigations, the collection from an electronic DB facilitates the centralization and access to them may be more profitable (Gearing et al., 2006).

When implemented correctly, the EHR has a great potential benefit to health systems and decision-making because they can improve the way the data of users are documented and organized. Consequently, the EHR provides better readability of the user data, simultaneous and remote access, and integration with other information sources (Powsner et al., 1998). Thereby, all of the points referred above contribute to improve the delivery of healthcare.

Fortunately, physicians and health professionals have been realizing the importance of the implementation of electronic records, verifying that they have benefits, such as accuracy, readability of data, complete information and reducing repetition of data entry (Munyisia et al., 2011).

Compared to the manual paper system, the electronic documentation resulted in improvements on users, i.e., greater usefulness of records to provide healthcare without compromising the results of users, which means that there are significant improvements in health (Rossi et al., 2014). Study results also show that the greatest benefit is the reduction in cost control and data management. Of course, the exact value depends on the estimation of parameters that affect the calculations (Pavlović et al., 2009).

Nevertheless, with both the manual records as the EHR, errors still occur. The failure of some EHR, already computerized, may be due to bad design information (Powsner et al., 1998). The existence of errors in medical documents is very common. The classification of these errors would help to understand their causes, their origin and, finally, develop support tools for understanding. The literature provides numerous examples of medical errors rating. These classifications are the basis for reporting errors and, therefore, to reflect the needs of specific areas of expertise. In addition to vary according to the area of specialization, error classification schemes differ in dimensions along which the classification is conducted (Tavakoli et al., 2011).

BUSINESS INTELLIGENCE

The implementation of Business Intelligence (BI) in healthcare organizations helps its managers and health professionals in their own decision-making processes through data analysis that provide relevant information about the processes and activities of those organizations. Thus, BI tools can improve the quality and safety in healthcare, and consequently the performance of the organizations (Bonney, 2013; Prevedello et al., 2010).

Many HIS as the EHR, contain large amounts of clinical information highly relevant for decision-making. Studies suggest that it is necessary to apply BI tools to ensure that the contents of the registers are efficiently used, since these tools allow the extraction of relevant information. Subsequently, the extracted data can be used by health professionals to support real-time decision, contributing to the improvement of healthcare (Bonney, 2013).

In most health organizations, data is stored in different systems and it is sometimes necessary to relate them. Typically, these systems are poorly integrated, making extraction a difficult operation. For this reason, there is interest in developing applications that make access and data extraction an easier process. BI tools are able to work efficiently with health data to generate information and knowledge in real time, this being the reason why these tools are used in the health sector. Over the years, the interest in the application of BI tools in the health sector has increased and different solutions have been created (Bonney, 2013).

Business Intelligence Systems

The term BI is assigned to an area of decision support systems that refers to the process of collection, compilation, integration, storage, analysis and presentation of data on the activities of a particular organization (Glaser & Stone, 2008; Prevedello et al., 2010). This type of representation of knowledge by the information submitted by BI systems can be relevant and strategic to support professionals in decision-making (Bonney, 2013). This technology provides the means to transform the data into relevant and strategic information, in order to constitute significant and important knowledge to support decisions of the organization's professionals. This allows the workers as executives, managers and analysts, to make better decisions quickly (Bonney, 2013; Loshin, 2013).

The main benefits of using BI systems are its flexibility and time reducing in data access and data analysis. Decision-making is supported by actual data, making it more likely that the assessment is correct and feasible (Bonney, 2013). The use of BI makes the quality of inputs increases. These systems have the ability to put the right information available to users at the right time, in order to help in the decision-making process (Mettler & Vimarlund, 2009). In this aspect, it becomes clear to identify the advantage in implementing these systems. BI systems must be able to integrate high amounts of data from various sources and, accordingly, providing analytical tools for data analysis, these being the two main tasks of the BI (Popovič et al., 2012).

BI systems provide tools relatively easy to use, which make this type of systems easily available to all its end users, revealing himself as an advantage for organizations that implement BI (Chaudhuri et al., 2011; Glaser & Stone, 2008; Prevedello et al., 2010).

Business Intelligence Steps

Throughout the recent years, it has been noticed a significant improvement in the development of BI tools. The speed of data collection has increased, as well as the sophistication and interactivity in handling the data and the report query in the tools used to present information. The BI technology includes various software features as Extraction, Transformation and Load (ETL), Data Warehouse, Online Analytical Process (OLAP), Data Mining (DM), reporting, query and virtualization of databases (Bonney, 2013). A BI system integrates data from heterogeneous sources, and converts them into a unified format to carry them to a DW. This process of extraction, transformation and loading of data, can be very complex and time consuming. After the implementation of the ETL process, the data stored in the DW can be used for analytical applications capable of aggregating them using OLAP (Prevedello et al., 2010).

ETL

Running the ETL process is one of the most difficult tasks for the settlement of a DW. It is complex, lengthy and consumes most of the time in the implementation of the DW. The process to populate a DW, running an ETL tool, consists of three steps. The first is extraction, where data are drawn from different sources. The second refers to transformation, which, as the name implies, consists in processing and cleaning the data. The third step commits the data to the load and DW is called by load. ETL tools are specialized in addressing issues of heterogeneity of information sources, and dealing with the cleaning and data transformation. The ETL is an essential step for loading large volumes of data and to ensure their quality and hence good results in the indicators presented by BI tools (Chaudhuri et al., 2011; El-Sappagh et al., 2011).

The ETL is a complex combination of processes and technologies that consume a significant amount of effort in the population of a DW. The ETL process is not a sporadic event. As the data sources vary, the DW will update itself periodically. That is, the DW will not change its structure, even if it is loaded with more information. For this, the ETL process will run again in order to maintain its value as a tool in aiding decision-making. Clearly, the ETL process must be designed to be easily modified (El-Sappagh et al., 2011).

As already mentioned, an ETL system consists of three consecutive steps, summarized in Figure 1:

- **Extraction:** It is the first step of the ETL process and it is responsible for extracting data from the different sources. Each data source has its specific features that have to be managed in order to effectively extract the data for the ETL process. The process should integrate the systems that may have different platforms, such as management systems with different databases, operating systems and communication protocols (El-Sappagh et al., 2011).

Figure 1. ETL processes (El-Sappagh et al., 2011 adapted)

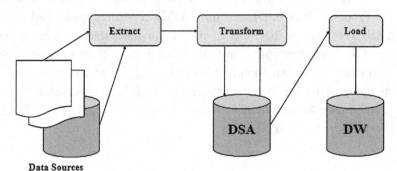

- **Transformation:** The second step of any ETL process includes cleansing, transforming and integrating data. This step cleans information, in order to obtain accurate data, i.e., correct, complete, consistent and unambiguous information. This process sets all the characteristics to which the data must obey (El-Sappagh et al., 2011).
- **Load:** Load data into the DW is the last of the three steps of the ETL process. It loads information into DW, which is a data structure prepared to receive the previously extracted and processed data (El-Sappagh et al., 2011).

Data Warehouse

The main component of a BI system is a DW; a repository of data from different sources that stores information about an organization activities (Loshin, 2013). The DW can store and consolidate data in a valid and consistent format for each organization. It also allows users to analyze and explore the data using other tools. The DW enables the integration of different data from heterogeneous sources. This allows an analysis of dimensions (properties). For the reasons above, the databases of DW are considered multi-dimensional and object-oriented to facilitate the use of information, the object being the set of information about a particular process in an organization. In addition to object-oriented, a DW has the ability to integrate data, which is one of its main features. Thus, the process of data entry enables the elimination of inconsistencies (Park & Kim, 2013).

The DW only performs two different operations, which are inserting and querying data. Because the data is loaded in a large DW volume, upgrading is not executed regularly. It can then be said that the DW is not volatile, i.e., the data are not deleted or updated. But the rate at which data is loaded, varies depending on the needs of each organization (Park & Kim, 2013). The storage of relevant data from different sources and formats can improve the speed and efficiency of knowledge discovery process, which makes the decision-making more correct and quickly due to the greater amount of information (El-Sappagh et al., 2011; Prevedello et al., 2010).

The data stored in DW is consistent and is available for analysis by BI tools in order to extract information and generate reports to apply in the decision-making process. The DW differs from those operational databases, because they are integrated, organized by theme and vary over time, which means that each entry in the DW corresponds to a specific point of time, allowing the temporal analysis of the data. In addition, the DW size is larger than the data marts and allows OLAP, being essentially used for decision support (El-Sappagh et al., 2011). Unlike operating systems, the DW was not designed for a quick and efficient transaction process, but rather for quick access to information for analysis and reporting purposes (Popovič et al., 2012).

The DW organizes its information depending on the dimensional model that the user defines. This model being the better and more efficient method to represent the data (Loshin, 2013). There are several different dimensional models, but the most common are as follow:

- **Star Schema:** In the star schema model, all tables are directly related to a central table, called by fact table, the others being referred as dimension tables. These links occur between the primary keys of dimension tables and foreign keys of fact table. The dimension tables contain the description of the measured facts, and these attributes are often used to identify headers in query results. This model is called Star Schema since the fact table is surrounded by the dimension tables, resembling a star. The fact table is the main element of the model and represents the events used to measure performance and outcomes of processes (Chaudhuri et al., 2011; Soler et al., 2008). The Star Schema model is shown in Figure 2 and can be constituted by more tables but they all have to be attached to the fact table.
- **Snow Flake:** In this model, the dimension tables also relate to the fact table, but there are some dimensions that are not directly related to the fact table but related to other dimension tables, relating only between them. This purposes the normalization of dimension tables in order to reduce the space occupied by these tables. In the Snow Flake model, there are auxiliary dimension tables that standardize the main dimension tables. Building the database in this way, started to use more tables to represent the same dimensions, but occupying less disk space than the Star Schema model (Chaudhuri et al., 2011; Soler et al., 2008). In the Figure 3, the model demonstrated is the Snow Flake one given that the model may consist of more tables linked together.

Figure 2. Star Schema model of a DW

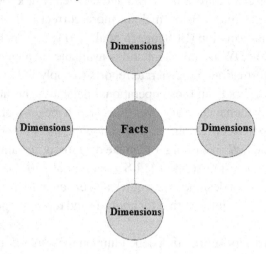

Figure 3. Snow Flake model of a DW

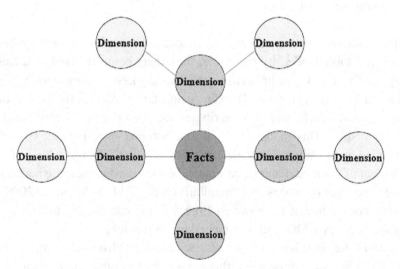

The Snow Flake model reduces the space required for storage of data, but increases the number of tables to the model, making it more complex. As more tables are used, the access to data through queries will be hampered and it will take longer to be implemented, i.e., data access is slower than the previous model.

On the other hand, the Star Schema model presents simpler and easier navigation through the software, but wastes space and can repeat the same descriptions along the boards.

Therefore, it is more advantageous to use a Star Schema model, because it provides a faster and easier access to data, creating auxiliary tables for specific dimensions only when strictly necessary, i.e., namely when it is shown a benefit to justify the loss of query performance, which is not so great depending on how the tables are built. That being said, most DW use Star Schema model for representation of the data (Kimball & Ross, 2002; Loshin, 2013; Pardillo et al., 2010).

In Figure 4 the architecture of a DW can be observed.

Data Mining

The DM in DB defines a process with a continuous set of activities that produce knowledge from DB. This set consists of five steps such as selection, pre-processing, processing, DM, and finally interpretation or evaluation (Heinrichs & Lim, 2003).

In the first step, there is a selection of key data to perform the DM. Secondly, comes pre-processing, including data cleaning and treating, in order to make them consistent and feasible for further processing. This cleaning process, also referred to as elimination of noise, noise reduction or elimination feature, can be made by ETL or other available techniques. According to the destination, the data is processed, this being the phase transformation. Finally, in the DM phase, the kind of result to be achieved and its purpose are defined. The interpretation or evaluation is the last step and consists in the interpretation and evaluation, as the name implies, of the patterns obtained. The validity of the results is checked by applying the standards found in new sets of data. In short, DM is the process of holding large amounts of data looking for consistent patterns as rules or time sequences, to detect relationships between information, thus finding new subsets of data (Heinrichs & Lim, 2003; Hema & Malik, 2011; PhridviRaj & GuruRao, 2014).

Figure 4. Architecture of a DW (Chaudhuri et al., 2011 Adapted)

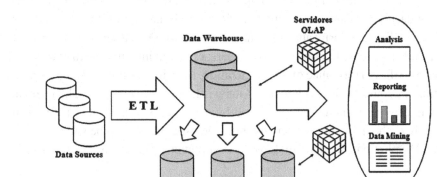

DM has evolved rapidly due to the introduction of new methods in various applications related to different fields including medicine (Heinrichs & Lim, 2003; PhridviRaj & GuruRao, 2014). As mentioned above, it is used to analyze the relationships between information and discover patterns from existing data. The main objective of DM is then to extract information from the data and make it understandable (Hema & Malik, 2011).

Pentaho Community

The software Pentaho Community was developed in 2004 by Pentaho Corporation and it consists in a BI tool that provides data integration, reporting, charts and dashboards based on data processing technologies. This software was created in the Java language and is the first with an open source version in the market of BI tools, this being the community edition version, but there is also another license, not free, which corresponds to the enterprise edition[2].

Most of the information presented by the Pentaho Community is shaped in dashboards that align the organization's strategy and the monitoring of their progress with the objectives of the different areas. The dashboards can have several uses ranging depending on the user. There are two types of dashboards: analytic and integral. The analytic allows obtaining reports and indicators from DM. This type of strategic dashboards are ways to analyze the areas surrounding unrelated environment, consisting in a query tool with the objective of presenting indicators (Sharma et al., 2012).

The BI tool, Pentaho Community, has different modules in the structure, among which, used in this work, CDE.

Pentaho CDE was created to simplify the processes of creating, editing and interpretation of dashboards. It is a powerful and complete tool that combines custom data sources and components with a visual interface to create a layout customized by the user, which can add several components from text boxes to graphics. These layouts of dashboards are simply created with a combination of rows and columns, *html* blocks, CSS, JavaScript and even images. Pentaho CDE has a graphical environment that allows access to information by users: essential information to understand and optimize the performance of an organization. Easy integration between Pentaho Reporting, Pentaho CDE and Pentaho Analysis modules is possible. The user can define the origins of the data represented by dashboards, that is, it is required to specify where the data comes from and how the user entails it to be shown[3].

The CDE plugin is divided into Layout, Components, Data Sources and Preview.

Layout

The layout section is defined by creating a framework for the user, formatting the dashboard structure through *html* code, allowing inserting functions in JavaScript or CSS. The CDE also has templates already defined that the user can choose to save time in creating the dashboard.

Components

It is in the components section that different components can be created and edited, to be inserted into the dashboard, and it is required in advance to assign a space for each component in the layout section. This section is divided into six categories, and it is through these that the user can choose the components that he wants to insert.

Data Sources

Each of these components, created in the previous section, will be associated with a DB in order to show its contents. This connection between the components and DB is made in this section, through which queries will only show the information that the user requires.

Preview

Finally, the preview section allows the users to preview the dashboard. However, for this to be possible, the user has to record the dashboard whenever making a change before the preview.

Advantages and Disadvantages of CDE

After the study of BI tools, it was possible to draw some conclusions regarding the module CDE of Pentaho Community such as:

- Flexible development options for the user;
- Allows connections to multiple data sources;
- The definition of the layout depends entirely on the user;
- Wide range of visual components, graphs, tables, text, selection, parameters, etc.;
- Interaction with the user in the solution itself;

- Share irreversibility;
- Do not need a DW, being chosen by the user to create one;
- Low technical documentation supporting the development.

CASE STUDY

This study applied data from CHP, a hospital in north of Portugal, covering thousands of people.

The Electronic Medical Prescription

The prescription of CDTP is a task of particular interest not only for screening of diseases but mainly in an attempt to find the cause of issues, presenting itself as a powerful task available to clinicians to the decision-making process and therefore the well-being of patients. The prescription of CDTP occupies a large percentage of consultation time, as well as a lot of the day-to-day of a healthcare professional. Thus, it is of major interest to minimize the time spent on prescription of CDTP, with a more rational and efficient use of all available resources to ensure the provision of healthcare with maximum efficiency and quality.

The generalization of the prescription process, in addition to promoting global dematerialization of the whole process of electronic prescribing and the adoption of electronic provision, also results in many benefits, for health professionals as well as users.

Among these benefits, there can be mentioned:

- Reduction in prescription errors;
- Orders placed in time;
- Streamlining and standardization of procedures;
- Reduced operating costs inherent in the process of prescribing CDTP.

Business Intelligence Platform

The business intelligence platform was developed in order to identify physicians who take longer in EMP processes. Nevertheless, to achieve this goal, the physicians' prescription time was not the only variable in study. It was also analyzed the number of requests among the numerous distinct specialties and sub-specialties, between

1st June 2013 and 31st March 2014. After the identification of these individuals, it was certainly essential to understand why such event occurs. One hypothesis is the unsuitable familiarization with the SAM platform that contains the application of CDTP prescription.

To obtain the final product of this study, the BI platform was carried out one series of steps, which are briefly described below.

Selection of Data

Understanding the data domain is the driver element to acquire knowledge in Database (DB), since existing knowledge can be complemented with the attained information in the discovery process. First of all, for this study, it was performed a selection and data collection at CHP, which required prior study to understand the outlook of this project so as to select the data you want to analyze, and finally collect them. The intent was to frame the dissertation project with the area of the organization, in this case the CHP, by defining the project goals, as well as acquiring fundamental concepts to perform it.

Before selecting the data, it is necessary to exploit it and understand it. However, access to tables does not imply that data is accessible to understanding the context of tables and the meaning of each attribute; hence, the need to understand all that is contained in the DB, since the designation of each table until the origin of the values of each attribute. After an understanding of the data, it will then be possible to select the relevant information to be used in the project.

Data Extraction

The data used in the study, corresponds to real data from CHP's DB, which was extracted after being selected. The application SAM aims to aid in medical activities allowing the integration of clinical applications, such as the EMP cited above. The SAM's DB contains various types of data spread across multiple tables.

Creating Tables

After the extraction of the CHP's data, the handling of DB was performed with Oracle SQL Developer, an integrated and free development environment. Several tables were created, with its primary keys and foreign keys. Subsequently, the data selected and extracted earlier, was loaded.

Creating Views

In order to create a Data Warehouse (DW), various views were built in aim to represent subsets of information existing in the created tables.

Data Warehouse

The finalization of DW was based essentially on SQL queries manipulation. After creating the views, they were loaded with the desired information. This step is carried out by crossing queries, shifting the data tables to views in order to obtain useful knowledge.

Platform Development

Initially, for the development of BI platform, it began by defining the structure in section layout of CDE (Community Dashboard Editor) from Pentaho Community, where is created a dashboard.

Then the best schemas were chosen to represent the information, which are bar graphs, point graphs and tables. Finally, so that these graphs contain information, it was necessary to establish a link between the data and the platform. That is, a connection between Oracle SQL Developer, to create queries, and module CDE of Pentaho Community.

Knowledge Extraction

During the study, it was performed the knowledge extraction (KE), in tables or graphs, from the platform built using the Pentaho Community software. This extraction was executed on the CDTP prescription orders, which allowed a better analysis and a broader view of the CHP's prescription service, in order to generate knowledge. This KE was carried out using the Oracle SQL Developer software. The aim is to analyze, through indicators, the average time registration for prescription of CDTP between the beginning of June 2013 and the end of March 2014. The indicators analyzed are:

- Number of requests by specialty;
- Number of requests by subspecialty;
- Number of requests by specialty per day;
- Average time tasks by subspecialty;

- Average time of each task by specialty and physician;
- Requests of CDTP by specialty;
- Requests of CDTP by physician.

Subspecialty relates to groups where each specialty is divided. It analyzed the average time applications in seconds and minutes, as well as the average time of tasks, knowing that a request may or may not have tasks. These analyzes are all made in seconds. Next, we analyzed the relationship between the time of application and the number of requests, time of the tasks and the number of applications. And, finally, it is possible to obtain the percentage of time that a physician uses in completing tasks on demand. This percentage value is obtained by the average ratio of the average of the tasks and applications. It should be noted that the analysis done by subspecialty is also made by physician. Ultimately, it allows identifying the physicians who spend more time in prescribing CDTP.

Comparison with Existing Studies

In the last years, a panoply of BI applications have been developed through BI tools, which are designed to store, retrieve, analyze, transform and present data for BI. In short, it corresponds to the analysis of data in order to provide useful information. The insertion of BI tools in healthcare environments assists managers and health professionals though decision-making, improving healthcare quality, safety, efficiency and delivery. These BI tools include spreadsheets, reporting and querying software, OLAP, digital dashboards, data mining, data warehousing and local information systems. In the market, there is a large set of application software that have been used to build BI applications including TACTIC, JasperReport, Zoho Reports, Palo, Tableau Software, BIRT and Pentaho, just to name a few.

The choice of the BI tool to use is an important decision which depends on what data is going to be analysed and how, so it can be provided with the right kinds of tools. Some of the basic needs that must be considered in the choice of a BI tool include speed, the kind of breadth expected out of the BI application and its usability, among others.

It is worth noting that the use of BI tools by industry widespread among all fields including engineering, mathematics, economics, computer science and, as already mentioned, healthcare. For instance, BI open-source tools were already applied in the field of Radiology to create a prototype model of a data warehouse for BI (Prevedello et al., 2010) and an HIV BI tool was used to provide a reporting system for population indicators, being an effective tool to monitor and further impact the epidemic (Snyder et al., 2014).

RESULTS

In this section, some of the results of the various case studies conducted through the platform are presented. They were obtained with the module CDE of Pentaho Community, which is a tool through which it is possible to treat and analyze data in order to provide useful information to extract knowledge and assist in decision-making. Several indicators were tested and they are displayed in the form of title's section of this chapter.

Number of Requests by Specialty

The chart in Figure 5 indicates to the platform users the amount of CDTP requests made in the period between 1st June 2013 and 31st March 2014, by specialty. Analyzing the graph, it shows that, during this period, applications of ten different specialties were made. If the study was carried out in a shorter time interval some of these specialty applications would not exist, and the number of graph bars would be lower. It can be verified that the radiology specialty, is, without any doubt, the one that has made most requests, with 37,614 requests. In contrast, the specialties of physiatry and genetics have only 18 and 6 requests, respectively.

Number of Requests for Subspecialty

In addition to the analysis of the number of requests by specialty, it was further done a more detailed analysis of the amount of orders. Therefore, it was used another indicator: the number of requests per subspecialty. This analysis was realized since

Figure 5. Number of requests by specialty

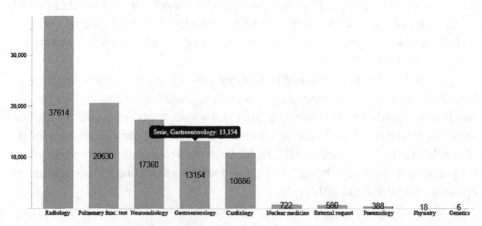

a specialty may or may not be divided into others, as can be seen in the table of Figure 6, where the cardiology specialty is divided into six different subspecialties, being noninvasive arrhythmology, echocardiography, electrocardiography, hemodynamics, pacing and electrophysiology, and HJU. While the specialty of physiatry, for instance, has none. As can be seen, more than 60 CDTP requests have been registered per subspecialties.

Number of Requests by Specialty per Day

To study the amount of orders per day, it was created a picker, which allows the platform users to choose the day, between 1st June 2013 and 31st March 2014 to get the information. The number of bars also varies depending on the chosen days. In the example, the picker is on July 7, 2013, as shown in Figure 7. In this graph,

Figure 6. Number of requests for subspecialty

SubSpecialty	NRequests
Cardiology - Noninvasive arrhythmology	732
Cardiology - Echocardiography	7146
Cardiology - Electrocardiography	1878
Cardiology - Hemodynamics	982
Cardiology - Pacing and electrophysiology	90
Cardiology - HJU	58
Genetics	6
Physiatry	18
Gastroenterology - Biofeedback	30
Gastroenterology - Liver biopsy	104

Show 10 entries   Search:

Showing 1 to 10 of 64 entries

Figure 7. Number of requests by specialty per day

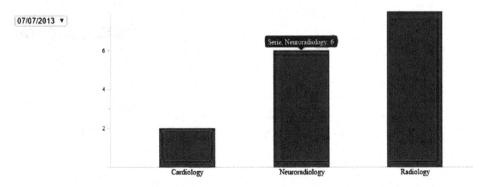

only CDTP of three different specialties were prescribed: cardiology with two applications, neuroradiology, and finally radiology with eight applications. Moving the cursor over the bars, the platform identifies the number of applications for the specialty in question. In this case, on July 7, 2013, six applications of neuroradiology specialty were recorded.

Average Time Tasks by Subspecialty

Each request of CDTP may or may not require health professionals to fill forms at each prescription. This process, which involves filling out surveys or forms, is called task. An application may have no associated task, only one, or can have several tasks. Therefore, an indicator was created to analyze the average time of the tasks for each of the subspecialties. This information is presented on the dot plot in Figure 8 where each dot represents a subspecialty.

Due to the high amount of subspecialties analysis, the names of each subspecialty overlap in the x-axis, preventing the user to see them. In order to understand the information and extract useful knowledge, the user can explore the various points with the cursor, and the platform will show both the subspecialty as well as the average time of the tasks. As this procedure can be unpractical, the table shown on Figure 9 was built. That being said, the graph presented in Figure 8 shows that the tasks of echocardiography cardiology specialty takes an average of 56.3 seconds to be performed. All this information is represented in a readable way in the table of

Figure 8. Average time tasks by subspecialty

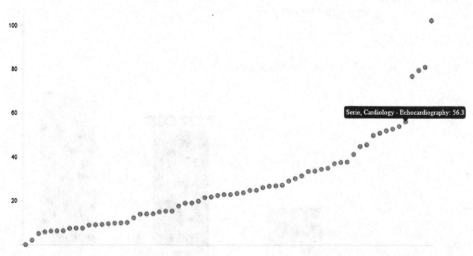

Figure 9. Average time tasks by subspecialty

SubSpecialty	AverageTime
Gastroenterology - HJU	125.6
Neuroradiology - Computed tomography	115.9
Cardiology - Hemodynamics	100.2
Gastroenterology - C.P.R.E.	95.5
Neuroradiology - Doppler ultrasound	94.9
Neuroradiology - Magnetic resonance imaging	92.7
Radiology - Computed tomography	91.9
Radiology/Neuroradiology - Magnetic resonance imaging	91.1
Gastroenterology - Liver biopsy	90.5
Gastroenterology - Upper endoscopy	90

Show 10 entries — Search: — Showing 1 to 10 of 76 entries

Figure 9, which identifies the subspecialty and the average time of the tasks associated with it. This table is sorted descendingly by the time consumption that every subspecialty spends carrying out its tasks.

It can be seen that the request whose tasks take, on average, more time to perform, refers to the specialty of gastroenterology and request for HJU.

Average Time of Each Task by Subspecialty and Physician

The following study is certainly the most relevant for this project. Through indicator analysis, the average time of each task by specialty and physician shows which physicians devote more time in the prescription process, compared to their colleagues who prescribe the same requests. Thereafter, a few examples will be presented, but the platform has the ability to analyze more than 60 different requests for various specialties.

Again, the platform uses a picker, where the user has the option of subspecialty, as can be seen in Figure 10.

For example, in the chart represented in Figure 10, where physicians who prescribed one pacing and electrophysiology are analyzed, it can be seen that there are clearly two physicians who take longer than their colleagues to prescribe the same examination of cardiology specialty. These two individuals are identifiable through their ID's, but for confidentiality reasons, they cannot be revealed. However, it is easily noticeable that they are, from left to right, the first and the sixth individuals, respectively. As already mentioned, it is possible to move the cursor to a desired point of the graphic and get information. It appears that the selected physician spends an average of 45.3 seconds on the performance of the tasks of pacing and electrophysiology.

Figure 10. Average time tasks by specialty and physician

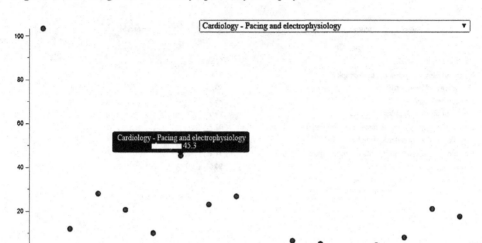

For examinations prescribed more often, the number of physicians who prescribe them is also higher. Thus, due to the large number of physicians who prescribe these tests, their ID's overlap in the x-axis, which makes it difficult to identify them, unless moving the cursor to the point where it is desired to get information. For this reason, once again, apart from the graph, a table that easily identifies the ID and the meantime was created, which is presented in Figure 11. This table is provided with a picker for the user to select the desired subspecialty. The average times are already ordered from highest to lowest, since the goal is to identify those that, on average, need more time in the prescription process.

Figure 11. Average time tasks by physician

Show 10 ▼ entries	Search:	Radiology - Computed tomography ▼
IDPhysician ⇕	**AverageTime** ⇕	
	704.3	
	573.5	
	445	
	377	
	325	
	298	
	216.8	
	186	
	184	
	179.5	

Showing 1 to 10 of 540 entries

Requests of CDTP by Specialty

In Figure 12, it is presented a detailed analysis of the average time in the log CDTP between 1st June 2013 and 31st March 2014. In this table the analysis is done by specialty, containing information on: the number of applications for each service; the total time spent in the prescription of all cases; the total time of the tasks of those requests; the average time in seconds of applications and tasks, respectively; the percentage of time that is spent on tasks during the prescription process; and finally, the total time applications in minutes, rounded to units.

Only to the top ten applications, it is possible to notice that electrocardiography is the request that occurs more often, with 9645 records. Despite being the examination with the greatest number of requests, the echocardiography, with only 5557 applications, takes longer to be prescribed, as the total time of applications of echocardiography is superior to the electrocardiographs. For the tasks' execution time, once again, echocardiography presents the highest total time, although it is not the examination with the greatest number of applications. Thus, it can be concluded from this information that applications for echocardiography involve filling in more forms than requests for electrocardiographs.

On the other hand, the prescription of liver biopsy, the gastroenterology specialty, takes longer in the forms of prescription. For about 22% of the time the prescription is spent in performing the tasks.

Figure 12. Average time on registration of CDTP by specialty

Specialty	SubSpecialty	NRequests	Time Requests (seg.)	Time Tasks (seg.)	AverageTime Request	AverageTime Task	% Tasks	Time Requests (min.)
Cardiology	Cardiology - Hemodynamics	793	116453	13250	146.85	16.71	11.378	1941
Cardiology	Cardiology - Pacing and electrophysiology	105	8160	328	77.71	3.12	4.02	136
Cardiology	Cardiology - HJU	248	4375	489	17.64	1.97	11.177	73
Cardiology	Cardiology - Electrocardiography	9645	103615	9858	10.74	1.02	9.514	1727
Cardiology	Cardiology - Noninvasive arrhythmology	2953	42035	2583	14.23	0.87	6.145	701
Cardiology	Cardiology - Echocardiography	5557	432083	36850	77.75	6.63	8.528	7201
Physiatry	Physiatry	1745	132	19	0.08	0.01	14.394	2
Gastroenterology	Gastroenterology - Liver biopsy	53	8712	1890	164.38	35.66	21.694	145
Gastroenterology	Gastroenterology - HJU	565	68139	5060	120.6	8.96	7.426	1136
Gastroenterology	Gastroenterology - Functional anorectal disorders	120	6145	727	51.21	6.06	11.831	102

Show 10 ▼ entries   Search:

Showing 1 to 10 of 64 entries

Requests of CDTP by Physician

In Figure 13, a detailed analysis is presented, which corresponds to the average time of a CDTP registration by a physician, between 1st June 2013 and 31st March 2014. As shown in Figure 12, this is the same information about the number of requests, but this time for each physician.

As can be seen, in this period, requests were prescribed for more than 40,000 physicians, bearing in mind that a physician prescribes various applications, i.e., that does not mean that there are over 40,000 health professionals. Although, in the example shown, all physicians have prescribed noninvasive arrhythmologys (cardiology specialty), some have superior times.

For instance, the third doctor presented prescribed 16 noninvasive arrythmologys, all in a total of 201 seconds, which amounts to an average of 13 seconds per request. Compared to their colleagues, this physician is much less time consuming than, for example, the sixth physician in the table that takes 53 seconds on average per request. This is not to say that the fastest physician is more effective in the electronic prescription process. On the contrary, it is shown that the faster individual has a percentage value of task below 1%, while the term used for comparison in

Figure 13. Average time on registration of CDTP by physician

Physician	SubSpecialty	NRequests	Time Requests (seg.)	Time Tasks (seg.)	AverageTime Request	AverageTime Task	% Tasks	Time Requests (min.)
	Cardiology - Noninvasive arrhythmology	4	174	8	44	2	4.598	3
	Cardiology - Noninvasive arrhythmology	2	242	3	121	2	1.24	4
	Cardiology - Noninvasive arrhythmology	16	201	2	13	0	0.995	3
	Cardiology - Noninvasive arrhythmology	4	163	7	41	2	4.294	3
	Cardiology - Noninvasive arrhythmology	2	421	10	211	5	2.375	7
	Cardiology - Noninvasive arrhythmology	2	105	8	53	4	7.819	2
	Cardiology - Noninvasive arrhythmology	4	55	7	14	2	12.727	1
	Cardiology - Noninvasive arrhythmology	6	111	17	19	3	15.315	2
	Cardiology - Noninvasive arrhythmology	4	143	6	36	2	4.196	2
	Cardiology - Noninvasive arrhythmology	4	401	10	100	3	2.494	7

Show 10 entries   Search:

Showing 1 to 10 of 40,107 entries

this example is about 8%. These values may cast doubt on the third doctor of the list, because only approximately 1% of the prescription of time is devoted to tasks. The question that arises is: does this physician correctly fills all matters of forms?

DISCUSSION

With a review of the audit platform for their potential users, it is possible identifying physicians who spend more time in CDTP prescription process. With that being said, it is also achievable identifying the reasons which cause those physicians to perform, on average, a lower number of consultations within a period of time. This is of upmost importance since the prescription is an existing task in much of the consultations carried out in this country. With the extracted information through the platform, the organization's administrators can make decisions such as imposing the optimization of the prescription process. Reducing the prescription time, they will be able to reduce the time of the consultations, consequently. On the other hand, to decrease the time of a query, physicians will be able to give more consultations a day, which will bring benefits to consumers, as the waiting times decrease. In addition, consultations, in private health organizations, are most likely to reduce their costs, which is another considerable advantage for users.

Nonetheless, the platform SAM, which owns the EMP platform, is minimally evaluated since, in addition to the prescription platform, it has many other features. Nevertheless, this evaluation is done through an analysis with the aim to improve through the implementation of changes.

CONCLUSION AND FUTURE RESEARCH

Nowadays, it is essential on the part of all organizations the use of ICT in their services. These technologies are provided with automated mechanisms for data processing. The use of BI systems allows users to access the right information in the shortest time possible, making effective decisions, correcting processes and anticipating the needs of the institutions.

It is important to note that the use of EHR systems encompasses several groups of professionals in a hospital setting. Thus, such systems should be developed to meet their requirements, developing the interaction between all healthcare providers, and presenting itself as an improvement and benefit in the workplace.

The use of a BI system for the construction of a platform has proved to be useful in knowledge extraction process. In addition, the platform itself has several advantages, among which the decrease in the prescription process and consequently the reduction of appointment duration (after the decision-making by managers of health organizations). This means that it is possible to perform more queries per day, i.e., the productivity of physicians' increases and reduce waiting lists, which will probably lower the cost of these same queries.

After the development of the platform, it is clear that it will bring plenty of benefits such as the time decrease of the prescription process and, consequently, the reduction of appointment duration. Ultimately, this means that it is possible to perform more consultations a day, which probably will lower the consultations' cost, i.e., it follows that you can improve and make more efficient the entire process of EMP.

Future Work

As future work, it is suggested to analyze the forms associated with each request (i.e. to examine the issues of jobs and consequently analyze the responses of health professionals) as there may be physicians who, even in mandatory, do not answer questions in the most correct way, which may cause the times of the tasks and applications to decrease. Consequently, the below average physicians, identified as outliers by this platform, may even be those who respond to all questions of the form, and correctly.

It is suggested to even perform fieldwork, and measure the times of applications and tasks in the very act of limitation, in the query. Most likely because, while the doctor is making his request for the CDTP, he will not be completely focused on completing the tasks since he could, for instance, be talking to the patient. That is, the process of prescription requests and the tasks will not be continuous, which makes the results a less viable platform since the data is measured automatically. Hence, it is important to perform measurements on the ground, to get a sense of the times and the physicians that the platform points out as the most accurate.

On the other hand, it is also possible to study the self-limitation platform SAM, in order to predict potential improvements. Nonetheless, it may be needed to reformulate the questions of the various tasks, as there may be questions difficult to interpret, even by health professionals, as they may be interfering with time spent on the EMP process. After following these suggestions, it can be possible to ascertain with any certainty who the slowest physicians are in prescribing CDTP.

Moreover, it could be interesting to execute this same study but with other BI tools or explore more features of Pentaho Community.

Finally, it is believed that, using as a basis the work presented throughout this dissertation and considering the proposals submitted previously, it is possible to improve the efficiency of the entire EMP of CDTP process.

ACKNOWLEDGMENT

This work is funded by National Funds through the FCT - *Fundação para a Ciência e Tecnologia* (Portuguese Foundation for Science and Technology) - within project PEst-OE/EEI/UI0752/2014.

REFERENCES

Allison, J. J., Wall, T. C., Spettell, C. M., Calhoun, J., Fargason, C. A., Kobylinski, R. W., & Kiefe, C. et al. (2000). The art and science of chart review. *The Joint Commission Journal on Quality Improvement*, *26*, 115–136. PMID:10709146

Ammenwerth, E., Schnell-Inderst, P., Machan, C., & Siebert, U. (2008). The Effect of Electronic Prescribing on Medication Errors and Adverse Drug Events: A Systematic Review. *Journal of the American Medical Informatics Association : JAMIA*, *15*(5), 585–600. doi:10.1197/jamia.M2667 PMID:18579832

Bonney, W. (2013). Applicability of Business Intelligence in Electronic Health Record. *Procedia: Social and Behavioral Sciences*, *73*, 257–262. doi:10.1016/j.sbspro.2013.02.050

Cassidy, L. D., Marsh, G. M., Holleran, M. K., & Ruhl, L. S. (2002). Methodology to improve data quality from chart review in the managed care setting. *The American Journal of Managed Care*, *8*, 787–793. PMID:12234019

Chaudhuri, S., Dayal, U., & Narasayya, V. (2011). An overview of business intelligence technology. *Communications of the ACM*, *54*(8), 88. doi:10.1145/1978542.1978562

Chiasson, M., Reddy, M., Kaplan, B., & Davidson, E. (2007). Expanding multi-disciplinary approaches to healthcare information technologies: What does information systems offer medical informatics? *International Journal of Medical Informatics*, *76*, 89–97. doi:10.1016/j.ijmedinf.2006.05.010 PMID:16769245

Duarte, J., Portela, C. F., Abelha, A., Machado, J., & Santos, M. F. (2011). Electronic health record in dermatology service. In *Communications in Computer and Information Science* (Vol. 221, pp. 156–164). CCIS; doi:10.1007/978-3-642-24352-3_17

Eder, C., Fullerton, J., Benroth, R., & Lindsay, S. P. (2005). Pragmatic strategies that enhance the reliability of data abstracted from medical records. *Applied Nursing Research*, *18*(1), 50–54. doi:10.1016/j.apnr.2004.04.005 PMID:15812736

El-Sappagh, S. H. A., Hendawi, A. M. A., & El Bastawissy, A. H. (2011). A proposed model for data warehouse ETL processes. *Journal of King Saud University - Computer and Information Sciences*. doi:10.1016/j.jksuci.2011.05.005

Gearing, R. E., & Mian, I. a, Barber, J., & Ickowicz, A. (2006). A methodology for conducting retrospective chart review research in child and adolescent psychiatry. *Journal de l'Académie Canadienne de Psychiatrie de L'enfant et de L'adolescent* [Journal of the Canadian Academy of Child and Adolescent Psychiatry], *15*, 126–34. Retrieved from http://www.pubmedcentral.nih.gov/articlerender.fcgi?artid=2277255&tool=pmcentrez&rendertype=abstract

Glaser, J., & Stone, J. (2008). Effective use of business intelligence. *Healthcare Financial Management : Journal of the Healthcare Financial Management Association*, *62*, 68–72. PMID:18309596

Gregory, K. E., & Radovinsky, L. (2012). Research strategies that result in optimal data collection from the patient medical record. *Applied Nursing Research*, *25*(2), 108–116. doi:10.1016/j.apnr.2010.02.004 PMID:20974093

Hasman, A. (1998). Education and health informatics. International Journal of Medical Informatics, 52(1-3), 209–216. doi:10.1016/S1386-5056(98)90133-3

Heeks, R. (2006). Health information systems: Failure, success and improvisation. *International Journal of Medical Informatics*, *75*(2), 125–137. doi:10.1016/j.ijmedinf.2005.07.024 PMID:16112893

Heinrichs, J. H., & Lim, J. S. (2003). Integrating web-based data mining tools with business models for knowledge management. *Decision Support Systems*, *35*(1), 103–112. doi:10.1016/S0167-9236(02)00098-2

Hema, R., & Malik, N. (2011). *Data Mining and Business Intelligence*. Bvicamacin.

Kawado, M., Hinotsu, S., Matsuyama, Y., Yamaguchi, T., Hashimoto, S., & Ohashi, Y. (2003). A comparison of error detection rates between the reading aloud method and the double data entry method. *Controlled Clinical Trials*, *24*(5), 560–569. doi:10.1016/S0197-2456(03)00089-8 PMID:14500053

Kimball, R., & Ross, M. (2002). *The data warehouse toolkit: the complete guide to dimensional modelling*. New York: Wiley. doi:10.1145/945721.945741

Loshin, D. (2013). Business Intelligence: The Savvy Manager's Guide. Morgan Kaufmann. Retrieved from http://scholar.google.com/scholar?hl=en&btnG=Search&q=intitle:Business+Intelligence:+The+Savvy+Manager's+Guide#4

Mettler, T., & Vimarlund, V. (2009). Understanding business intelligence in the context of healthcare. *Health Informatics Journal*, *15*(3), 254–264. doi:10.1177/1460458209337446 PMID:19713399

Munyisia, E. N., Yu, P., & Hailey, D. (2011). The changes in caregivers' perceptions about the quality of information and benefits of nursing documentation associated with the introduction of an electronic documentation system in a nursing home. *International Journal of Medical Informatics*, *80*(2), 116–126. doi:10.1016/j.ijmedinf.2010.10.011 PMID:21242104

Murray, M. D., Smith, F. E., Fox, J., Teal, E. Y., Kesterson, J. G., Stiffler, T. A., & McDonald, C. J. et al. (2003). Structure, functions, and activities of a research support informatics section. *Journal of the American Medical Informatics Association*, *10*(4), 389–398. doi:10.1197/jamia.M1252 PMID:12668695

Pan, L., Fergusson, D., Schweitzer, I., & Hebert, P. C. (2005). Ensuring high accuracy of data abstracted from patient charts: The use of a standardized medical record as a training tool. *Journal of Clinical Epidemiology*, *58*(9), 918–923. doi:10.1016/j.jclinepi.2005.02.004 PMID:16085195

Pardillo, J., Mazón, J. N., & Trujillo, J. (2010). Extending OCL for OLAP querying on conceptual multidimensional models of data warehouses. *Information Sciences*, *180*(5), 584–601. doi:10.1016/j.ins.2009.11.006

Park, T., & Kim, H. (2013). A data warehouse-based decision support system for sewer infrastructure management. *Automation in Construction*, *30*, 37–49. doi:10.1016/j.autcon.2012.11.017

Paul, J., Seib, R., & Prescott, T. (2005). The internet and clinical trials: Background, online resources, examples and issues. *Journal of Medical Internet Research*, *7*(1), e5. doi:10.2196/jmir.7.1.e5 PMID:15829477

Pavlović, I., Kern, T., & Miklavčič, D. (2009). Comparison of paper-based and electronic data collection process in clinical trials: Costs simulation study. *Contemporary Clinical Trials*, *30*(4), 300–316. doi:10.1016/j.cct.2009.03.008 PMID:19345286

PhridviRaj, M. S. B., & GuruRao, C. V. (2014). Data Mining – Past, Present and Future – A Typical Survey on Data Streams. *Procedia Technology*, *12*, 255–263. doi:10.1016/j.protcy.2013.12.483

Popovič, A., Hackney, R., Coelho, P. S., & Jaklič, J. (2012). Towards business intelligence systems success: Effects of maturity and culture on analytical decision making. *Decision Support Systems, 54*(1), 729–739. doi:10.1016/j.dss.2012.08.017

Powsner, S. M., Wyatt, J. C., & Wright, P. (1998). Opportunities for and challenges of computerisation. *Lancet, 352*(9140), 1617–1622. doi:10.1016/S0140-6736(98)08309-3 PMID:9843122

Prevedello, L. M., Andriole, K. P., Hanson, R., Kelly, P., & Khorasani, R. (2010). Business intelligence tools for radiology: Creating a prototype model using open-source tools. *Journal of Digital Imaging, 23*(2), 133–141. doi:10.1007/s10278-008-9167-3 PMID:19011943

Rossi, M., Campbell, K. L., & Ferguson, M. (2014). Implementation of the nutrition care process and international dietetics and nutrition terminology in a single-center hemodialysis unit: Comparing paper vs electronic records. *Journal of the Academy of Nutrition and Dietetics, 114*(1), 124–130. doi:10.1016/j.jand.2013.07.033 PMID:24161368

Saleem, J. J., Russ, A. L., Justice, C. F., Hagg, H., Ebright, P. R., Woodbridge, P. A., & Doebbeling, B. N. (2009). Exploring the persistence of paper with the electronic health record. *International Journal of Medical Informatics, 78*(9), 618–628. doi:10.1016/j.ijmedinf.2009.04.001 PMID:19464231

Sharma, S., Osei-Bryson, K.-M., & Kasper, G. M. (2012). Evaluation of an integrated Knowledge Discovery and Data Mining process model. *Expert Systems with Applications, 39*(13), 11335–11348. doi:10.1016/j.eswa.2012.02.044

Snyder, L., Mcewen Dean, L., Davidson, A., Thrun, M., Mccormick, E., & Mettenbrink, J. C. (2014). Integrating Data into Meaningful HIV Indicators Using Business Intelligence. *2014 Council of State and Territorial Epidemiologists Annual Conference.*

Soler, E., Trujillo, J., Fernández-Medina, E., & Piattini, M. (2008). Building a secure star schema in data warehouses by an extension of the relational package from CWM. *Computer Standards & Interfaces, 30*(6), 341–350. doi:10.1016/j.csi.2008.03.002

Tavakoli, N., Jahanbakhsh, M., Mokhtari, H., & Tadayon, H. R. (2011). Opportunities of electronic health record implementation in Isfahan. Procedia Computer Science (Vol. 3, pp. 1195–1198). doi:10.1016/j.procs.2010.12.193

Waegemann, C. (2003). EHR vs. CPR vs. EMR. *Healthcare Informatics Online.*

Worster, A., & Haines, T. (2004). Advanced Statistics: Understanding Medical Record Review (MRR) Studies. *Academic Emergency Medicine*, *11*(2), 187–192. doi:10.1111/j.1553-2712.2004.tb01433.x PMID:14759964

ADDITIONAL READING

Coiera, E., Westbrook, J., & Wyatt, J. (2006). The safety and quality of decision support systems. *Yearbook of Medical Informatics*, 2006, 20–25. PMID:17051290

Fayyad, U., Piatetsky-shapiro, G., & Smyth, P. (1996). *Data Mining and Knowledge Discovery*, *17*(3), 37–54.

Ferreira, J., Miranda, M., Abelha, A., & Machado, J. (2010). O Processo ETL em Sistemas Data Warehouse. *INForum 2010 - II Simpósio de Informática* (pp. 757–765).

Inmon, W. H. (2002). *Building the Data Warehouse* (3rd ed.). New York, NY, USA: John Wiley & Sons, Inc.

Koh, H. C., & Tan, G. (2005). Data mining applications in healthcare. *Journal of Healthcare Information Management : JHIM*, *19*(2), 64–72. PMID:15869215

KEY TERMS AND DEFINITIONS

Business Intelligence (BI): Set of technologies capable of treating and analyzing data in order to present relevant and strategic information, helpful in the decision-making process of an organization.

Data Mining (DM): Process of discovering interesting and relevant patterns in large datasets.

Data Warehouse (DW): Component of a BI system that stores and consolidates data into a valid and consistent format and allows the analysis and exploration of that data using other tools.

Electronic Health Record (EHR): HIS that covers the different services and units of a healthcare institution and consists of a set of standardized documents for the registration of the medical procedures provided to a particular patient.

Extraction, Transformation and Load (ETL): Process that transforms and converts data coming from several sources to a unified format, fitted to the DW schema where these data will be stored.

ENDNOTES

1   http://www.min-saude.pt/portal
2   http://www.pentaho.com/product/product-overview; http://www.pentaho.com/solutions/healthcare
3   http://www.webdetails.pt/ctools/cde/

Chapter 12
Clinical Business Intelligence to Prevent Stroke Accidents

Nuno Gonçalves
University of Minho, Portugal

Cesar Quintas
Centro Hospitalar do Porto, Portugal

José Machado
University of Minho, Portugal

ABSTRACT

Stroke is considered the third main cause of death among all population, without distinguishing genders, led by heart diseases in first place. In other hand, despite representing a significant number of mortality, these diseases are the causes for a long-term disability in all countries with a vast recovery time going parallel with its costs. However, leaving aside this facts, stokes and heath diseases can also be easily prevented considering the outcome. This paper presents a new methodology to prevent these events to happen by using segmentation methods, which allows distinguishing and aggregating clusters of historical records, classification methods, such as Artificial Neural Networks, capable of classifying a new record according to its distribution among the clusters. A Multi-Agent Case Based Reasoning system is also proposed to evaluate solutions based in a similar case.

DOI: 10.4018/978-1-4666-9882-6.ch012

1. INTRODUCTION

Stroke is a blood supply interruption that occurs in the brain. This interruption happens when an artery, which is a blood vessel responsible for carrying the blood, is blocked, causing an ischaemic stroke, or bursts, causing an haemorrhagic stroke. Being a major factor related with mortality this disease is also closely followed with the main purpose of preventing it from happen since, when diagnosed, it becomes less dangerous and more treatable comparing with other similar diseases. There are several risk factors associated with stroke, however there are those who represent a major influence relating this event. Some risk factors can be treated or controlled like high blood pressure, as being a leading cause of stroke and the most controllable risk factor, cigarette smoking, the nicotine and carbon monoxide can damage the cardiovascular system therefore can augment the probability of stroke, diabetes mellitus, having this kind of diabetes also increases the risk of stroke since can cause blood vessels diseases, high blood cholesterol, being the main cause of ischaemic strokes, and physical inactivity. Despite this risk factors there are those who can't be controlled such as age, older people have more tendency to stroke, gender, stroke is more common in men then in women though more women die from strokes than men, and the mere fact of having suffered a previous stroke represents an increased risk factor not controlled by any means. Knowing this risk factors is already is an advantage if well considered and treat when so. Consequently this document emphasis the cluster prediction of a giving record, according with an historical dataset with different cases of stroke, which is used to retrieve a similar case from a Case Based Reasoning Multi-Agent System. Yet, the objective is not to predict if an input, composed of several symptoms, will suffers from a stroke or not but in case it does retrieve a better treatment according with similarity among other records. Supporting this decision process is a logic programing based approach to knowledge and reasoning with a special focus on the Degree of Confidence defined by a mathematical expression with a normalization background.

2. METHODOLOGY

Previously mentioned throughout this analysis there are three kinds of concepts that are worth to understand and explain. The concept behind this system is to identify clusters in a multi-agent system. Each agent has its own data knowledge, making them different from each other, which affects the decision support during case processing. The first method applied to every agent's dataset it's a cluster method. This method involves the identification e segmentation of identical records given, or not, an attribute to relate in a distance function. Hence, a cluster is a group of records identical between them and consequently different among other groups. Once segmented, each record is associated with its corresponding cluster, defining the class attribute in the record. The second methodology consists in a classification technique using Artificial Neural Networks. This ANN receives n tuples, where n is the number of inputs, and each tuple is composed with three measures where one of them is the Degree of Confidence of the corresponding input. The purpose of this method is to classify the new symptom with a number of cluster with a model generated based on the data knowledge of each agent. This methodology integrates the first step of the Case Based Reasoning allowing the system to identify with more accuracy clusters with similar cases. The retrieved case is obtained with the application of a mathematical expression calculating the similarity within the cluster. After this process the system is able to present the user a solution suiting, as close as possible, a similar treatment which can make a difference on the patient's recovery.

3. KNOWLEDGE REPRESENTATION

In this approach we represent data in two different ways, understandable to the user and normalized increasing classification performance. This views allows perception at different levels improving the retrieval of significant cases to be applied as relevant, or not, to a case study. There are a few main aspects that must be drilled in other to understand attributes influence and their importance in this approach.

Attribute Analysis

The dataset holds information about risk factors considered critical in the prediction and diagnosis of stroke disease. Composed by fifteen attributes this multivariate dataset has 1899 records with missing values. As the table I shows, attributes data type can be numeric or nominal and all of them must have a corresponding domain. Intervals are represented with a new attribute where new attribute's name is a merge of the attribute's name to represent and "Range".

Symptoms aggregate a variety of attributes, who can be characterized by their occurrence in the symptom. Focusing in real scenarios attributes can be optional or defined by an interval within its domain. Domains are set according with requirements analysis, considering their ranges, maximum and minimum, with the population and some standards pre-defined by health specialists. Hence, a given attribute can be defined in four different ways. Attributes with numeric values can be represented as

$$x \in [a,b] \tag{1}$$

Table 1. Identification and attribute features

Attribute	Description	Data Type	Min	Max
Name	Patient's name	Nominal	-	-
Gender	Patient's gender	Nominal	0	1
Age	Patient's age (min)	Numeric	0	100
Age Range	Patient's age (max >Age)	Numeric	0	100
Hypertension	Is hypertensive	Nominal	0	1
Headache	Has headache	Nominal	0	1
Diabetes	Has mellitus diabetes	Nominal	0	1
Activity	Physical activity frequency	Nominal	0	100
Smoker	Is smoker	Nominal	0	1
Systolic	Systolic pressure (min)	Numeric	70	200
Systolic Range	Systolic pressure (max >= Systolic)	Numeric	70	200
Previous Stroke	Had previous stroke	Nominal	0	1
Medication	Taking any medication	Nominal	0	1
Cholesterol HDL	HDL cholesterol value (min)	Numeric	20	90
Cholesterol HDL Range	HDL cholesterol value (max >= Cholesterol HDL)	Numeric	20	90
Cholesterol LDL	LDL cholesterol value (min)	Numeric	50	250
Cholesterol LDL Range	LDL cholesterol value (max, >= Cholesterol LDL)	Numeric	50	250
Cholesterol Tri	Triglycerides cholesterol value (min)	Numeric	90	600
Cholesterol Tri Range	Triglycerides cholesterol value (max, >= Cholesterol Tri)	Numeric	90	600
Vomiting	Has vomiting	Nominal	0	1

Attributes with nominal or interval values with are represented as

$$[x,y] \subseteq [a,b], a < x < y \wedge y < b \tag{2}$$

Finally attributes unknown are represented as

$$\perp = [a,b] \tag{3}$$

Normalization

Frequently data provided or obtained are incomplete, with noise (values with wrong values), the simple fact that it is not significant or needed for analysis attributes with low predictive influence, besides data inconsistency. These data are designated as raw data with a level of quality that can be improved using some techniques. Compared with a typical data mining process this method would be incorporated in data transformation since all previous phases were already validated phase.

Normalization is particularly useful for classification algorithms involving neural networks and its main purpose is to map data according with a certain scale. Therefore, this system has implemented a *Min-Max* normalization technique, which consists in performing a linear alteration on the original data normalizing it within a given range. With this technique is also possible to determinate the *Degree of Confidence* for each attribute and for the whole symptom as a combination of mul-

Figure 1. Conceptual model representing whole data mining process

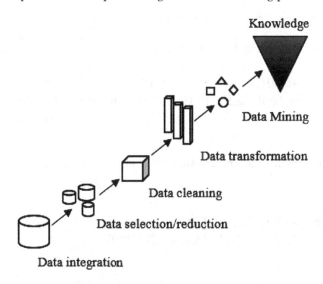

tiple attributes. Example demonstrated in Box 1 represents an extraction of some attributes with four different cases regarding their occurrence in a symptom. Attributes selected were Age, Hypertension, Physical Activity and Systolic Pressure.

As it is represented in Box 1, the first interaction is to transform the original data into continuous intervals, which in this case have its minimum established in zero and its maximum in one. Attributes previously represented in continuous interval are left in the same interval however unknown values, like Hypertension (*Hyp*) in the example above, is replaced for its corresponding domain. Nominal attributes must have a corresponding domain for each nominal value being replaced for that same interval. Numeric values are transformed in an interval composed with *min=max=value* With this method all attributes fits in the same range interval proceeding with calculation of *DoC* for each attribute and for the entire symptom.

Degree of Confidence

Data provided in a given input can be noisy and contain missing values reducing the level of truth and certainty for that same case. If all attributes are to be considered, giving missing data or uncertain data may influence the result. However to represent, as a measures, this level of truth in a record it is necessary to calculate, after normalization, de *Degree of Confidence*. This measure is represented with a numeric value between zero and one, in other words $DoC \in [0,1]$ The *Degree of Confidence* is obtained through the equation where Δl stands for the length between the extremes of a given normalized attribute's interval. Obviously numeric attributes

Box 1.

$$\{$$
$$sym(A, Hyp, Pa, Sp) :: 0.65 \equiv$$

$$sym([45,50], \quad \perp, \quad Medium, 130) \quad \longleftarrow \quad \text{term}$$
$$[0,100] \quad [0,1] \quad [0,100] \quad [70,200] \quad \longleftarrow \quad \text{domain of}$$
$$\text{term's}$$
$$\text{argument}$$

$\Downarrow$ 1st interaction: transition to continuous intervals

$$sym([45,50], \quad \perp, \quad [40,70], \quad 130)$$
$$[0,100] \quad [0,1] \quad [0,100] \quad [70,200]$$

$\Downarrow$ 2nd interaction: normalization $\dfrac{Y - Y_{min}}{Y_{max} - Y_{min}}$

$$sym\left(\left[\frac{45-0}{100-0}, \frac{50-0}{100-0}\right], \left[\frac{0-0}{1-0}, \frac{1-0}{1-0}\right], \left[\frac{40-0}{100-0}, \frac{70-0}{100-0}\right], \left[\frac{130-70}{200-70}, \frac{130-70}{200-70}\right]\right)$$

$$sym([0.45,0.5], \quad [0,1], \quad [0.4,0.7] \quad [0.46,0.46])$$
$$[0,1] \quad [0,1] \quad [0,1] \quad [0,1]$$
$$\}$$

Figure 2. Relation, and calculation between normalized attribute's interval and the Degree of Confidence. First quadrant of a unit circle of radius one is centered at origin (0,0)

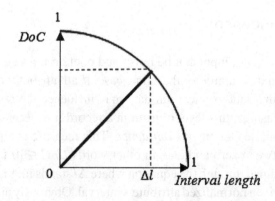

are more accurate, precise and reliable then attributes represented by intervals. Consequently the greater the distance between extremes less reliable is the data in the corresponding attribute.

Shown in Box 2, normalized attributes are used to calculate de DoC.

Based on this measure it is possible to understand data quality and, in a certain way, provide a level of confidence, truth, which the system or any other user may rely to answer to a given case.

Clustering

Within a dataset there are relationships and characteristics similar to different records. Considering these facts, clustering is a technique used to group data in different groups

Box 2.

$$
\begin{aligned}
&\{ \\
&sym([0.45,0.5], \quad [0,1] \quad [0.4,0.7] \quad [0.46,0.46]) \\
&\qquad\quad [0,1] \qquad\quad [0,1] \quad [0,1] \qquad [0,1]
\end{aligned}
$$

1st interaction: calculate interval length (Δl)

$$
\begin{aligned}
&sym(0.05, \quad 1, \quad 0.3, \quad 0) \\
&\qquad\quad [0,1] \quad [0,1] \quad [0,1] \quad [0,1]
\end{aligned}
$$

2nd interaction: apply the expression $DoC = \sqrt{1 - \Delta l^2}$ for each attribute

$$
\begin{aligned}
&sym(0.998, \quad 0, \quad 0.953, \quad 1) \\
&\qquad\quad [0,1] \quad [0,1] \quad [0,1] \quad [0,1]
\end{aligned}
$$

3rd interaction: calculate global DoC

$$
DoC = \frac{0.998 + 0 + 0.953 + 1}{4} = 0.737
$$

}

according with record's characteristics. This method allows distinguishing different cases and excluding those who don't gather the requirements or the same characteristics compared with the new case submitted. To accomplish this unsupervised learning process the system uses The *Expectation Maximization* (EM) algorithm, ideal for solving parameter estimation problems for neural networks; moreover, EM algorithm has great performance where problems provide partial information or missing values. This algorithm follows two alternating steps, E-step where hidden data is re-estimated resulting in expected values, M-step which maximizes the likelihood between data re-estimating model parameters. The integration of such technique is considered as an optimization improving selection method used in Case Based Reasoning systems reducing the number of cases to consider.

Artificial Neural Network

Artificial Neural Network are computational systems of connectionist base to solve problems. This system are designed based on a simplified model of humans' central nervous systems defined by a connected structured of computation units called neurons with learning capabilities. A neuron is identified by its network position and characterized by state value using an axon as communication channel, which connects to other neurons or to itself. Considering different problems with different

Figure 3. Agent's representation of dataset according with different clusters

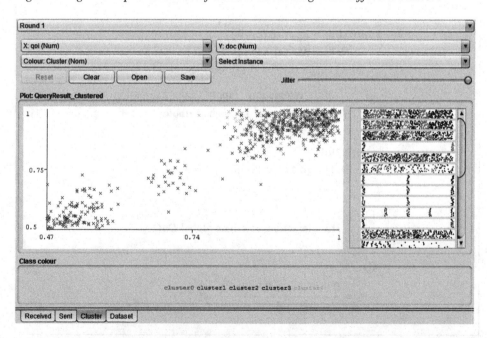

scenarios, frequently, one node is not enough, regardless the number of inputs. A neural network is also characterized by is architecture which are distinct in the way that neuron are displayed or connected. This system has implemented a *feedforward network*; hence, it is composed by artificial neuron organized by layers where the connection, communication, is made in a unidirectional way with the next layers. Also depending on the dataset the neural network is composed with multiple layers. To provide an efficient result and model the artificial neural network receives normalized data with the corresponding clusters previously defined. The input is composed by n tuples, where n is the number of attributes. Each tuple has three inputs relating an attribute, the minimum and maximum values from the normalized result, and the *DoC* of each attributes. The output is a numeric value indicating the best suitable cluster for the submitted input.

4. CASE BASED REASONING

A problem solving methodology consisting in finding and justifying the solution for a given problem with the integration of similar historical cases, reprocessing or adapting knowledge from those same retrieved cases. This historical situation, cases, had their occurrence in the past in a problem resolution. This document en-

Figure 4. Conceptual representation of the artificial neural network architecture

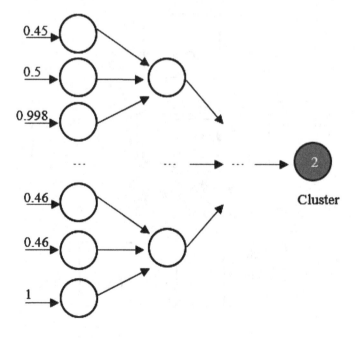

hances the retrieval process in the CBR using previews data mining techniques to reduce data, clustering the dataset in their different groups to identity the one that best describes the new case.

However, reducing cases with clustering and assigning a cluster to the new input was not enough to retrieve one case. To achieve a similar a function was used to calculate the similarity within a cluster for each case returning the one with less difference. The gap between the new cases and the cases in the cluster is given by the following function, where *IS* represents the input case, *HS* the historical case, *n* the number of attributes and *Max* and *Min* representing the attributes' normalized maximum and minimum values.

$$sim = \sum_{n}^{1} \frac{\frac{\left(ISAttrMax_i - HSAttrMax_i\right) + \left(ISAttrMin_i - HSAttrMin_i\right)}{2} * w_i}{n}$$

(4)

A weight is associated with each attribute representing the impact of that attribute on a symptom. The weight depends on the risk and the level of influence in a stroke disease.

Figure 5. Case Based Reasoning model

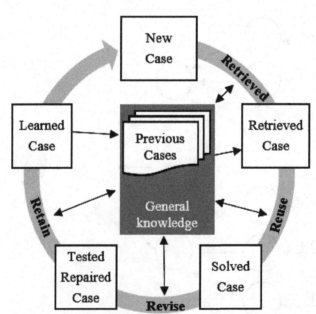

Table 2. Attribute weight

Attribute	Weight
Gender	1
Age	$\dfrac{age * 6}{100}$
Hypertension	5
Headache	3
Diabetes	5
Activity	5
Smoker	5
Systolic	6
Previous stroke	4
Medication	1
Cholesterol HDL	5
Cholesterol LDL	5
Cholesterol Tri	3
Vomiting	

5. MULTIAGENT SYSTEM

Interoperability can be accomplished through many methodologies that allow communication between all different scenarios and environments. A multi agent system (MAS) comprehends a group of entities that cooperates in order to solve a given problem, which, usually is towards individual capabilities. Those entities, also designated as intelligent agents, act upon their environment, producing a certain effect being characterized by their flexibility develop for an environment and its autonomy capacity. Agents, in this multi agent system react upon a given input handling perceptions through input reception provide by different entities. However all selection process mentioned above indicates execute their action based on rules containing predicative or symbolic models explicit of their environment, whose state of knowledge may modify, in a certain way, the logical-mathematical reasoning, making this MAS architecture deliberative. Because the idea of an ideal, for this system, is to combine both reactive and deliberative characteristics, agent were developed to answer as quite as possible to a given input but also process the information as a deliberative agent, granting the reasoning characteristics capabilities of decision. Agents were divided according with their functionality and task processing resulting in four agents entirely different, Monitor Agent, Decision Agent, Process Agent and Resource Agent. Agents can be more reactive then deliberative or vice versa, for instances, A Monitor Agent has a condition / action relationship in the system, building dynamic symptoms with inputs provided by users sending them to the Decision Agent.

A Decision Agent is responsible for the process decision making evaluation all involving Process Agent, in a certain round, and deciding which result should go through and sent back to the Monitor Agent.

Figure 6. Monitor Agent

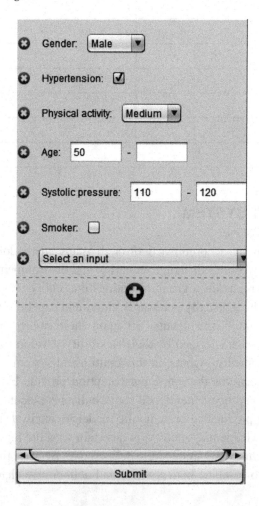

All deliberative process and all reasoning is implemented in Process Agents using Resource Agents to retrieve information from their own database, using it to choose the best answer possible for a given symptom.

Communication is established with a specific ontology implemented via a TCP/ IP channel using sockets. To insure data flow, an acknowledgement message was implemented in every action involving two or more different agents. This kind of

Figure 7. System monitoring by Decision Agent

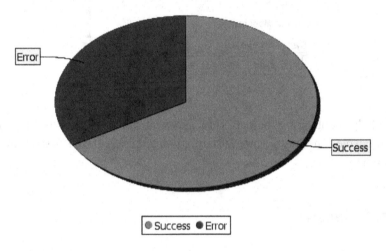

Figure 8. Agents monitoring by Decision Agent

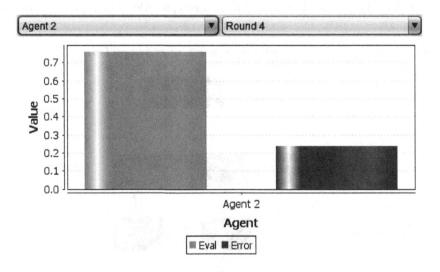

Figure 9. Process Agent

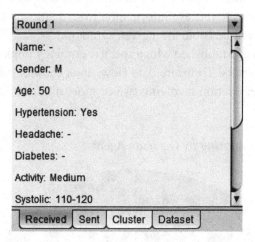

message helps controlling the data flow and controlling agent's enrollment in the system lifecycle. The multi agent system architecture can be visualized in the following image.

6. CONCLUSION

Nowadays healthcare organizations have handle a considered large amount of information, making them incapable of fully analyze relationships and other aspects between data. The use of data mining techniques provides and improves better per-

Figure 10. Architecture representation of multi agent system here

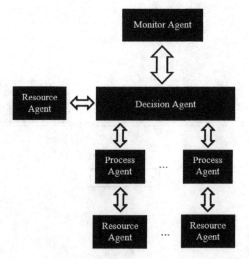

formance relating this information and process decision-making. When presented to this process, every historical record represents a part of knowledge relationships whose existence may influence the outcome of new cases. As demonstrated in this document, symptoms can be different according with data quality and even with its value allowing clustering all records in order to distinguish the most appropriate to analysis. With the classifier implemented, Artificial Neural Network, the new cases can be properly classified considering the model previously trained with the historical cases. Results from this system were satisfactory since all agents retrieve answer to a new case with a similarity very close when it comes to symptoms attributes.

REFERENCES

American Heart Association. (2009). *Heart Disease and Stroke Statistics 2009 Update*. Dallas, Texas.

Chambless, L. E., Heiss, G., Shahar, E., Earp, M. J., & Toole, J. (2004). Prediction of ischemic stroke risk in the atherosclerosis risk in communities study. *American Journal of Epidemiology, 160*(3), 259–269. doi:10.1093/aje/kwh189 PMID:15257999

Longstreth, W. T. Jr, Bernick, C., Fitzpatrick, A., Cushman, M., Knepper, L., Lima, J., & Furberg, C. (2001, February). Frequency and predictors of stroke death in 5,888 participants in the Cardiovascular Health Study. *Neurology, 56*(3), 368–375. doi:10.1212/WNL.56.3.368 PMID:11171903

Lumley, T., Kronmal, R. A., Cushman, M., Manolio, T. A., & Goldstein, S. (2002, February). A stroke prediction score in the elderly: Validation and web-based application. *Journal of Clinical Epidemiology, 55*(2), 129–136. doi:10.1016/S0895-4356(01)00434-6 PMID:11809350

Machado, J. (2002). *Agentes Inteligentes como Objectos dum Sistema Distribuído de Realidade Virtual*. Braga.

Neves, J., Ribeiro, J., Pereira, P., Alves, V., Machado, J., Abelha, A., Novais, P., Analide, C., Santos, M., Fernández-Delgado, M. (2012). Evolutionary intelligence in asphalt pavement modeling and quality-of- information. Progress in Artificial Intelligence. *Progress in Artificial Intelligence, 1*(1), 119-135.

Zhang, X.-F., Attia, J., D'este, C., Yu, X.-H., & Wu, X.-G. (2005). A risk score predicted coronary heart disease and stroke in a Chinese cohort. *Journal of Clinical Epidemiology, 58*(9), 951–958. doi:10.1016/j.jclinepi.2005.01.013 PMID:16085199

Chapter 13
Applying Soft Computing to Clinical Decision Support

José Machado
Universidade do Minho, Portugal

Luís Barreiro
Universidade do Minho, Portugal

Lucas Oliveira
Universidade do Minho, Portugal

Serafim Pinto
Universidade do Minho, Portugal

Ana Coimbra
Universidade do Minho, Portugal

ABSTRACT

This article aims to explain the construction process of the learing systems based on Artificial Neural Networks and Genetic Algorithms. These systems were implemented using R and Python programming languages, in order to compare results and achieve the best solution and it was used Diabetes and Parkinson datasets with the purpose of identifying the carriers of these diseases.

INTRODUCTION

Clinical Decision Support is a process whose main goal is to improve heath and healthcare delivery by supporting health-related decisions and actions. (Healthcare Information and Management Systems Society, n.d.) (HealthIT.gov, n.d.)

Nowadays, there is a huge supply of data in Internet through abundant data sources in several areas of knowledge, such as commerce, science and society. Often, is difficult to analysis, obtain conclusions and/or predict future results in this

DOI: 10.4018/978-1-4666-9882-6.ch013

data. Through the use of some tools and techniques it is possible realize a more specify and objective analysis of data, with this analysis it is possible to find results, determine which are the most relevant results of the analysis, and interprets them in order to decide on how they may be useful in the context of the data analyzed.

This way, through Neural Networks and Genetic Algorithms, in this work were analyzed two sets of different data. It was used one dataset about the Diabetes disease and another about Parkinson, which will be explained later. The main goal was to create many different scenarios, make several tests, and then find the best possible solution for these learning systems. Always with the goal of optimize the problem and be able to make a prediction of results with the lowest possible error.

DATASETS

For this work it was select two datasets of public domain, available for download in https://archive.ics.uci.edu/ml/datasets.html. The first is about the Diabetes disease, more particularly in female individuals with at least 21 years old and Pima Indian descent. It is composed by 9 attributes and 768 instances, to know:

1. Number of times pregnant
2. Plasma glucose concentration a 2 hours in an oral glucose tolerance test
3. Diastolic blood pressure (mm Hg)
4. Triceps skin fold thickness (mm)
5. 2-Hour serum insulin (mu U/ml)
6. Body mass index (weight in kg/(height in m))^2)
7. Diabetes pedigree function
8. Age (years)
9. Class variable (0 or 1)

The second dataset analyzes various biomedical measures corresponding to Parkinson disease or not. The main goal of the information is discriminate the people that are Parkinson patients. The information is divided in 23 attributes and 197 instances, to know:

1. Name - ASCII subject name and recording number
2. MDVP:Fo(Hz) - Average vocal fundamental frequency
3. MDVP:Fhi(Hz) - Maximum vocal fundamental frequency
4. MDVP:Flo(Hz) - Minimum vocal fundamental frequency
5. MDVP:Jitter(%),MDVP:Jitter(Abs),MDVP:RAP,MDVP:PPQ,Jitter:DDP - Several measures of variation in fundamental frequency

6. MDVP:Shimmer,MDVP:Shimmer(dB),Shimmer:APQ3,Shimmer:APQ5,MD VP:APQ,Shimmer:DDA - Several measures of variation in amplitude
7. NHR, HNR - Two measures of ratio of noise to tonal components in the voice
8. Status - Health status of the subject (one) - Parkinson's, (zero) - healthy
9. RPDE, D2 - Two nonlinear dynamical complexity measures
10. DFA - Signal fractal scaling exponent
11. spread1, spread2, PPE - Three nonlinear measures of fundamental frequency variation

This two datasets fit perfectly in the project goal. They have a considerable number of attributes and instances, and studies disease cases that can be applied a results forecast.

Data Normalization

The data normalization allows to assign one new scale to an attribute so that the values of this attribute fall into the new scale, such as between, -1.0 a 1.0 or from 0.0 to 1.0. It is a relevant technique since it allows, without loss of information, assign an equal scale for all the attributes of the dataset. It is of particular importance when using neural networks, once, without attribute normalization some would have more weight than others for being naturally bigger. With this in mind, all the attributes, excluding the class variables, were normalized for the scale that ranges between -1.0 and 1.0. All this process allows to create a faster and with less error learning system that if the data were not normalized.

Beyond this normalization, all the not numerical attributes were removed from the datasets, since they do not have any relevance for the development of the Neural Networks and the Genetic Algorithms.

ARTIFICIAL NEURAL NETWORKS

An Artificial Neural Network (ANN) is a computational system of connectionist base. It is based on a model on the central nervous system of human beings. One ANN is defined by a interconnected structure of computational units, named neurons, with capacity of learning. (Dayhoff & DeLeo, 2001)

The artificial neuron is a mathematical logic structure, which seeks to simulate the shape, the behavior and functions of a biological neuron. (Dayhoff & DeLeo, 2001) Therefore, the dendrites were replaced by inputs, whose links with the artificial cell body are performed by elements designated weight (simulating synapses).

The stimulus caught by the inputs is processed by the sum function, and the trigger threshold of the biological neuron was replaced by the transfer function. (Dayhoff & DeLeo, 2001) (Krenker et al., 2011)

An ANN is a combination of a several artificial neurons. The inputs, simulating one area of capture of stimulus, can be connected in several neurons, thus resulting, a series of outputs, where each neuron represents the output. This connections, in comparison with the biological system, represents the contact of the dendrites with the others neurons, forming the synapses. The function of the connection is to transform the output signal of a neuron in an input signal of another, or yet, guide the output signal for the external world (real world). The different possibilities of connections between the neurons layers can generate N numbers of different structures. An example of an ANN can be seen on Figure 2.

A neuronal network can have many variations, so, combining them, the architecture can be changed according to the needs of the application. Basically, the items which constitute a neural network and, therefore, subject to change, are the following:

- Connections between layers
- Intermediate layers
- Amount of neurons
- Transfer function
- Learning algorithm

Figure 1. Artificial Neuron

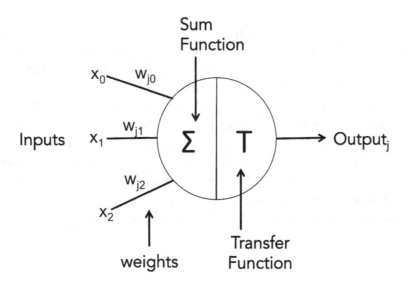

Figure 2. Example of an ANN

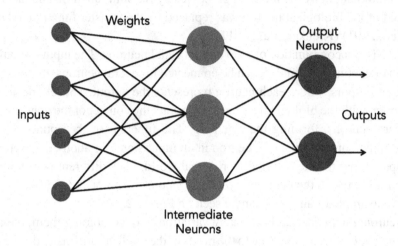

With the available datasets, were created several networks, with multiple different scenarios, to minimize the error, and then predict the best possible way the final result (if the patient have or not the disease).

R Programming Language

R is a powerful scripting language, especially used for statistical analysis, data mining, and learning systems. (The R Foundation, n.d.)

Diabetes

It was obtained really positive results for the Diabetes *dataset*, it was even able to the network predict with a great hit rate, and so a really small error. In table can be seen different scenarios that were used, the obtained results and the optimal solution.

Some scenarios with really low error can be observed in Table 1, however, some have advantages compared to other, once, the time of execution, the RMSE, and the steps are differents. With this in mind, the best solution for the ANN used in this work is the one whose intermediate nodes are 20-15-10-5. With this solution, it is possible to get a fairly accurate prediction as the patient has Diabetes or not. In Figure 3 is represented the final Neuronal Network. And in Figure 4 can be seen the tests with the prediction model working. This ANN could be even more precise, but for that it would be necessary more training and data test.

Table 1. Results obtained from ANN in R with the Diabetes dataset.

Intermediate Nodes	Error	Steps	RMSE	Time (s)
5-3	25.62030536	13934	0.5289252355	6.145
10-6	11.08546208	52163	0.7237468645	40.253
15-9	2.256872287	51921	0.6172133998	60.816
20-12	0.3623852806	63432	0.7237468645	101.676
20-15	0.1012991681	89516	0.8091735937	180.201
20-15-10	0.02361959633	19021	0.6546536707	48.721
20-15-15	0.03124205135	19427	0.7598558761	53.555
20-15-10-5	0.01261599756	6517	0.5232681185	18.515
20-15-15-10-5	0.008367339333	4820	0.5669467095	19.630

Figure 3. Final ANN for Diabetes

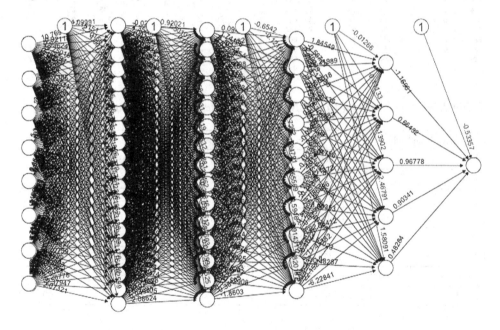

Parkinson

For this dataset, the results were also positive. Taking into account all the variables, as it can be seen in Table 2, the best solution for the ANN used in this work is the one whose intermediate nodes are 20-15-15. With this solution, even with few data test, it is possible to have an effective forecast. This ANN is not optimized as the

Figure 4. Prediction Model with test data

```
                        630  0      0  660  1      0  690  1      0  720  1   1
   actual prediction    631  1      0  661  0      1  691  0      0  721  0   0
601    0    0           632  0      0  662  1      1  692  1      0  722  0   0
602    0    0           633  0      0  663  1      1  693  0      1  723  1   0
603    0    0           634  0      0  664  1      1  694  1      0  724  0   0
604    1    0           635  0      1  665  1      1  695  0      0  725  0   0
605    1    1           636  1      1  666  0      1  696  1      0  726  0   0
606    0    1           637  0      1  667  1      0  697  1      1  727  0   0
607    1    1           638  0      0  668  1      1  698  0      0  728  0   1
608    0    0           639  1      0  669  0      0  699  0      1  729  0   0
609    0    0           640  0      0  670  0      0  700  0      0  730  0   0
610    0    0           641  0      0  671  0      1  701  0      0  731  1   0
611    0    0           642  0      0  672  0      0  702  1      0  732  1   1
612    1    1           643  1      1  673  0      1  703  1      0  733  1   1
613    1    1           644  0      0  674  0      0  704  0      1  734  0   0
614    0    1           645  0     -1  675  0      0  705  0      0  735  0   0
615    1    1           646  0      0  676  1      1  706  0      0  736  0   1
616    0    0           647  1      0  677  1      1  707  1      0  737  0   0
617    0    0           648  1      1  678  0      0  708  0     -1  738  0   0
618    0    0           649  1      0  679  1      0  709  1      1  739  0   0
619    1    0           650  0      0  680  0      0  710  0      0  740  1   0
620    1    1           651  0      0  681  0      0  711  0      0  741  1   1
621    0    1           652  0     -1  682  1      1  712  0      1  742  0  -1
622    0    0           653  0      1  683  0      0  713  1      1  743  0   0
623    0    1           654  0      0  684  1      1  714  0      0  744  1   1
624    0    0           655  0     -1  685  0      0  715  0      0  745  0   1
625    0    1           656  1      1  686  0      0  716  1      1  746  0   1
626    0    1           657  0      0  687  0      0  717  1      1  747  1   0
627    0    0           658  0      0  688  0      1  718  0      0  748  0   1
628    0    1           659  0      0  689  0      0  719  0      0  749  1   1
629    0    1           660  1      0  690  1      0  720  1      1  750  1   1
```

Table 2. Results obtained from ANN in R with the Parkinson dataset.

Intermediate Nodes	Error	Steps	RMSE	Time (s)
5-3	0.03427546852	977	0.714920353	0.260
10-6	0.03388269913	1039	0.6666666667	0.433
15-9	0.005496716113	2492	0.6831300511	1.391
15-9-5	0.01840487369	477	0.6831300511	0.335
20-12	0.0586598929	1075	0.6497862897	0.845
20-15	0.7551364078	811	0.6666666667	0.789
20-15-10	0.02026826017	439	0.6666666667	0.459
20-15-15	0.0174758063	328	0.6666666667	0.400

previous, and present values of high RMSE, which is not very good. This is due to the fact that is a small *dataset*, and consequently there are few data to train the network. In Figure 5 can be seen the final ANN.

Python

Python is an high level programming language that contains a huge standard library with plenty of methods, class and functions to multitask. One of these tasks is to train

Figure 5. Final ANN for Diabetes

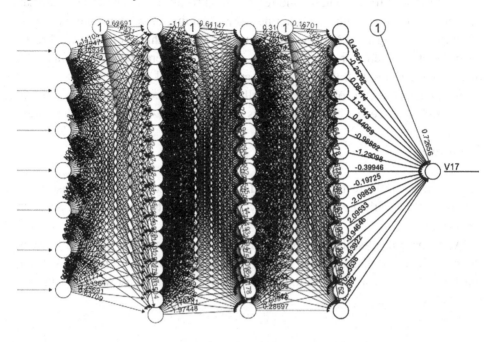

Figure 6. Prediction Model with test data

	actual	prediction			
151	1	1	173	0	1
152	1	1	174	0	1
153	1	1	175	0	1
154	1	1	176	0	1
155	1	1	177	0	1
156	1	1	178	1	1
157	1	1	179	1	1
158	1	1	180	1	1
159	1	1	181	1	1
160	1	1	182	1	1
161	1	1	183	1	1
162	1	1	184	0	1
163	1	1	185	0	1
164	1	1	186	0	1
165	1	1	187	0	1
166	0	0	188	0	1
167	0	0	189	0	1
168	0	0	190	0	1
169	0	1	191	0	1
170	0	1	192	0	1
171	0	0	193	0	1
172	0	1	194	0	1
173	0	1	195	0	1

a neural network from a dataset and reach a final result. It was used the NeuroLab library because it contains neuronal networks, training algorithms and structures capable of creating and exploring other networks. Within this library is available the nweff function where, for each input node, are created several intermediate neurons, once or more times, to train the network and reach a final result.

It was also used an older library, called PyBrain. Several tests were done in several different scenarios, and the results approached the same used by NeuroLab.

Diabetes

For this data set, the results shows that the more intermediate neurons exist in the network, along with the selected library, it is possible to achieve more accurate final results.

After these results, the node that has the lowest error is the 25-25-25, but on the other hand it takes too long to execute and consumes more resources to the machine. Therefore, is possible to present a fairly strong forecast whether a patient has Diabetes or not.

Figure 7. Final graphic for intermediate nodes 5-3

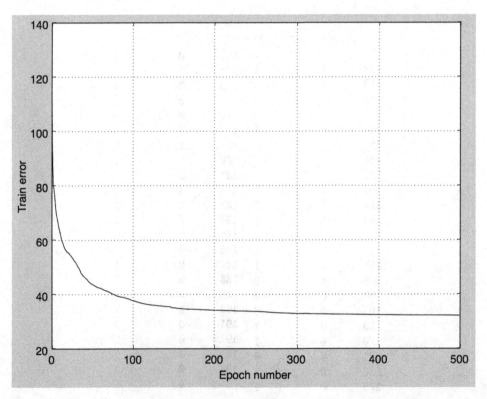

Figure 8. Final graphic for intermediate nodes 20-10-15

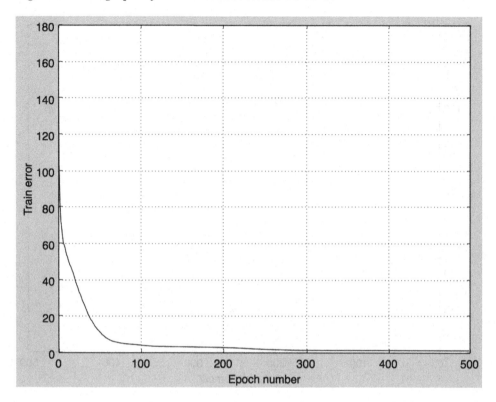

Table 3. Summary of the graphs with final results.

Intermediate Nodes	Error	Epochs
5-3	32.4077128878	500
20-10-15	1.53903083728	500
20-25-25	0.0500219411684	500

Parkinson

For this dataset the results represented in Table 4 shows that worse results are obtained if intermediate neurons are increased, this happens because either all the tests do not converge to the defined maximum Epochs or the obtained graphic is blank which shows that it was not possible to train the network.

After an analysis of the figures and it can be concluded that a final result can be achieved using few neurons, but with a very big error. However the more the

Figure 9. Final graphic for intermediate nodes 25-25-25

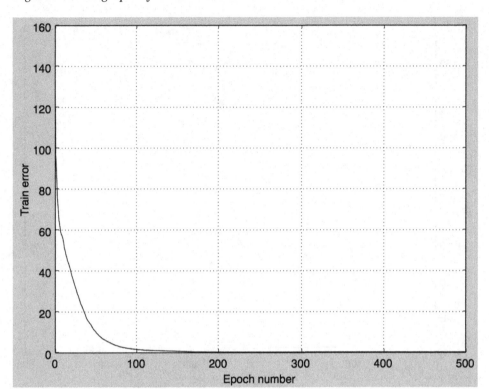

Table 4. Summary of the graphs with final results.

Intermediate Nodes	Error	Epochs
4-4-4	0.499999924644	500
15-10-10	1.53903083728	100

intermediate neurons are increased, or the more intermediate layers exist for the network to be trained, required iterations are rarely made. The fact that this dataset has inconclusive results is because this dataset has few test instances.

GENETIC ALGORITHMS

Genetic Algorithms form adaptive processes of search in space solutions by applying modeled operators according to the concept of inheritance, inherent in the theory of

Figure 10. Final graphic for intermediate nodes 5-3

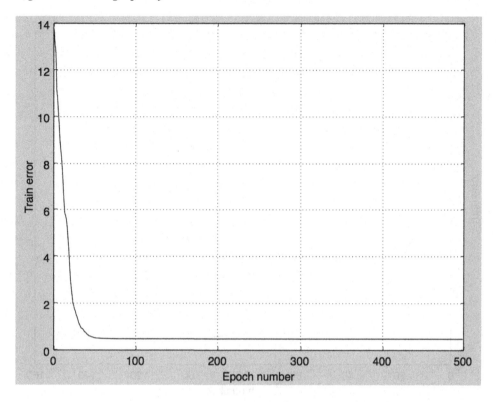

evolution, by Charles Darwin. They belong to the class of probabilistic algorithms, distinguished by search method that they use and by the specific treatment of great places. In general they are applied to problems that involve solutions improvement and problems where the solutions computation is hard or even impossible. For a genetic algorithm the environment, the inputs and the outputs are represented by sets of symbols with fixed size, for example the binary {0,1}. The basic entities for the knowledge representation are the chromosome, compound by genes which in turn are compounded by individual values present in the alphabet. (Mitchell, 1999)

The execution cycle can be seen in Figure 12, where:

- The initial population is randomly chosen.
- The reproduction is compound by the application of the evaluation function to all individuals of the population and by the choice of the next generation that should ensure the choice of the structure with better performance.

Figure 11. Final graphic for intermediate nodes 15-10-10

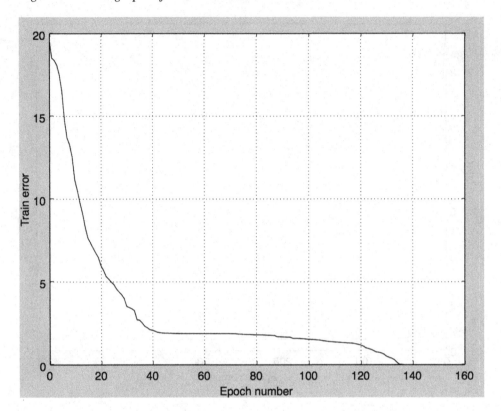

- The crossing consists in the crossing of values between a pair of elements, as the name implies.
- The mutation change one or more values of the elements of the population. This allows the possibility to reach any solution of the problem.

R

The Genetic Algorithms, as indicated before, are indicated to improve solutions and find solutions closer to the optimum in difficult problems. The fitness function is a function that evaluates the potential quality of a solution in relation to others potential solutions. Based on this principle, was produced a random fitness solution that allows to analyze the results produced by the GA library of R.

In Figure 13 it is called the GA function from the GA library. They are used real values that ranges between -1 and 1, and are realized 500 iterations, taking into account that fitness function is just one sum of past values multiplied by *dataset* values. As this algorithm is created to minimize this value, the call of the function is negative becoming maximizer.

Figure 12. Execution cycle of Genetic Algorithm

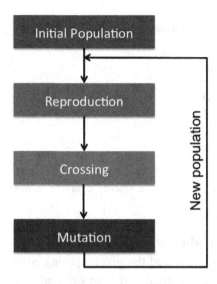

Figure 13. Call to the library GA that runs the genetic algorithm

```
ga.fitness <- ga(   type='real-valued',
                    min=c(-1,-1,-1, -1,-1,-1, -1,-1),
                    max=c(1,1,1, 1,1,1, 1,1),
                    popSize=500,
                    maxiter=500,
                    keepBest=T,
                    fitness = function(b) -fitness(data, b[1],b[2], b[3],
                                            b[4], b[5], b[6], b[7], b[8])
                )
ga.model <- summary(ga.fitness)
ga.model
```

Table 5. Obtained results for Diabetes

Iteraction	Mean	Best
1	-0.0114103	3.461928
2	0.624003	3.461928
3	1.172053	3.580189
…	…	…
498	4.904897	5.136926
499	4.913023	5.136926
500	4.914153	5.136926

Figure 14. Information summary of the Genetic Algorithm

```
GA settings:
Type                    = real-valued
Population size         = 500
Number of generations = 500
Elitism                 = 25
Crossover probability = 0.8
Mutation probability  = 0.1
Search domain
     x1 x2 x3 x4 x5 x6 x7 x8
Min -1 -1 -1 -1 -1 -1 -1 -1
Max  1  1  1  1  1  1  1  1

GA results:
Iterations              = 500
Fitness function value = 5.136926
Solution                =
          x1         x2         x3         x4        x5         x6         x7         x8
[1,] -0.952538 -0.9651945 -0.8637909 -0.9581028 0.985579 -0.9153922 -0.9536537 -0.9796359
```

The best solution (maximum) eventually stabilizes.

In the Figure 14 are presented the given options when calling the function or default options, as well as the final optimum solution.

CONCLUSION

With this work, it was found that for the same datasets the results were worst when Python was used instead of R, despite different Python libraries have been tried. It can be concluded that for this type of systems it is better to use R language. Once the datasets were not in the order of thousands instances the used neural network might not be the best, thus, therefore they can be improved. Genetic Algorithms were not implemented in python because an accessible and stable library that make it possible to explore and get good results was not found. The formulation of a coherent fitness function was a complicated task. However, despite this limitation, it was possible to perform an example in R, which allowed us to understand how to apply this type of algorithms to any dataset, as long as it was possible to develop a fitness function.

REFERENCES

Dayhoff, J. E., & DeLeo, J. M. (2001). Artificial neural networks. *Cancer Supplement, 91*(8), 1615–1635. doi:10.1002/1097-0142(20010415)91:8+<1615::AID-CNCR1175>3.0.CO;2-L PMID:11309760

HealthIT.gov. (n. d.). *Clinical Decision Support (CDS)*. Retrieved from http://www.healthit.gov/policy-researchers-implementers/clinical-decision-support-cds

Healthcare Information and Management Systems Society. (n. d.). *Clinical Decision Support*. Retrieved from http://www.himss.org/library/clinical-decision-support

Krenker, A., Bešter, J., & Kos, A. (2011). *Artificial Neural Networks - Methodological Advances and Biomedical Applications*. InTech.

Mitchell, M. (1999). *An Introduction to Genetic Algorithms*. MIT Press.

The R Foundation. (n. d.). *What is R?* Retrieved from https://www.r-project.org/about.html

Chapter 14
A Multiplatform Decision Support Tool in Neonatology and Pediatric Care

Tiago Guimarães
Universidade do Minho, Portugal

Simão Frutuoso
Centro Hospitalar do Porto, Portugal

Ana Coimbra
Universidade do Minho, Portugal

António Abelha
Universidade do Minho, Portugal

ABSTRACT

As regards the dosage of drug, children are a much more vulnerable population than the adults. With this in mind it is extremely important the administration of the correct dosage. For this purpose, it was develop a framework, based on a prototype already tested in a real environment, with the main concern to help pediatricians in their daily tasks. Thus, this framework includes tools that can help in the preparation of Total Parenteral Nutrition prescriptions, table pediatric and neonatal emergency drugs, medical scales of morbidity and mortality, anthropometry percentiles (weight, length/height, head circumference and BMI), utilities for supporting medical decision on the treatment of neonatal jaundice and anemia and other calculators. This paper presents the architecture, their functionalities and a SWOT analysis of the solution proposed.

DOI: 10.4018/978-1-4666-9882-6.ch014

INTRODUCTION

The paediatric and neonatal patients are the most vulnerable population in respect to drug administration. Therefore, a dosage error can leave serious consequences and even be fatal. As it can be seen in Literature, 8% of the medication errors are from paediatric specialty, this may happen because to determine the medication dosages for each paediatrics patients the paediatricians have to take in count several factors, such as patient age, body weight, and in some cases body surface. The constant calculations and the numerous times that healthcare professionals have to check tables, may delay the medical consultation and also makes human error more likely to happen in the overly execution of those tasks. (Kaushal, et al., 2001; Rosse, et al., 2009)

The automation of these tasks available through an e-health and a m-health application will aim to make the professional life easier, saving their time, reducing the human error risks during calculations and improving the quality of healthcare delivery.

Artificial Intelligence in Medicine (AIM) appear with the need of introducing computers into medical practice for aid the physicians decisions using Artificial Intelligence based medical diagnostic reasoning, making possible to solve complex decision models in real time. Nowadays it is more common to describe them as clinical decision support systems (CDSS) instead of AIM systems. However this first CDSS generation was often inaccurate or irrelevant due to the fact that these systems were not integrated with other computerized systems making it impossible to support hospital operation and patient data management. (Zheng, 2010; Coiera, 2003)

The CDSS are computer based information systems that are interactive, flexible and adaptable, developed with the purpose of improving decision-making processes, providing this way to the physicians and other individuals with knowledge and specific, individualized information, intelligently filtered and presented at appropriate times. An example of a commonly used CDSS is the laboratory systems that generate alerts for abnormal values. (Zheng, 2010; Ramnarayan & Britto, 2002)

The most precious resource in a medical practice is clinical time, this is extremely limited, a physician in a medical consultation have to examine the patient, review historical data, make decisions, document new findings and prescribe treatments and drugs if necessary, with all this the CDSS could not be a distraction, or occupy more time than usual to perform all these tasks. Furthermore a CDSS should help the physicians by reducing the wasted time in useless things and reducing the time to perform a simple task, for example finding the patient historical data or even in the calculation of the drug dosages. (Zheng, 2010)

Another thing that has to be taken into consideration is the interaction between physician and patient. If the physician spends too much time looking at the computer, the patient may consider it rude. (Zheng, 2010)

Currently CDSS is found more commonly supporting medication prescribing, making the prescription more legible than handwritten ones, and still lead to a better structured and more complete medication prescriptions by forcing the physicians to include dose, route of administration, and frequency before the final authorizing. Another advantage of having an electronic prescription is that the software can warn the physicians if they are contra-indications about that type of drug that he is trying to prescribe for that patient by accessing to the patient background information through a connection to the Hospital database, being capable of generating warning alerts against drug-drug interactions and drug-allergy interactions. (Rosse, et al., 2009; Zheng, 2010; Ramnarayan & Britto, 2002)

With all this in mind, it was developed a prototype called "Sabichão", that was tested in the Units of Paediatrics and Neonatology and on the Intensive Care Unit of Paediatrics of the *Centro Hospitalar do Porto*, the *Centro Materno-Infantil do Norte* and the *Centro Hospitalar Tâmega e Sousa*.

STATE OF ART

The work in this area of the clinical decision support systems (CDSS) and also in the neonatal and pediatric medicine has already begun. Examples of that are the INTCARE and the INTCARE II projects that introduce a new perspective in Intensive Care units. These projects make use of the new technologies of Artificial Intelligence to build an Intelligent Decision Support System that is able to predict the organ failure and patient outcome, using data collected and processed in real-time with adaptive data mining models. (Portela, et al., 2014; Portela, et al., 2014; Peixoto, Santos, Abelha, & Machado, 2012; Cardoso, et al., 2014)

The "Sabichão" prototype was developed based on an existing tool, with the same name, that already has a big impact in medical area. This tool was developed by a paediatrician (Dr. Simão Frutuoso) through language such as *Visual Basic* to applications and the *Microsoft Excel 2007*. It has a set of tools that facilitate the paediatricians work. However, it has some limitations such as competition, availability, scalability, and interoperability.

Typically, in the Hospital pharmacy there is only one system that processes all orders from all Units in the hospital, so, when a paediatrician orders a medication that order it is blended with others, and because the paediatric and neonatal patients need a special attention in terms of drug dosage the need arose to also create an framework to be used in the hospital pharmacy that only process the orders from this medical area. (Miller, Gardner, Johnson, & Hripcsak, 2005)

WORK MOTIVATION, OBJECTIVES AND EXPECTED RESULTS

Despite the first "Sabichão" created by Dr. Simão Frutuoso already had a big impact and a good adherence it has some limitation and problems:

- **Competition:** All forms are stored in a single Excel file, if this file is open in another device it is impossible to the pharmacy to execute the requests.
- **Availability:** It is only functional for specific version of Excel within Office from Microsoft, not working on other widely used and free alternatives of the program from OpenOffice or LibreOffice.
- **Efficiency:** Is a high size document that result of the complex application leading to an increase of opening and usage time.
- **Scalability:** When the number of record become significant the performance is limited.
- **Interoperability:** It can not be directly integrated with any Electronic Health Records or Health Information System.

With all this identified problems a set of objectives were defined such as kept the same efficiency in terms of intelligent decision support on therapies and procedures in neonatal and paediatric care that already existed in the Excel "Sabichão" version; ensure the high availability, scalability and portability of the system; assure the integration and interoperability of the system; and provide a version available outside of the hospital to be used by students. With this, is expected to extend the use of the tool to more hospital units and provide a mobile version of the system.

RESEARCH METHODOLOGIES

The work methodology is based on an investigation methodology *action research* that consists in continued attempt, systematically and empirically grounded to improve practice describing any process that follows a cycle in which it enhances the practice by the oscillation between acting on the practice field and investigate about it.

MULTIPLATFORM OF CLINICAL DECISION SUPPORT

The platform can be divided in two parts, the components associated to a Web Server, and the components that can be associated and integrated in any Heath Institution as it can be seen in Figure 1.

However, the developed architecture has four main requirements: scalability, scalable within the medical facilities and in the number of medical facilities that can connect to the main webserver; availability, availability solutions like offline login and late dispatching of the anonymous information; adaptability, through the use of web services, the application can be adapted to any HIS; and ubiquity, the system is always available anywhere and in any device.

Figure 1. Architecture of the developed platform

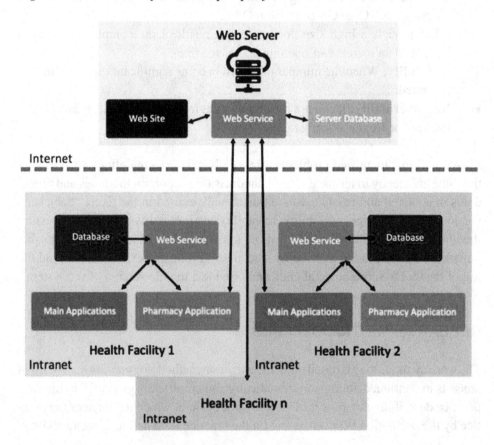

Components on the Intra-Institution of Health

To an integrated operation and without limitation of the application in the health institution it was necessary a set of components, an application in the hospital pharmacy, a medical application and two support components.

The support components are the database and the Web Service, and they as the name says, support the application. The database stores the forms made in medical application and the requests made to the pharmacy. The communication between medical applications, database, pharmacy, and hospital database is mediated by the Web Service, as it can be seen in Figure 2.

The application for the hospital pharmacy emerged from the need to simplify and organize the reception process of the requests of *total parenteral nutrition* made by the paediatricians. These requests are stored in the local database and it can be accessed by the pharmacists and they can even be elaborate nutrition bags, request print and even the print of labels to be placed in bags.

The Medical Application contain tools belonging to five modules:

- **Total Parenteral Nutrition (TPN):** TPN consists in intravenous nutrition. This module aims to provide the necessary support for the TPN individualized prescription, decreasing the time and the human error associated.
- **Emergency Sheets:** This module aims to help the filling of the dosages prescriptions sheets in emergencies.

Figure 2. Communication between the applications in a Heath Institution and the Web Server

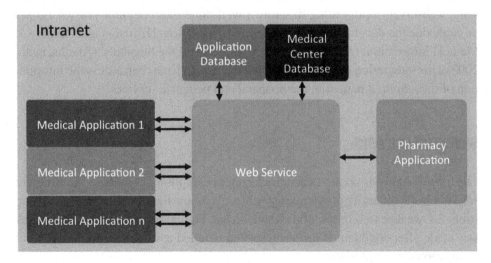

- **Dosages:** This module aims to help the paediatricians in prescribing infusions of drugs, according to the patient weight and wanted dosage. It is divided in: Dopamine and Dobutamine, Adrenalin and Noradrenaline, Morphine and Midazolam and finally, Fentanyl and Vecuronium.
- **Scales:** This module provides a range of Scales and probabilistic scores automatically calculated:
- **Anthropometry:** This module contains tools associated to the anthropometry percentiles.

Web Server

It was extremely important to set up a Web Server for the application to be fully scalable and independent from the Institution. The Web Server supports a *Web Application*, a *Database* and a *Web Service.*

The Database on the Web Server storages the users confidential.

The Web Service mediate the communications between the Web Application and the Database and even between the Medical Applications housed in Institutions and the Database on Server.

The Web Application is divided into two sections, one for the users and other for the administrators. Once the user authentication is not automatic, because patient data must be protected and can not be accessed by anyone, it was essential the creation of an area were the administrators can validate new users and when necessary change information of the already existing users, for these reasons it was created the administration area. In the user area, the users can register, and after administrator validation, download the Medical Application.

In this platform what stands is the fact that all the hospitals are connected to the same webserver, representing this way a well-done interoperability witch is only possible due the development of Agency for Integration, Diffusion and Archive of Medical Information (AIDA), already deployed in all the hospitals. (Abelha, et al., 2003) This integration is necessary so that the pediatricians can access the information of the admitted patient in the neonatal and pediatric services.

SWOT ANALYSIS

The SWOT Analysis allows to acquire a better perception of reality of the structure solution and so, identify problems, as well as overcome them. This consists in group strengths, weaknesses, opportunities and threats. The analysis of this different points was made after conducting various tests and detailed assessments to the different applications in the platform.

Strengths of the application:

- Scalability
- Easy access to a large number of tools in the paediatric and neonatal areas
- Easy adaptability to different health institutions
- Easy access to the data of patients admitted in neonatal and paediatric ICU, and even in the paediatric services, in the health institutions
- Easy in the requests delivery and management to the Hospital Pharmacy
- Easy use of the different application of the platform
- Maintaining a common historical of the TPN requests within each Health Institution
- Easy user management by the administrator
- Security ensured by authentication and the use of the cryptographic hash functions

Weaknesses of the application:

- Requires connection to the hospital intranet (to access history and to send requests to the Hospital Pharmacy)
- Requires internet connection, at least during the first authentication of the paediatrician
- Some features of the application, for its complexity, have a slower performance
- Lack of redundancy in the accommodation of the Web Service compromising the availability of the application

Opportunities of the application:

- Modernization and organizational development
- Increasing expectation of the patients to obtain faster and reliable responses of clinical services
- Provide the tool to help the daily tasks of the paediatricians
- Medical Error Reduction
- The platform will be provided for free

Threats of the application:

- Competition/market pressure
- Lack of acceptance to resort to new technologies by healthcare professionals

Technology Acceptance Model (TAM)

The evaluation of the technological applications is crucial to measure the users satisfaction levels. One of the most used models is the TAM. The TAM is an adaptation of the Theory of Reasoned Action directed to information technology. TAM main objective is to present an approach to evaluate and explain the individuals behaviour in relation to the information technologies, providing and justifying the acceptance or the not acceptance of one system by their users. This model aims to provide a theoretical basis to map the impact of the external variables in the sense of the users personal beliefs, attitudes and intentions. (Novo, et al., 2015) (Legris, Ingham, & Collerette, 2003)

In TAM perspective, people tend to use or not an application or technology according to the possibility of improving their performance at work, this is called Perceived Usefulness. However, even if the user understand that a particular application is useful, their effective use can be impaired if the use is considered too complicated, so that the benefits of the new technology does not compensate for the stress of using it. This concept is called Perceived Ease-of-use. (Ferreira & Queiroz, 2010)

Both Perceived Ease-of-use as Perceived Usefulness influence the attitude that users have on the system, and this is a determinant factor on how the system will be evaluated, positively or negatively. Within the TAM concept, by the Perceived Usefulness and by the Attitude Toward Use, determine the Intent of Use. It is the intended that determine the real use of the system.

It has been proposed two extensions to the TAM, the TAM 2 and the TAM 3. The TAM 2 identifies the determinants factors for the Perceived Usefulness and the TAM 3 combines the TAM 2 with the determinants of Perceived Ease.

USABILITY STUDY

To improve the developed platform it was subjected a study of usability. With the help of Dr. Simão Frutuoso, a pediatrician at the Centro Hospitalar do Porto (CHP), the interface and the features of different applications on the platform were adjusted.

Apart from this, it was created a questionnaire for the users, with the purpose of ascertain their views about the developed work.

Questionnaires are a method widely used when it comes to the users evaluation of interfaces, existing features, and even about features that they think that are missing. (Root & Draper, 1983)

For that reason, it was developed a questionnaire that aims to get a better perception about the tool already in use, developed in Microsoft Office Excel and realize what advantages or disadvantages the new application exposed.

It is divided into three sections: Information about the person being questioned, information about the use of the tool in Excel and finally were placed some statements about the new tool on which the users would have to validate their agreement with this statement. The selected questions concerning the developed application are developed based on the four constructs of MAT 3. For now, the answers were still being accepted.

CONCLUSION

The main purpose of the creation of the application "Sabichão" was the development of a platform that helped the paediatricians in their daily tasks, bridging the older system adding other functionalities.

With the SWOT analysis it could be concluded that this platform is able to improve quality of service in medical practices, because it has all the strengths previously explained that are a which are an asset, however, the platform weakness could not be forgotten.

Hereafter, it could be developed a *Business Intelligence* system, for better interpretation of the data taken from the platform usage, leading to an improvement of the application from structural changes in interfaces to removal features if necessary.

The creation of the same modules that already exist in the Medical application in the users area in the Web site would be an advantage because the functionalities that exists in the Medical Application could thus be used for example in colleges where the future paediatricians could practice wherever they want. Which leads to the translation of the platform for wider core users can use it.

REFERENCES

Abelha, A., Machado, M., Santos, M., Sollari, A., Rua, F., Paiva, M., & Neves, J. (2003). Agency for archive, integration and diffusion of medical information. *Proceeding of AIA*.

Cardoso, L., Marins, F., Portela, F., Santos, M., Abelha, A., & Machado, J. (2014, May). The next generation of interoperability agents in healthcare. *International Journal of Environmental Research and Public Health*, *11*(5), 5349–5371. doi:10.3390/ijerph110505349 PMID:24840351

Coiera, E. (2003). Clinical Decision Support Systems. In E. Coiera (Ed.), Guide to Health Informatics (2nd ed., Ch. 25). CRC Press. doi:10.1201/b13618-34

Ferreira, J., & Queiroz, S. (2010). Avaliação da aceitação de um ambiente virtual de aprendizagem em uma disciplina de comunicação científica. *Revista Latinoamericana de Tecnología Educativa RELATEC*, 9(2), 187205.

Kaushal, R., Bates, D., Landrigan, C., McKenna, K., Clapp, M., Frederico, F., & Goldmann, D. (2001). Medication errors and adverse drug events in pediatric inpatients. *Journal of the American Medical Association, 285*(16), 2114–2120. doi:10.1001/jama.285.16.2114 PMID:11311101

Legris, P., Ingham, J., & Collerette, P. (2003, January). Why Do People Use Information Technology?: A Critical Review of the Technology Acceptance Model. Inf. & Manage., 40(3), 191-204.

Miller, R., Gardner, R., Johnson, K., & Hripcsak, G. (2005, July). Clinical Decision Support and Electronic Prescribing Systems: A Time for Responsible Thought and Action. *Journal of the American Medical Informatics Association, 12*(4), 403–409. doi:10.1197/jamia.M1830 PMID:15905481

Novo, A., Duarte, J., Portela, F., Abelha, A., Santos, M., & Machado, J. (2015). *Information systems assessment in pathologic anatomy service.* In A. Rocha, A. M. Correia, S. Costanzo, & L. P. Reis (Eds.), New Contributions in Information Systems and Technologies (Vol. 2, pp. 199–209). doi:10.1007/978-3-319-16528-8_19

Peixoto, H., Santos, M., Abelha, A., & Machado, J. (2012). Intelligence in Interoperability with AIDA. In L. Chen, A. Felfernig, J. Liu, & Z. Ras, (Eds.), Foundations of Intelligent Systems SE (Vol. 7661, pp. 264-273).

Portela, F., Cabral, A., Abelha, A., Salazar, M., Quintas, C., Machado, J., & Santos, M. (2014). Knowledge Acquisition Process for Intelligent Decision Support in Critical Health Care. *In Healthcare Administration: Concepts, Methodologies, Tools, and Applications: Concepts, Methodologies, Tools, and Applications.* Hershey, PA, USA: IGI Global.

Portela, F., Santos, M., Silva, Á., Machado, J., Abelha, A., & Rua, F. (2014). *Pervasive and Intelligent Decision Support in Intensive Medicine – The Complete Picture.* Springer. doi:10.1007/978-3-319-10265-8_9

Ramnarayan, P., & Britto, J. (2002). Paediatric clinical decision support systems. *Archives of Disease in Childhood, 87*(5), 361–362. doi:10.1136/adc.87.5.361 PMID:12390900

Root, R. W., & Draper, S. (1983). Questionnaires as a software evaluation tool.

van Rosse, F., Maat, B., Rademaker, C. M. A., van Vught, A. J., Egberts, A. C. G., & Bollen, C. W. (2009). The Effect of Computerized Physician Order Entry on Medication Prescription Errors and Clinical Outcome in Pediatric and Intensive Care: A Systematic Review. *Pediatrics*, *123*(4), 1184–1190. doi:10.1542/peds.2008-1494 PMID:19336379

Zheng, K. (2010). Clinical Decision-Support Systems. In Encyclopedia of Library and Information Sciences (Vol. 3).

Chapter 15

Evolutionary Intelligence and Quality–Of–Information
A Specific Case Modelling

Eliana Pereira
University of Minho, Portugal

Ana Pereira
University of Minho, Portugal

Eva Silva
University of Minho, Portugal

Bruno Fernandes
University of Minho, Portugal

José Neves
University of Minho, Portugal

ABSTRACT

The strategy of making predictions for a specific case or problem, in particular regarding scenarios with incomplete information, should follow a dynamic and formal model. This chapter presents a specific case concerning the employment of professionals for a health institution, as technicians and physicians, to demonstrate a model that requires the Quality-of-Information and the Degree-of-Confidence of the extensions of the predicates that model the universe of discourse. It is also mentioned a virtual intellect, or computational model, in order to maximize the Degree-of-Confidence that is associated with each term in the extensions of the predicates, according to the approximate representation of the universe of discourse. This model is prepared to be adopted by a Business Intelligence platform in order to increase the Quality-of-Information and the Degree-of-Confidence of the extensions in healthcare.

DOI: 10.4018/978-1-4666-9882-6.ch015

INTRODUCTION

Decision-support systems appeared in the early 1970s in contrast to transaction-processing or operational applications, such as order entry, inventory control and payroll systems. Over the years, the decision-support domain has widely expanded until the concept of Business Intelligence (BI) appears, in the early 1990s (Watson & Wixom, 2007).

A business collects and acquires an enormous amount of data every day and recent surveys confirm that over 93% of this data is not usable in the business decision-making process today (Reinschmidt & Francoise, 2000).

Nowadays, BI is extensively used to describe analytic applications as a strategic initiative in driving business effectiveness and innovation (Watson & Wixom, 2007).

Data organization can lead to a competitive advantage and learning how to uncover and leverage this advantage is what BI is all about (Reinschmidt & Francoise, 2000).

Knowledge Representation is the area of Artificial Intelligence (AI) concerned with how knowledge can be represented symbolically and manipulated in an automated way by reasoning programs. There are many different ways to approach and study the area of Knowledge Representation. One might think in terms of a representation language like that of symbolic logic, and concentrate on how logic can be applied to problems in AI (Brachman & Levesque, 2003).

Many approaches for Knowledge Representation and Reasoning have been proposed using the Logic Programming (LP) paradigm (Kakas, Kowalski, & Toni, 1998) (Gelfond & Lifschitz, 1988) (Pereira L. a., 2009). Here, the authors follow the proof theoretical approach and an extension to the logic programming language, to Knowledge Representation and Reasoning as represented in the article "Evolutionary intelligence in asphalt pavement modeling and Quality-of-Information" (Neves, et al., 2012).

In practical terms, at the end of this process the authors expect to get a set of theories (or scenarios) that correspond to the best models of the universe of discourse. It will be possible to apply the program in various scenarios of the case that is being studied and, in each of these scenarios, obtain a set of predicates and each attribute of these predicates will be represented in the form of slices of a pie chart.

This model of Knowledge Representation can be generalized and applied to any problem in any knowledge domain in which the concepts of Quality-of-Information (QoI) and Degree-of-Confidence (DoC) must be considered for the decision-making process to get a good diagnosis.

BACKGROUND

BI systems are rapidly being adopted to provide enhanced analytical capabilities to previously existing systems that manage and integrate a very large array of information. BI systems are defined as specialized tools for data analysis, query, and reporting that support organizational decision-making that potentially enhances the performance of a range of business processes. BI systems are also complemented by specialized IT infrastructure (including Data Warehouses, Datamarts and Extract Transform and Load (ETL) tools) which is necessary for their deployment and effective use (Elbashir, Collier, & Davern, 2008).

In order to improve the QoI comes the implementation of BI strategies. This is a major step since it provides actionable information delivered at the right time, at the right location, and in the right form to assist the decision-making process. By improving the timeliness and quality of inputs, only valuable information is considered and the final models are the most accurate possible (Negash, 2004).

Some non-classical techniques to model the universe of discourse and reasoning procedures of intelligent systems have been proposed and many of them based on logic with probability theory (Kakas, Kowalski, & Toni, 1998) (Pereira & Lopes, 2007) (Subrahmanian, 2001).

Logic programming has emerged as an attractive formalism for Knowledge Representation and Reasoning tasks, introducing an efficient mechanism for solving search problems (Neves, et al., 2012).

In AI, one promising approach for Knowledge Representation and Reasoning, in particular in scenarios with defective information, is a measure of the QoI associated to a logic program or theory, which may allow one to access the confidence on how much that theory or logic program models the universe of discourse (Neves, et al., 2012).

Due to the growing need to offer user support in decision-making processes, some studies have been presented related to the qualitative models and qualitative reasoning in Database Theory and in AI research (Kovalerchuk, 2010) (Halpern, 2003). Concerning the problem of Knowledge Representation and Reasoning mechanisms in LP, a measure of QoI of such programs has been object of some work with encouraging results.

EVOLUTIONARY INTELLIGENCE AND QUALITY-OF-INFORMATION

Knowledge Representation and Reasoning

As mentioned, the proof theoretical approach in terms of an extension to the LP language to Knowledge Representation was followed. That said, an Extended Logic Program (ELP) is defined as a finite set of clauses in the form:

$$q \leftarrow p_1 \wedge p_n \wedge not\ q_1 \wedge ... \wedge not\ q_m$$

$$?\ p_1 \wedge ... \wedge p_n \wedge not\ q_1 \wedge ... \wedge not\ q_m\ (n, m \geq 0)$$

where *?* is a domain atom denoting falsity, the *pi*, *qj*, and *p* are classical ground literals, i.e., either positive atoms or atoms preceded by the classical negation sign (Neves, A logic interpreter to handle time and negation in logic data bases, 1984).

In this representation formalism, every program is associated with a set of abducibles, given here in the form of exceptions to the extensions of the predicates that make the program.

It is considered a procedure given in the terms of the extension of a predicate denoted as demo to demonstrate the body of knowledge that considers incomplete information. This meta predicate is given by the signature demo: *T,V → {true, false, unknown}*, according to the following set of terms:

$$demo(T, true) \leftarrow T$$
$$demo(T, false) \leftarrow \neg T$$
$$demo(T, unknown) \leftarrow not\ T, not\ \neg T$$

The first clause in this meta predicate defines that the response to a question T is true (1) if it's possible develop a test T from the positive information in the existing knowledge base. The second clause denotes that the response to a question T return false (0) if it's possible to prove the ¬T . The third and last clause in the meta predicate demo defines that the response of a question T returns a truth-value of type unknown if there is no proof of ¬T neither proof of T (Neves & Analide, Representação de Informação Incompleta, 1996). The result of this clause belongs to the interval]0,1[.

In AI, one promising approach for Knowledge Representation and Reasoning, in particular in scenarios with defective information, is a measure of the QoI associated to a logic program or theory, which may allow one to access the confidence on how much that theory or logic program models the universe of discourse (Neves, A logic interpreter to handle time and negation in logic data bases, 1984).

The QoI for a predicate *i* will be given by a truth-value in the interval [0,1], i.e., if the information is known (positive) or false (negative) the QoI for the extension of predicate *i* is 1.

For situations where the information is unknown, the QoI is given by:

$$QoI_i = \lim_{N \to \infty} \frac{1}{N} = 0 \, (N \gg 0)$$

where *N* denotes the cardinality of the set of terms or clauses of the extension of predicate *i* that stand for the incompleteness under consideration.

For situations where the extension of predicate *i* is unknown but can be taken from a set of values, the QoI is given by:

$$QoI_i = \frac{1}{Card}$$

where Card denotes the cardinality of the abducibles set for *i*, if the abducibles set is disjoint. If the abducibles set is not disjoint, the QoI is given by:

$$QoI_i = \frac{1}{C_1^{Card} + ... + C_{Card}^{Card}}$$

where C_{Card}^{Card} is a card-combination subset, with *Card* elements.

The next element of the model to be considered is the relative importance that a predicate assigns to each of its attributes under observation, i.e., which stands for the relevance of attribute *k* in the extension of predicate *i*. It is also assumed that the weights of all the attribute predicates are normalized, i.e.:

$$\sum_{1 \le k \le n} w_i^k = 1, \forall i$$

where, $\forall$ denotes the universal quantifier. It is now possible to define a predicate's scoring function $V_i(x)$ so that, for a value $x = (x_1, ..., x_n)$ in the multi-dimensional space, defined in terms of the attributes of predicate *i*, one may have:

$$V_i(x) = \sum_{1 \le k \le n} w_i^k \times \frac{QoI(x)}{n}$$

It is now feasible to rewrite the extensions of the predicates referred to above, in terms of a set of possible scenarios, according to productions of the type:

$$predicate_i(QoI, x_1, ..., x_n, DoC)$$

where $DoC = V_i(x_1, ..., x_n)$ denotes the one's confidence on a particular term of the extension of predicate *i*.

In practical terms, at the end of this process a set of theories (or scenarios) that correspond to the best models of the universe of discourse is expected. The program above can be applied in various scenarios of the case that is being studied and, in each of these scenarios, results a set of predicates and each attribute of these predicates will be represented in the form of slices in a pie chart.

Evolving Systems

Evolving systems are in constant development and they require the learning process. According to Herbert Simon, "learning denotes changes in a system that enable the system to do the same task more efficiently next time". Basically, the idea behind learning is that percepts should be used not only for acting, but also for improving the agent's ability to act in the future. Learning takes place as a result of the interaction between the agent and the world, and from observation by the agent of its own decision-making processes (Russel & Norvig, 1995).

The evolving systems can be represented by a computational model, named virtual intellect, which is constituted by a set of entities denoted as symbolic neurons. Each neuron is associated with a logic program or theory that models the view that such entities have of the whole system, given by the extensions of the predicates that make their corpus. The list of sub-problems to be solved, according to the diverse scenarios, is the input of each neuron. Indeed, the evolutionary process starts with an approximate representation of the universe of discourse and proceeds in order to maximize the DoC that is associated with each term in the extensions of the predicates. If the output layer has more than one neuron, it means that there are different theories that model the universe of discourse, being selected the one that presents the best DoCs in each term in the extensions of the predicates (Neves, et al., 2012).

An Evolutionary Algorithm (EA) is made of a set of computational mechanisms inspired by the fundamentals of the Darwinist Theory, and often used to solve optimization problems. During the process of evolution of an EA, the phenotype is the basis for the assessment of an individual (Neves, et al., 2012).

Each neuron in the intellect is coded with two types of genes, namely processing genes that specify how each neuron will evaluate its output, i.e., they determine how each neuron translates the input in output, and a set of connection genes which specify the potential connections to other neurons, built in terms of the extensions of the remaining predicates that model the universe of discourse. The processing genes are formed by the extensions of the predicates, invariants, structural and relationship dependencies, and inference mechanisms that make the realm of each neuron (Neves, et al., 2012).

Using the evolutionary programming, the candidate solutions for the problems are seen as evolutionary logic programs or theories and a measure of the DoC carried out by those logical theories or programs is used to test whether a solution is optimal.

The virtual intellect can be demonstrated in Figure 1.

Initially, an inference that represents a particular problem or question about the case being studied will be created. This problem will be processed in the form of a conjunction of the existing predicates and this process constitutes the input layer in our virtual intellect. This input layer can be exemplified by the following inference:

$$? \, demo((p_1(X), p_2(Y), p_3(Z), p_4(V)), S)$$

Figure 1. A schematic representation of a virtual intellect

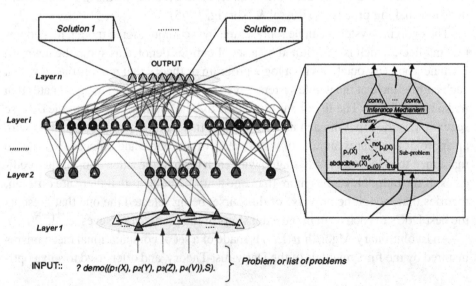

The computational model begins from the nodes in the input layer and goes other nodes that belong to the next layer. This layer is an intermediate layer and between the input and the output layer there may be several intermediate layers. The model continues until reaching the output layer. The nodes constituting each layer (input, intermediate or output) change according to the inference imposed.

An artificial intellect (or "artilect"), according to Dr. Hugo de Garis, is a computer intelligence superior to that of humans in one or more spheres of knowledge together with an implicit will to use the intelligence (De Garis, 2005).

The intellect learns from a past situations and self organizes itself, allowing to answer questions considering past experience. Over the time, when a new invariant is presented to the system, the intellect will be the same as the intellect used by the previous question, with addition to the new links discovered with new relationships.

For a better understanding of the subject discussed above the authors considered the application of the model in a practical case to exemplify the Knowledge Representation applied to a virtual intellect. Therefore, this example is about a company in the health field that is employing individuals and for this task it is considered that the individuals have the following attributes: IDEmploy, Age, Sex, Job, Qualifications, Experience and Clinical history. This example is illustrated in Figure 2.

Figure 2. An extension of the relational database model

#	IDEmploy	Age	Sex	Height	Job	Qualifications	Experience	Clinical_history
1.	1	25	1	[155,170]	4	3	0	
2.	2	40	0	[170,180]	5	4	1	
3.	3	33	1	[164,170]	{1,2}	1	1	
4.	4	29	0	[167,172]	3	2	⊥	

Jobs

#	IDJob	Job	Weekly hours
1.	1	Cleaning	40
2.	2	Receptionist	30
3.	3	Technician	35
4.	4	Nurse	40
5.	5	Physician	36

Qualifications

#	IDQualification	Qualification	ISCED
1.	1	High School	3
2.	2	Bachelor	5
3.	3	Master	5
4.	4	Specialist	6

It's considered that in the case of the attribute Qualifications, the classification can have four designations (1 – 4) and each designation represents the value of the attribute IDQualifications in the table Qualifications. In the case of the attribute Job, is also considered that can have five designations (1 – 5) and each of them represent the value of the attribute IDJob in table Job. This information is represented on a graphically where the respiratory rate was evaluated for a 5 days period for each candidate.

For this example, the relations represented in Figure 2 were rewritten as the following predicates:

$$jobs : IDJob \times Job \times Weekly\_hours \leftarrow 0...1$$
$$qualifications : IDQualification \times Qualification \times ISCED \leftarrow 0...1$$
$$employment : IDEmploy \times Age \times Sex \times Height \times Job \times Qualification \times Experience$$
$$\times Clinical\_history \leftarrow 0...1$$

It is now possible to exemplify the extensions of the predicates declared above in the form of programs.

Program 1: The extended logic program for predicate Employment

$$employment\{$$
$$\neg employment(IDEmploy, Age, Sex, Height, Job, Qualifications, Experience,$$
$$Clinical\_history) \leftarrow$$
$$not\ employment(IDEmploy, Age, Sex, Height, Job, Qualifications, Experience,$$
$$Clinical\_history),$$
$$not\ abducible_{employment}(IDEmploy, Age, Sex, Height, Job, Qualifications, Experience,$$
$$Clinical\_history).$$

$$abducible_{employment}(IDEmploy, Age, Sex, Height, Job, Qualifications, Experience,$$
$$Clinical\_history) \leftarrow$$
$$employment(IDEmploy, Age, Sex, Height, Job, Qualifications, \bot, Clinical\_history).$$

$abducible_{employment}(1, 25, 1, Height, 4, 3, 0, graphic1) \leftarrow 155 \leq Height \leq 170.$

$abducible_{employment}(2, 40, 0, Height, 5, 4, 1, graphic2) \leftarrow 170 \leq Height \leq 180.$

$abducible_{employment}(3, 33, 1, Height, 1, 1, 1, graphic3) \leftarrow 164 \leq Height \leq 170.$

$abducible_{employment}(3, 33, 1, Height, 2, 1, 1, graphic\ 3) \leftarrow 164 \leq Height \leq 170.$

$abducible_{employment}(4, 29, 0, Height, 3, 2, \bot, graphic\ 4) \leftarrow 167 \leq Height \leq 172.$

$?((abducible_{employment}(IDEmploy1, Age1, Sex1, Height1, Job1, Qualifications1, Experience1,$
$\qquad\qquad Clinical\_history1) \vee$

$abducible_{employment}(IDEmploy2, Age2, Sex2, Height2, Job2, Qualifications2, Experience2,$
$\qquad\qquad Clinical\_history2) \wedge$

$\neg(abducible_{employment}(IDEmploy1, Age1, Sex1, Height1, Job1, Qualifications1, Experience1,$
$\qquad\qquad Clinical\_history1) \wedge$

$abducible_{employment}(IDEmploy2, Age2, Sex2, Height2, Job2, Qualifications2, Experience2,$
$\qquad\qquad Clinical\_history2))).$

}

In this program the first clause denotes the closure of the predicate Employment. In the second and third clauses, the symbol $\bot$ stands for a null value, that subsumes that variable Experience stands for any value in the its domain. The next four clauses exemplify the other cases referred in the table Employment. Specifying two of these clauses, the seventh and eighth clauses denotes that the Job of a female employee 1 with 33 years, with a height greater than 155 and less than 170, a qualification and experience of 1 and a clinical history with a specific graph, is either 1 or 2. Finally, the last clause states that the value of Job is either 1 or 2, but not both.

Program 2: The extended logic program for predicate Jobs

$jobs\{$

$\neg jobs(IDJob, Job, Weekly\_hours) \leftarrow not\ jobs(IDJob, Job, Weekly\_hours),$

$not\ abducible_{jobs}(IDJob, Job, Weekly\_hours),$

$jobs(1, Cleaning, 40).$

$jobs(2, \text{Re}cepcionist, 30).$

$jobs(3, Technician, 35).$

$jobs(4, Nurse, 40).$

$jobs(5, Physician, 36).$

}

In this program the first clause denotes the closure of the predicate Jobs. The next five clauses exemplify each case referred in the table Jobs.

Program 3: The extended logic program for predicate Qualifications

$qualifications\{$
$\neg qualifications(IDQualification, Qualification, ISCED) \leftarrow$
  $not\ qualifications(IDQualification, Qualification, ISCED),$
$not\ abducible_{qualifications}(IDQualification, Qualification, ISCED).$
$qualifications(1, HighSchool, 3).$
$qualifications(2, Bachelor, 5).$
$qualifications(3, Master, 5).$
$qualifications(4, Specialist, 6).$

In this program the first clause denotes the closure of the predicate Qualifications. The next four clauses exemplify each case referred in the table Qualifications.

SOLUTIONS AND RECOMMENDATIONS

After the representation of the existing predicates, it is now possible to engender any possible scenarios to represent the universe of discourse, based on the information given in the logic program above. This way, it is easier for the reader to understand the purpose and the practical application of this method.

Scenario 1 for Employee 1

For Scenario 1, please consider Figures 3 to 6 and their designation.

$employment(1, 25, 1, [155; 170], 4, 3, 0, Graphic\ X1)$

1. $\underbrace{[1; 1], [25; 25], [1; 1], [155; 170], [4; 4], [3; 3], [0; 0], [48; 49]}_{attribute's\ domains}$

$employment(1, 25, 1, [155; 170], 4, 3, 0, Graphic\ Y1)$

2. $\underbrace{[1; 1], [25; 25], [1; 1], [155; 170], [4; 4], [3; 3], [0; 0], [49; 49]}_{attribute's\ domains}$

Figure 3. Clinical History - Graphic X1

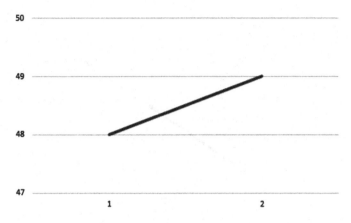

Figure 4. Clinical History - Graphic Y1

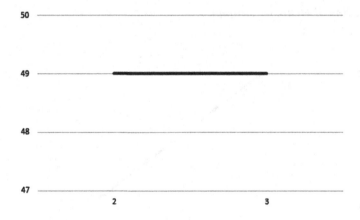

3.

$$employment(1, 25, 1, [155; 170], 4, 3, 0, Graphic\,W1)$$

$$\underbrace{[1;1], [25;25], [1;1], [155;170], [4;4], [3;3], [0;0], [49;52]}_{attribute's\,domains}$$

4.

$$employment(1, 25, 1, [155; 170], 4, 3, 0, Graphic\,Z1)$$

$$\underbrace{[1;1], [25;25], [1;1], [155;170], [4;4], [3;3], [0;0], [52;48]}_{attribute's\,domains}$$

As shown, the employment function for employee 1 can be represented in various ways due to the graphic concerning the clinical history of a particular candidate.

Then, to calculate the DoC for the considered predicates, a reference interval for each attribute in the predicate must be set:

Figure 5. Clinical History - Graphic W1

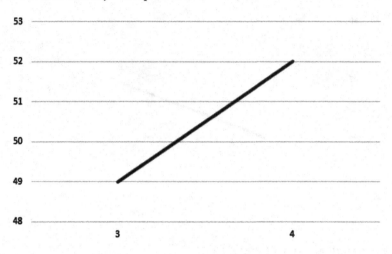

Figure 6. Clinical History - Graphic Z1

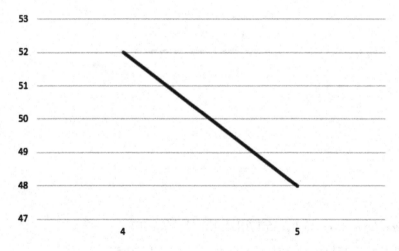

- **IDEmploy:** [0;50]
- **Age:** [18;65]
- **Sex:** [0;1]
- **Height:** [150;200]
- **Job:** [1;5]
- **Qualifications:** [1;4]
- **Experience:** [0;1]
- **Clinical History:** [45;55]

All the values for each attribute of the predicate employment were discretized. For example, Scenario 1 was discretized considering the following intervals:

$$employment([1;1],[25;25],[1;1],[155;170],[4;4],[3;3],[0;0],[48;49])$$

To calculate the DoC for each attribute in the predicate was necessary to normalize the information using Equation 1.9:

$$Normalization = \frac{UL - LL}{ULR - LLR}$$

where UL corresponds to the upper limit of the attribute interval, LL corresponds to the lower limit of that interval, ULR is the upper limit of the reference interval and LLR is the lower limit of the reference interval of the attribute.

For example, the normalization value for the attribute Height for Scenario 1 is given by:

$$N = \frac{170 - 155}{200 - 150} = 0.3$$

Once the normalization values for each attribute is obtained, one can calculate the DoC for each attribute considering the relation given in Figure 7.

Figure 7. Relationship between DoC and the normalized value (N)

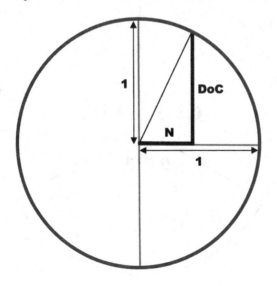

For the attribute Height the DoC can be calculated as:

$$1^2 = N^2 + DoC^2 \Leftrightarrow 1^2 = 0.3^2 + DoC^2 \Leftrightarrow DoC = 0.9539$$

This procedure is also applied to the other attributes in Scenario 1, resulting in a set of DoCs. The DoC for the scenario is obtained calculating the average of the DoCs obtained for each attribute in that scenario. For Scenario 1 the result is:

$$DoC(1,1,1,0.9539,1,1,0,0,0.9950) :: 0.8686$$

Therefore, the DoC for Scenario 1 is 0.8686.

The last procedure is to calculate the QoI and from this parameter it is possible to create a pie chart for the considered scenario.

For Scenario 1, the pie chart is represented in Figure 8.

In this case, there isn't any unknown value neither a set of specific values. Then, it is considered that the value of QoI for an interval of values is 1 because in the case of an interval of values there is always the certainty that the value belongs to the range defined by the limits of the interval, so the QoI is given by:

$$QoI = 1 \times 1 = 1$$

Figure 8. A representation of Scenario1

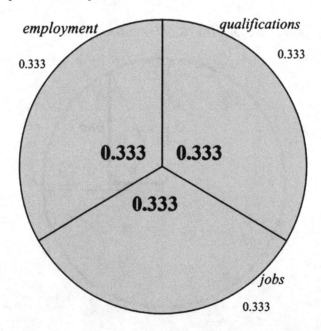

Since there is a total of three predicates in this scenario and, as mentioned above, there are no unknown values neither a set of specific values, each slice of the pie is $1 \times 1 / 3 = 0.333$.

The value of QoI for the slices in the pie corresponding to the predicates jobs and qualifications is always the same for each scenario since there are no unknown values or a set of specific values. However, this does not occur with the predicate employment, as will be exemplified later on.

It is now possible to rewrite the extensions of the predicate employment according to productions of the type:

$$predicate_i(QoI, x_1, \ldots x_n, DoC)$$

Performing the calculations described above, the results obtained are:

$employment(0.333, 1, 25, 1, [155; 170], 4, 3, 0, Graphic\ X1, 0.8686)$

$employment(0.333, 1, 25, 1, [155; 170], 4, 3, 0, Graphic\ Y1, 0.8692)$

$employment(0.333, 1, 25, 1, [155; 170], 4, 3, 0, Graphic\ W1, 0.8635)$

$employment(0.333, 1, 25, 1, [155; 170], 4, 3, 0, Graphic\ Z1, 0.8588)$

Scenario 2 for Employee 2

For Scenario 2, please consider Figures 9 to 12 and their designation.

$employment(2, 40, 0, [170; 180], 5, 4, 1, Graphic\ X2)$

1. $\underbrace{[2; 2], [40; 40], [0; 0], [170; 180], [5; 5], [4; 4], [1; 1], [51; 50]}_{attribute's\ domains}$

$employment(2, 40, 0, [170; 180], 5, 4, 1, Graphic\ X2)$

2. $\underbrace{[2; 2], [40; 40], [0; 0], [170; 180], [5; 5], [4; 4], [1; 1], [50; 50]}_{attribute's\ domains}$

$employment(2, 40, 0, [170; 180], 5, 4, 1, Graphic\ X2)$

3. $\underbrace{[2; 2], [40; 40], [0; 0], [170; 180], [5; 5], [4; 4], [1; 1], [50; 48]}_{attribute's\ domains}$

$employment(2, 40, 0, [170; 180], 5, 4, 1, Graphic\ X2)$

4. $\underbrace{[2; 2], [40; 40], [0; 0], [170; 180], [5; 5], [4; 4], [1; 1], [48; 47]}_{attribute's\ domains}$

Figure 9. Clinical History - Graphic X2

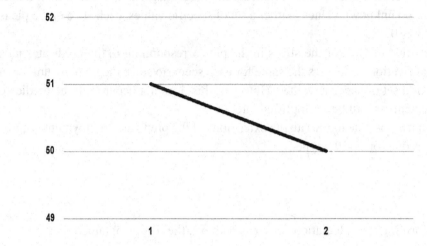

Figure 10. Clinical History - Graphic Y2

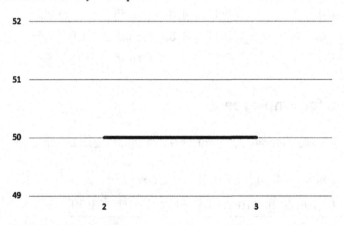

Figure 11. Clinical History - Graphic W2

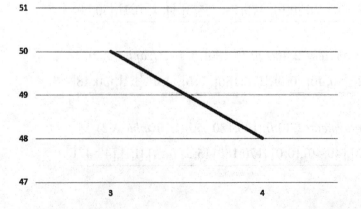

Figure 12. Clinical History - Graphic Z2

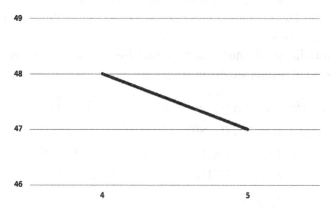

Performing the same calculations described in the previous scenario to obtain the value of QoI:

$$QoI = 1 \times 1 = 1$$

Then, the representation of Scenario 2 is obtained as represented in Figure 13.

Figure 13. A representation of Scenario 2

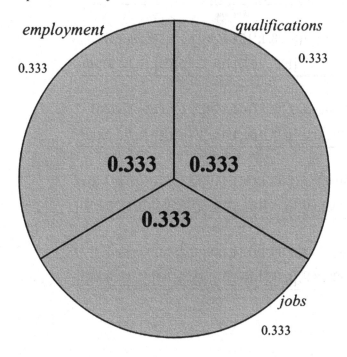

As can be seen, this representation is the same as the representation of Scenario 1 due to the fact that both cases don't have any case with unknown values or a set of specific values.

After performing all the necessary calculations to obtain the values of QoI and DoC, the following results are obtained:

$employment(0.333, 2, 40, 0, [170; 180], 5, 4, 1, Graphic\, X2, 0.995)$

$employment(0.333, 2, 40, 0, [170; 180], 5, 4, 1, Graphic\, Y2, 0.9975)$

$employment(0.333, 2, 40, 0, [170; 180], 5, 4, 1, Graphic\, W2, 0.995)$

$employment(0.333, 2, 40, 0, [170; 180], 5, 4, 1, Graphic\, Z2, 0.9969)$

Scenario 3 for Employee 3

For Scenario 3, please consider Figures 14 to 17 and their designation.

$employment(3, 33, 1, [164; 170], 1, 1, 1, Graphic\, X3)$

1. $\underbrace{[3; 3], [33; 33], [1; 1], [164; 170], [1; 1], [1; 1], [1; 1], [52; 50]}_{attribute's\, domains}$

$employment(3, 33, 1, [164; 170], 1, 1, 1, Graphic\, Y3)$

2. $\underbrace{[3; 3], [33; 33], [1; 1], [164; 170], [1; 1], [1; 1], [1; 1], [50; 51]}_{attribute's\, domains}$

$employment(3, 33, 1, [164; 170], 1, 1, 1, Graphic\, W3)$

3. $\underbrace{[3; 3], [33; 33], [1; 1], [164; 170], [1; 1], [1; 1], [1; 1], [51; 49]}_{attribute's\, domains}$

$employment(3, 33, 1, [164; 170], 1, 1, 1, Graphic\, Z3)$

4. $\underbrace{[3; 3], [33; 33], [1; 1], [164; 170], [1; 1], [1; 1], [1; 1], [49; 49]}_{attribute's\, domains}$

$employment(3, 33, 1, [164; 170], 2, 1, 1, Graphic\, X3)$

5. $\underbrace{[3; 3], [33; 33], [1; 1], [164; 170], [2; 2], [1; 1], [1; 1], [52; 50]}_{attribute's\, domains}$

$employment(3, 33, 1, [164; 170], 2, 1, 1, Graphic\, Y3)$

6. $\underbrace{[3; 3], [33; 33], [1; 1], [164; 170], [2; 2], [1; 1], [1; 1], [50; 51]}_{attribute's\, domains}$

Figure 14. Clinical History - Graphic X3

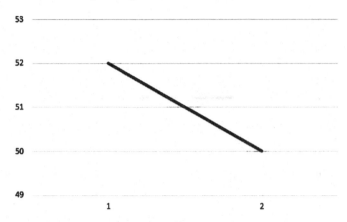

Figure 15. Clinical History - Graphic Y3

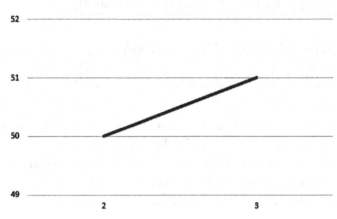

Figure 16. Clinical History - Graphic W3

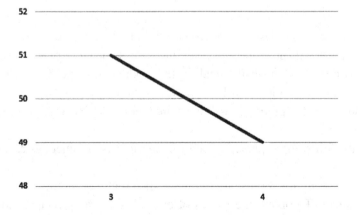

Figure 17. Clinical History - Graphic Z3

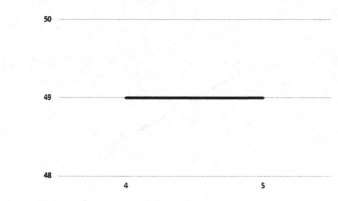

$$employment(3, 33, 1, [164; 170], 2, 1, 1, Graphic\,W3)$$

7. $\underbrace{[3; 3], [33; 33], [1; 1], [164; 170], [2; 2], [1; 1], [1; 1], [50; 51]}_{attribute's\,domains}$

$$employment(3, 33, 1, [164; 170], 2, 1, 1, Graphic\,Z3)$$

8. $\underbrace{[3; 3], [33; 33], [1; 1], [164; 170], [2; 2], [1; 1], [1; 1], [50; 51]}_{attribute's\,domains}$

In this case there is an attribute that as a set of possible values in the predicate employment, as can be seen in Figure 2. Here is considered that employee 3 can have job 1 or job 2, because this jobs (cleaning and receptionist) don't require a qualification above 1, so the candidate can be selected to job 1 or job 2, but not both. This fact changes the calculation of QoI, so it is:

$$QoI = 1 \times \frac{1}{2} = 0.5$$

Here, the two hypotheses for attribute job must be considered to calculate the QoI. For example, if the employee could have job 1, or job 2 or job 1 and 2, there would be 3 options. So, instead of making the product of it would be the product of .

Considering the value of QoI for the predicate employment, it is so, the slice corresponding to this predicate will have another circle divided into two slices of the same size.

Then, the following representation of Scenario 3 is obtained, as represented in Figure 18.

As can be seen, this representation has a slice that has another pie divided into two other slices. To obtain the values of each slice of the principal pie the same

Figure 18. A representation of Scenario 3

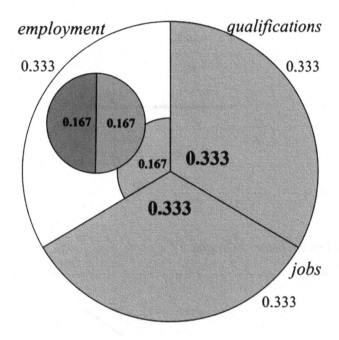

procedures are performed as in Scenario 1 and Scenario 2. Inside the *employment* slice, the secondary pie has two slices, each one equal to $1 \times 1 / 3 \times 1 / 2 = 0.167$.

After performing all the necessary calculations to obtain the values of QoI and DoC, the following results are obtained:

$employment(0.165, 3, 33, 1, [164; 170], \{1; 2\}, 1, 1, Graphic\ X3, 0.934)$
$employment(0.165, 3, 33, 1, [164; 170], \{1; 2\}, 1, 1, Graphic\ Y3, 0.9985)$
$employment(0.165, 3, 33, 1, [164; 170], \{1; 2\}, 1, 1, Graphic\ W3, 0.934)$
$employment(0.165, 3, 33, 1, [164; 170], \{1; 2\}, 1, 1, Graphic\ Z3, 0.999)$

Scenario 4 for Employee 4

For Scenario 4, please consider Figures 19 to 22 and their designation.

$employment(4, 29, 0, [167; 172], 3, 2, \perp, Graphic\ X4)$

1. $\underbrace{[4; 4], [29; 29], [0; 0], [167; 172], [3; 3], [2; 2], [0; 1], [50; 50]}_{attribute's\ domains}$

Figure 19. Clinical History - Graphic X4

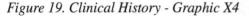

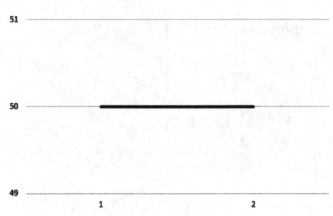

Figure 20. Clinical History - Graphic Y4

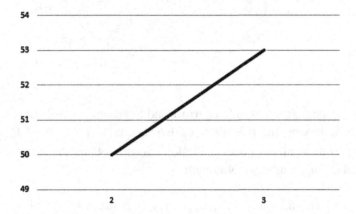

2. $employment(4, 29, 0, [167; 172], 3, 2, \perp, Graphic\, Y4)$
$$\underbrace{[4; 4], [29; 29], [0; 0], [167; 172], [3; 3], [2; 2], [0; 1], [50; 53]}_{attribute's\, domains}$$

3. $employment(4, 29, 0, [167; 172], 3, 2, \perp, Graphic\, W4)$
$$\underbrace{[4; 4], [29; 29], [0; 0], [167; 172], [3; 3], [2; 2], [0; 1], [53; 51]}_{attribute's\, domains}$$

4. $employment(4, 29, 0, [167; 172], 3, 2, \perp, Graphic\, Z4)$
$$\underbrace{[4; 4], [29; 29], [0; 0], [167; 172], [3; 3], [2; 2], [0; 1], [51; 47]}_{attribute's\, domains}$$

Figure 21. Clinical History - Graphic W4

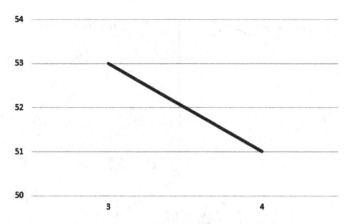

Figure 22. Clinical History - Graphic Z4

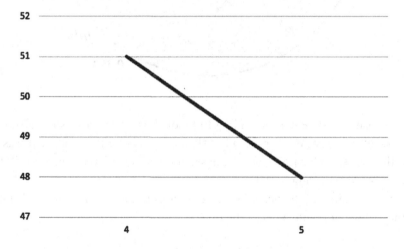

In this case there is an attribute that as an unknown value in the predicate employment. Then, it is considered that employee 3 can have any value for the attribute experience, which means that he/she can have 0 or 1, or, in other words, he/she can have experience (1) or not (0). Thus, the QoI is obtained:

$$QoI = 1 \times 0 = 0$$

Considering this value of QoI for the predicate employment the slice corresponding to this predicate will be 0. Then, the following representation of Scenario 4 is obtained, as represented in Figure 23.

Figure 23. A representation of Scenario 4

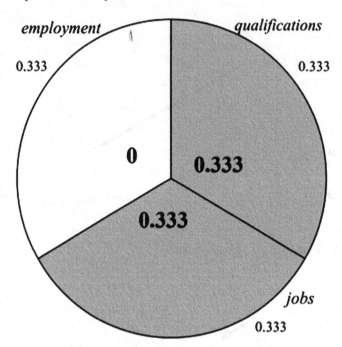

In this case, the slice corresponding to predicate employment should be 0, but this would affect the values for the other slices. To avoid this situation, it was considered that the slice for predicate employment has the value 0, but overall it still has a value corresponding to 0.333.

After performing all the necessary calculations to obtain the values of QoI and DoC, the following results are obtained:

$employment(0.333, 4, 29, 0, [167; 172], 3, 2, \perp, Graphic\ X4, 0.8744)$

$employment(0.333, 4, 29, 0, [167; 172], 3, 2, \perp, Graphic\ Y4, 0.8686)$

$employment(0.333, 4, 29, 0, [167; 172], 3, 2, \perp, Graphic\ W4, 0.8719)$

$employment(0.333, 4, 29, 0, [167; 172], 3, 2, \perp, Graphic\ Z4, 0.8686)$

Evolving Systems

In evolving systems, the application of this method follows a different representation.

Submitting questions to the system and express it in logic terms is done in the following form:

$$\forall (A, B, C, D, E, F, G, H, I, J, K, L, M, N, S).$$
$$? demo((employment(A, B, C, D, E, F, G, H), jobs(I, J, K), qualifications(L, M, N)), S).$$

The representation of the virtual intellect is shown in Figure 24.

In this representation the virtual intellect is constituted by three neurons associated to a logic program given by the extensions of the predicates employment, jobs and qualifications. These three neurons make the corpus of the virtual intellect, that is, the question presented to the system.

Each of these neurons have a list of sub-problems to be solved introduced as an input, according to their diverse scenarios.

After that, the evolutionary process starts by an approximated scenario in the memory of cases from the universe of discourse and then proceeds in order to maximize the DoC associated to each term in the extension of the predicates. As the input layer has more than one neuron, it means that there are different theories that model this universe of discourse and not just one. Hereafter, is selected the scenario in the memory of cases that can be used to answer the problem and, at the same time, maximizes the values of DoC and QoI.

Figure 24. A Representation of the Virtual Intellect for the Practical Case Being Studied

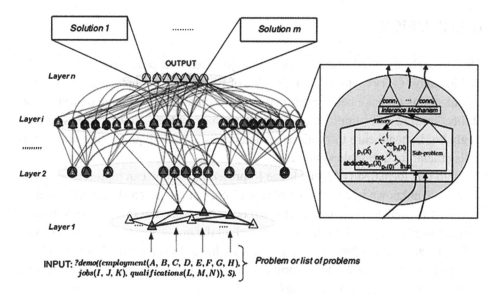

FUTURE RESEARCH DIRECTIONS

As new procedures and techniques arise every day, investigations over Knowledge Representation and Reasoning never stop developing. The importance of this type of models and their eminent advantages over BI systems, especially the ones applied to healthcare, make them an evolving area.

As for this specific model, any improvements may and should be applied in order to fix any possible unsolved issues. Making an evaluation of the model in different contexts might help finding not addressed situations and, therefore, not resolved by the model. This way, the application of the system would be evaluated and its viability would be tested for future efforts.

The application of the model in healthcare systems would be of major importance as the system could bring new possibilities in the decision-making process. That said, the QoI and the DoC, two of the most important measures in healthcare, would be improved and, therefore, the quality of the whole system.

In this manner, this model will be first applied to an healthcare unit located in Portugal – Centro Hospital do Porto – for evaluation and further validation to ease the process of making-decision in decision-support systems (Brandão, et al., 2014) (Portela, et al., 2014) (Pereira, Portela, & Abelha, 2016 (accepted for publication)). The whole implementation should be done in phases so the system is not compromised.

CONCLUSION

The applicability of BI, itself, is more than justified as it proves to be an essential tool in almost every system. The real value of BI systems lies in their use to support organizations to make better informed decisions that will lead to increased profitability, lowered costs, improved efficiency or whatever the goals of the organization might be. In healthcare institutions, efficiency is a main requisite that makes this tools crucial for a reliable system.

With this formalism of Knowledge Representation, one can represent exact information, unknown information, unknown information that can be taken from a set of values, as well as information represented as intervals. For this system to work it is necessary to represent all the attributes of all the predicates in a continuous way. In fact, even if the attribute is not continuous it has to be represented as continuous.

The cases represented in this form can be used as a case memory that represents each scenario in the universe of discourse.

To decide a solution to a problem presented to the system, the virtual intellect searches for the relationships between the attributes, knowing that the attributes values must be in an interval previously defined. The relationships chosen by the intellect are the ones that maximize the DoC and the QoI. In other words, the relationships maximize one's confidence in the attributes.

The intellect uses the evolutionary programming paradigm, therefore, the solutions are seen as evolutionary logic programs or theories and the system tests whether solution is optimal based on a measure of the DoC and the QoI carried out by those logical theories or programs.

This model of Knowledge Representation can be generalized and applied to any problem in any knowledge domain, in which may be necessary to consider a QoI and a DoC in the decision-making task in order to have a good diagnosis.

The implementation of the model mentioned above can improve the Quality-of-Information, a major requisite in healthcare BI systems, as well avoiding loss of information.

The computational framework followed is based on symbolic, evolutionary and connectionist paradigms for problem solving. The architecture that underlies this evolutionary system is defined as versatile, creative and powerful enough to engender a practically infinite variety of data processing and analysis capabilities, adaptable to any conceived task in the case to be modelled.

Presenting the full extension of the predicate demo, in terms of its functionalities, the users can foresee the emergency of learning machines under a symbolic and mathematical approach to computing, being a great opportunity to study the real nature of intelligence.

REFERENCES

Brachman, R., & Levesque, H. (2003). *Knowledge representation and reasoning.* San Francisco: Morgan Kaufmann Publishers Inc.

Brandão, A., Pereira, E., Portela, F., Santos, M., Abelha, A., & Machado, J. (2014). Real-time Business Intelligence platform to maternity care. *Proceedings of the IEEE Conference on Biomedical Engineering and Sciences IECBES '14* (pp. 379-384). IEEE.

De Garis, H. (2005). *The Artilect War: Cosmists vs. Terrans: A bitter controversy concerning whether humanity should build godlike massively intelligent machines.* Palm Springs: ETC Publications.

Elbashir, M., Collier, P., & Davern, M. (2008). Measuring the effects of business intelligence systems: The relationship between business process and organizational performance. *International Journal of Accounting Information Systems, 9*(3), 135–153. doi:10.1016/j.accinf.2008.03.001

Gelfond, M., & Lifschitz, V. (1988). *The stable model semantics for logic programming*. ICLP/SLP.

Halpern, J. a. (2003). *Reasoning about uncertainty*. MIT press Cambridge.

Kakas, A., Kowalski, R., & Toni, F. (1998). The Role of Abduction in Logic Programming. Handbook of logic in artificial intelligence and logic programming (pp. 235-324).

Kovalerchuk, B. R. (2010). Agent-based uncertainty logic network. *Proceedings of the 2010 IEEE International Conference on Fuzzy Systems (FUZZ)* (pp. 1-8). IEEE. doi:10.1109/FUZZY.2010.5584836

Negash, S. (2004). Business Intelligence. *Communications of the Association for Information Systems*, 13, 54.

Neves, J. (1984). A logic interpreter to handle time and negation in logic data bases. In J. Pottmyer, R. Muller, B. Mikelskas, & A. Roth (Eds.), *Proceedings of the 1984 annual conference of the ACM on The fifth generation challenge* (pp. 50-54). New York: ACM. doi:10.1145/800171.809603

Neves, J., & Analide, C. (1996). *Representação de Informação Incompleta*. Braga, Portugal.

Neves, J., Ribeiro, J., Pereira, P., Alves, V., Machado, J., Abelha, A., . . . Fernández-Delgado, M. (2012). Evolutionary intelligence in asphalt pavement modeling and quality-of-information. *Progress in Artificial Intelligence* (pp. 119-135).

Pereira, E., Portela, F., & Abelha, A. (n. d.). A Clinical Recommendation System to Maternity Care. In *Applying Business Intelligence to Clinical and Healthcare Organizations*. IGI Global.

Pereira, L. a. (2009). Evolution prospection. In K. Nakamatsu, G. Phillips-Wren, L.C. Jain, & R.J. Howlett (Eds.), New Advances in Intelligent Decision Technologies (pp. 51–63). Springer. doi:10.1007/978-3-642-00909-9_6

Pereira, L., & Lopes, G. (2007). Prospective logic agents. In J. Neves, M.F. Santos, & J.M. Machado (Eds.), Progress in Artificial Intelligence (pp. 73–86). Springer. doi:10.1007/978-3-540-77002-2_7

Portela, F., Santos, M., Machado, J., Abelha, A., Silva, Á., & Rua, F. (2014). Pervasive and intelligent decision support in intensive medicine - the complete picture. In M. Bursa, S. Khuri, & M.E. Renda (Eds.), Information Technology in Bio-and Medical Informatics (pp. 87–102). Springer. doi:10.1007/978-3-319-10265-8_9

Reinschmidt, J., & Francoise, A. (2000). *Business intelligence certification guide.* IBM International Technical Support Organisation.

Russel, S., & Norvig, P. (1995). *Artificial Intelligence: A Modern Approach.* New Jersey: Prentice-Hall, Inc.

Subrahmanian, V. (2001). Probabilistic databases and logic programming. In P. Codognet (Ed.), Logic Programming (p. 10). Springer. doi:10.1007/3-540-45635-X_8

Watson, H., & Wixom, B. (2007, September). The Current State of Business Intelligence. *Computer, 40*(9), 96–99. doi:10.1109/MC.2007.331

KEY TERMS AND DEFINITIONS

Degree-of-Confidence: Parameter that measures one's confidence on the list of characteristics presented by a specific case, set in terms of the attributes or variables that make the argument of its predicates.

Quality-of-Information: Measure of the confidence on how much a theory or logic program models the universe of discourse.

Universe of Discourse: Aggregate of the extensions of the predicates described within a case that might be represented by scenarios.

Virtual Intellect: The architecture of the computational model which is structured in terms of a set of entities denoted as symbolic neurons.

Compilation of References

Abelha, A., Machado, J., Santos, M., Allegro, S., & Paiva, M. (2002). Agency for integration, diffusion and archive of medical information. *Proceedings of theThird IASTED International Conference - Artificial Intelligence and Applications.* IASTED International Conference.

Abelha, A., Pereira, E., Brandão, A., Portela, C. F., Santos, M. F., & Machado, J. (2014). Simulating a multi-level priority triage system for Maternity Emergency. *Proceedings of ESM - 28th European Simulation and Modelling Conference*, Porto, Portugal. EUROSIS.

Abelha, A., Analide, C., Machado, J., Neves, J., Santos, M., & Novais, P. (2007). Ambient Intelligence and Simulation in Health Care Virtual Scenarios. In L. M. Camarinha-Matos, H. Afsarmanesh, P. Novais, & C. Analide (Eds.), *Establishing the Foundation of Collaborative Networks* (pp. 461–468). Boston, MA: Springer US. doi:10.1007/978-0-387-73798-0_49

Abelha, A., Machado, M., Santos, M., Sollari, A., Rua, F., Paiva, M., & Neves, J. (2003). Agency for archive, integration and diffusion of medical information.*Proceeding of AIA*.

Abelha, A., Pereira, E., Brandão, A., Portela, F., Santos, M. F., Machado, J., & Braga, J. (2015). Improving Quality of Services in Maternity Care Triage System. *International Journal of E-Health and Medical Communications, 6*(2), 10–26. doi:10.4018/IJEHMC.2015040102

Abelha, A., Pereira, E., Brandão, A., Portela, F., Santos, M. F., Silva, Á., & Braga, J. (2014). Improving Quality of Services in Maternity Care Triage System. *International Journal of E-Health and Medical Communications, 6(2), 10-26.*

Acampora, G., & Loia, V. (2008). A proposal of ubiquitous fuzzy computing for Ambient Intelligence. *Inf. Sci., 178*(3), 631–646. doi:10.1016/j.ins.2007.08.023

Adler-Milstein, J., & Bates, D. W. (2010). Paperless healthcare: Progress and challenges of an IT-enabled healthcare system. *Business Horizons, 53*(2), 119–130. doi:10.1016/j.bushor.2009.10.004

Agrawal, R., Grandison, T., Johnson, C., & Kiernan, J. (2007). Enabling the 21st century health care information technology revolution. *Communications of the ACM, 50*(2), 34–42. doi:10.1145/1216016.1216018

Compilation of References

Allison, J. J., Wall, T. C., Spettell, C. M., Calhoun, J., Fargason, C. A., Kobylinski, R. W., & Kiefe, C. et al. (2000). The art and science of chart review. *The Joint Commission Journal on Quality Improvement, 26*, 115–136. PMID:10709146

American Heart Association. (2009). *Heart Disease and Stroke Statistics 2009 Update*. Dallas, Texas.

Ammenwerth, E., Schnell-Inderst, P., Machan, C., & Siebert, U. (2008). The Effect of Electronic Prescribing on Medication Errors and Adverse Drug Events: A Systematic Review. *Journal of the American Medical Informatics Association : JAMIA, 15*(5), 585–600. doi:10.1197/jamia. M2667 PMID:18579832

Annoni, E., Ravat, F., Teste, O., & Zurfluh, G. (2006). Towards Multidimensional Requirement Design.*Proceedings of the 8th International Conference Data Warehousing and Knowledge Discovery (DaWaK)* (pp. 75-84). doi:10.1007/11823728_8

Araújo, S., Faria, J., & Cruz, J. (2007). *Propostas de Melhoria da Segurança dos Sistemas de Informação Clínica em Portugal*. Portugal: Faculdade da Universidade do Porto.

Atallah, L., Lo, B., & Yang, G.-Z. (2012). Can pervasive sensing address current challenges in global healthcare? *Journal of Epidemiology and Global Health, 2*(1), 1–13. doi:10.1016/j. jegh.2011.11.005 PMID:23856393

Atzori, L., Iera, A., & Morabito, G. (2010). The Internet of Things: A survey. *Computer Networks, 54*(15), 2787–2805. doi:10.1016/j.comnet.2010.05.010

Avison, D., Gregor, S., & Wilson, D. (2006). Managerial IT unconsciousness. *Communications of the ACM, 49*(7), 89–93. doi:10.1145/1139922.1139923

Azevedo, A., & Santos, M. F. (2008). KDD, SEMMA and CRISP-DM: A parallel overview. *Proceedings of the IADIS European Conference on Data Mining*Amesterdam, Netherlands (pp. 182-185).

Aztiria, A., Izaguirre, A., & Augusto, J. C. (2010). Learning patterns in ambient intelligence environments: A survey.*Artificial Intelligence Review, 34*(1), 35–51. doi:10.1007/s10462-010-9160-3

Banek, M., Tjoa, A. M., & Stolba, N. (2006). Integrating Different Grain Levels in a Medical Data Warehouse Federation. In A. M. Tjoa & J. Trujillo (Eds.), *DaWak, LNCS* (Vol. 4081, pp. 185–194). Heidelberg: Springer. doi:10.1007/11823728_18

Barua, S., Islam, M. M., & Murase, K. (2013). ProWSyn: Proximity weighted synthetic oversampling technique for imbalanced data set learning. In J. Pei, V. S. Tseng, L. Cao, H. Motoda, & G. Xu (Eds.), *Advances in Knowledge Discovery and Data Mining* (pp. 317–328). Berlin: Springer Berlin Heidelberg. doi:10.1007/978-3-642-37456-2_27

Bennett, W., Boone, E., Parker, D., Thorpe, A., Wang, M., & White, P. T. (2009). *Data Warehousing a New Focus in Healthcare Data Management*. Retrieved from http://www.himss.org/ files/HIMSSorg/content/files/EHR/DataWarehousing.pdf

315

Berbner, R., Grollius, T., Repp, N., Heckmann, O., Ortner, E., & Steinmetz, R. (2005). *An approach for the management of Service-oriented Architecture (SoA) based Application Systems* (pp. 208–221). EMISA.

Berger, S., & Ciotti, G. (1993). HIS (healthcare information systems) consultants: when are they necessary, and why? *Health Finance Management*, 47(6), 44-49.

Berg, M. (2001). Implementing information systems in health care organizations: Myths and challenges. *International Journal of Medical Informatics*, 64(2-3), 143–156. doi:10.1016/S1386-5056(01)00200-3 PMID:11734382

Berndt, D. J., Fisher, J. W., Hevner, A. R., & Studnicki, J. (2001). Healthcare Data Warehousing and Quality Assurance. *IEEE Computer*, 34(12), 56–65. doi:10.1109/2.970578

Berndt, D. J., Hevner, A. R., & Studnicki, J. (2003). The Catch Data Warehouse: Support for Community Health Care Decision-Making. *Decision Support Systems*, 35(3), 367–384. doi:10.1016/S0167-9236(02)00114-8

Bhatt, G. D., & Emdad, A. F. (2001). An analysis of the virtual value chain in electronic commerce. *Logistics Information Management*, 14(1/2), 78–85. doi:10.1108/09576050110362465

Biron, C., Ivers, H., Brun, J.-P., & Cooper, C. L. (2006). Risk assessment of occupational stress: Extensions of the Clarke and Cooper approach. *Health Risk & Society*, 8(4), 417–429. doi:10.1080/13698570601008222

Bizarro, P., & Madeira, H. (2002). Adding a Performance-Oriented Perspective to Data Warehouse Design.*Proceedings of 4th International Conference Data Warehousing and Knowledge Discovery* (pp. 232-244). doi:10.1007/3-540-46145-0_23

Bonney, W. (2013). Applicability of Business Intelligence in Electronic Health Record. *Procedia: Social and Behavioral Sciences*, 73, 257–262. doi:10.1016/j.sbspro.2013.02.050

Börger, E. (1998). High Level System Design and Analysis using Abstract State Machines. In D. Hutter, W. Stephan, P. Traverso, & M. Ullmann (Eds.), Current Trends in Applied Formal Methods FM-Trends '98, LNCS (Vol. 1641, pp. 1-43). Springer-Verlag.

Brachman, R., & Levesque, H. (2003). *Knowledge representation and reasoning*. San Francisco: Morgan Kaufmann Publishers Inc.

Brændeland, G., & Stølen, K. (2006). Using model-based security analysis in component-oriented system development. Paper presented at the *QoP '06: Proceedings of the 2nd ACM Workshop on Quality of Protection*, Alexandria, Virginia, USA (pp. 11-18). doi:10.1145/1179494.1179498

Brandão, A., Pereira, E., Portela, F., Santos, M., Abelha, A., & Machado, J. (2014). Real-time Business Intelligence platform to maternity care. *Proceedings of IECBES 2014 - IEEE Conference on Biomedical Engineering and Sciences*, Sarawak, Malaysia (pp. 379-384). IEEE.

Compilation of References

Brandão, A., Pereira, E., Portela, F., Santos, M., Abelha, A., & Machado, J. (2014). Real-time Business Intelligence platform to maternity care. Proceedings of IECBES 2014 IEEE Conference on Biomedical Engineering and Sciences, Sarawak, Malaysia (pp. 379-384). IEEE.

Brandão, A., Pereira, E., Portela, F., Santos, M., Abelha, A., & Machado, J. (2014). Real-time Business Intelligence platform to maternity care. *Proceedings of the IEEE Conference on Biomedical Engineering and Sciences IECBES '14* (pp. 379-384). IEEE.

Brandão, A., Pereira, E., Portela, F., Santos, M. F., Abelha, A., & Machado, J. (2014). Managing Voluntary Interruption of Pregnancy Using Data Mining. *Procedia Technology, 16*, 1297–1306. doi:10.1016/j.protcy.2014.10.146

Cabral, A., Abelha, A., Salazar, M., Quintas, C., Portela, F., Machado, J., . . . Santos, M. F. (2013). *Knowledge acquisition process for intelligent decision support in critical health care.* IGI Global Book. Retrieved from http://repositorium.sdum.uminho.pt/handle/1822/21710

Cabral, A., Pina, C., Machado, H., Abelha, A., Salazar, M., & Quintas, C. et al.. (2011). Data Acquisition Process for an Intelligent Decision Support in Gynecology and Obstetrics Emergency Triage. In M. M. Cruz-Cunha, J. Varajão, P. Powell, & R. Martinho (Eds.), *Enterprise Information Systems* (Vol. 221, pp. 223–232). CCIS.

Caldeira, A. T., Martins, M. R., Cabrita, M. J., Ambrósio, C., Arteiro, J., Neves, J., & Vicente, H. (2010). *Aroma Compounds Prevision using Artificial Neural Networks Influence of Newly Indigenous Saccharomyces SPP in White Wine Produced with Vitis Vinifera Cv Siria.*

Campbell, K. E., & Giannangelo, K. (2007). Language barrier: Getting past the classifications and terminologies roadblock. *Journal of American Health Information Management Association, 78*(2), 44–46, 48. PMID:17366992

Cardoso, L., Marins, F., Portela, F., Abelha, A., & Machado, J. (2014). Healthcare interoperability through intelligent agent technology. *Procedia Technology, 16*, 1334–1341. doi:10.1016/j.protcy.2014.10.150

Cardoso, L., Marins, F., Portela, F., Santos, M., Abelha, A., & Machado, J. (2014). The Next Generation of Interoperability Agents in Healthcare. *International Journal of Environmental Research and Public Health, 11*(5), 5349–5371. doi:10.3390/ijerph110505349 PMID:24840351

Carneiro, D., Novais, P., Andrade, F., Zeleznikow, J., & Neves, J. (2013). Using case-based reasoning and principled negotiation to provide decision support for dispute resolution. *Knowledge and Information Systems, 36*(3), 789–826. doi:10.1007/s10115-012-0563-0

Cassidy, L. D., Marsh, G. M., Holleran, M. K., & Ruhl, L. S. (2002). Methodology to improve data quality from chart review in the managed care setting. *The American Journal of Managed Care, 8*, 787–793. PMID:12234019

Cavanaugh, B., Garland, H., & Hayes, B. (2000). Upgrading legacy systems for the integrating the healthcare enterprise (IHE) initiative. *Journal of Digital Imaging, 13*(S1), 180–182. doi:10.1007/BF03167655 PMID:10847393

Chambless, L. E., Heiss, G., Shahar, E., Earp, M. J., & Toole, J. (2004). Prediction of ischemic stroke risk in the atherosclerosis risk in communities study. *American Journal of Epidemiology, 160*(3), 259–269. doi:10.1093/aje/kwh189 PMID:15257999

Chan, M., Estève, D., Fourniols, J.-Y., Escriba, C., & Campo, E. (2012). Smart wearable systems: Current status and future challenges. *Artificial Intelligence in Medicine, 56*(3), 137–156. doi:10.1016/j.artmed.2012.09.003 PMID:23122689

Chapman, P., Clinton, J., Kerber, R., Khabaza, T., Reinartz, T., Shearer, C., & Wirth, R. (2000). *CRISP-DM 1.0 Step-by-step data mining guide.* SPSS. Retrieved from ftp://ftp.software.ibm.com/software/analytics/spss/support/Modeler/Documentation/14/UserManual/CRISP-DM.pdf

Chapman, P., Clinton, J., Kerber, R., Khabaza, T., Reinartz, T., Shearer, C., & Wirth, R. (2000). *The CRISP-DM User Guide.* NCR Systems Engineering Copenhagen.

Chaudhuri, S., Dayal, U., & Narasayya, V. (2011). An overview of business intelligence technology. *Communications of the ACM, 54*(8), 88. doi:10.1145/1978542.1978562

Chen, P. P. S. (1976). The Entity-Relationship Model-Toward a Unified View of Data. *ACM Transactions on Database Systems, 1*(1), 9–36. doi:10.1145/320434.320440

Chiasson, M., Reddy, M., Kaplan, B., & Davidson, E. (2007). Expanding multi-disciplinary approaches to healthcare information technologies: What does information systems offer medical informatics? *International Journal of Medical Informatics, 76*, 89–97. doi:10.1016/j.ijmedinf.2006.05.010 PMID:16769245

Choi, J., Ahmed, B., & Gutierrez-Osuna, R. (2000). Ambulatory Stress Monitoring with Minimally-Invasive Wearable Sensors. *Comput. Sci. and Eng., Texas A&M.* Retrieved from http://citeseerx.ist.psu.edu/viewdoc/download?doi=10.1.1.188.4605&rep=rep1&type=pdf

Chute, C. G., Cohn, S. P., & Campbell, J. R. (1998). A framework for comprehensive health terminology systems in the United States: Development guidelines, criteria for selection, and policy implications. *Journal of the American Medical Informatics Association, 5*(6), 503–510. doi:10.1136/jamia.1998.0050503 PMID:9824798

Cios, K., Pedrycz, W., Swiniarski, R., & Kurgan, L. (2007). *Data Mining. A knowledge Discovery Approach.* Springer.

Clean Care is Safer Care Team (2011). *Report on the burden of endemic health care-associated infection worldwide: Clean care is safer care.* Geneva: World Health Organization. Retrieved from http://apps.who.int/iris/bitstream/10665/80135/1/9789241501507_eng.pdf?ua=1

Coiera, E. (2003). Clinical Decision Support Systems. In E. Coiera (Ed.), Guide to Health Informatics (2nd ed., Ch. 25). CRC Press. doi:10.1201/b13618-34

Comissão Nacional de Saúde Materna da Criança e do Abolescente. (2013). *Triagem Obstétrica-modelo de Triagem.* Lisboa: Direção Geral de Saúde.

Compilation of References

Commission recommendation of 2 July 2008 on cross-border interoperability of electronic health record systems. (2008). Off. J. Eur. Union.

Cortez, P., Rocha, M., & Neves, J. (2004). Evolving Time Series Forecasting ARMA Models. *Journal of Heuristics, 10*(4), 415–429. doi:10.1023/B:HEUR.0000034714.09838.1e

Crain, D. W., & Abraham, S. (2008). Using value-chain analysis to discover customers' strategic needs. *Strategy and Leadership, 36*(4), 29–39. doi:10.1108/10878570810888759

Currie, G., & Procter, S. (2002). Impact of MIS/IT upon middle managers: Some evidence from the NHS. *New Technology, Work and Employment, 17*(2), 102–118. doi:10.1111/1468-005X.00097

Damani, N. N. (2003). *Manual of infection control procedures* (2nd ed.). New York, NY: Greenwich Medical Media.

Darmont, J. (2008). Entreposage de Données Complexes pour la Medicine d'Anticipation Personalisée. *Proceedings of the 9th International Conference on System Science in Health Care* (p. 75).

Dayhoff, J. E., & DeLeo, J. M. (2001). Artificial neural networks. *Cancer Supplement, 91*(8), 1615–1635. doi:10.1002/1097-0142(20010415)91:8+<1615::AID-CNCR1175>3.0.CO;2-L PMID:11309760

De Garis, H. (2005). *The Artilect War: Cosmists vs. Terrans: A bitter controversy concerning whether humanity should build godlike massively intelligent machines.* Palm Springs: ETC Publications.

De Paola, A., Gaglio, S., Lo Re, G., & Ortolani, M. (2012). Sensor 9 k : A testbed for designing and experimenting with WSN-based ambient intelligence applications. *Pervasive and Mobile Computing, 8*(3), 448–466. doi:10.1016/j.pmcj.2011.02.006

Delone, W., & McLean, E. (2003). The DeLone and McLean Model of Information Systems Success: A Ten-Year Update. *Journal of Management Information Systems, 19(4), 9-30.*

Diamond, C., & Shirky, C. (2008). Health information technology: A few years of magical thinking? *Health Affairs, 27*(5), W383. doi:10.1377/hlthaff.27.5.w383 PMID:18713827

Duarte, J., Pontes, G., Salazar, M., Santos, M., Abelha, A., & Machado, J. (2013). Stand-alone electronic health record. *Proceedings of the 2013 IEEE International Conference on Industrial Engineering and Engineering Management IEEEM2013,* Bangkok, Thailand.

Duarte, J., Portela, C. F., Abelha, A., Machado, J., & Santos, M. F. (2011). Electronic health record in dermatology service. M. M. Cruz-Cunha, J. Varajão, P. Powell, & R. Martinho, (Eds.), Communications in Computer and Information Science, 221 (pp. 156-164).

Duarte, J., Salazar, M., Quintas, C., Neves, J., Santos, M., Neves, J., . . . Machado, J. (2010). Data quality evaluation of electronic health records in the hospital admission process. *Proceedings of the 2010 IEEE/ACIS 9th International Conference on Computer and Information Science ICIS* (pp. 201-206).

Duarte, J., Portela, C. F., Abelha, A., Machado, J., & Santos, M. F. (2011). Electronic health record in dermatology service. In *Communications in Computer and Information Science* (Vol. 221, pp. 156–164). CCIS; doi:10.1007/978-3-642-24352-3_17

Dutta, R. (2013). Health care data warehouse system architecture for influenza (flu) diseases. Proceedings of ACER (pp. 77–89).

Eder, C., Fullerton, J., Benroth, R., & Lindsay, S. P. (2005). Pragmatic strategies that enhance the reliability of data abstracted from medical records. *Applied Nursing Research*, *18*(1), 50–54. doi:10.1016/j.apnr.2004.04.005 PMID:15812736

Eichelberg, M., Aden, T., Riesmeier, J., Dogac, A., & Laleci, G. B. (2005, December). A survey and analysis of electronic healthcare record standards. *ACM Computing Surveys*, *37*(4), 277–315. doi:10.1145/1118890.1118891

Einbinder, J. S., Pates, R. D., & Reynolds, R. E. (2001). Case Study: A Data Warehouse for an Academic Medical Center. *Journal of Healthcare Information Management*, *15*(2), 165–175. PMID:11452578

Elbashir, M., Collier, P., & Davern, M. (2008). Measuring the effects of business intelligence systems: The relationship between business process and organizational performance. *International Journal of Accounting Information Systems*, *9*(3), 135–153. doi:10.1016/j.accinf.2008.03.001

El-Sappagh, S. H. A., Hendawi, A. M. A., & El Bastawissy, A. H. (2011). A proposed model for data warehouse ETL processes. *Journal of King Saud University - Computer and Information Sciences*, *23*(2), 91–104. doi:10.1016/j.jksuci.2011.05.005

European Community. (2009). Semantic interoperability for better health and safer healthcare. *Deployment and research roadmap for Europe.*

Fadlalla, A., & Wickramasinghe, N. (2004). An integrative framework for HIPAA-compliant I*IQ healthcare information system. *International Journal of Health Care Quality Assurance*, *17*(2/3), 65–74. doi:10.1108/09526860410526673 PMID:15301262

Fanger, P. O. (1970). *Thermal comfort: Analysis and applications in environmental engineering.* Danish Technical Press. Retrieved from http://books.google.pt/books?id=S0FSAAAAMAAJ

Fayyad, U., Piatetsky-shapiro, G., & Smyth, P. (1996). From Data Mining to Knowledge Discovery in Databases. American Association for Artificial Intelligence, 37–54.

Fayyad, U., Piatetsky-Shapiro, G., & Smyth, P. (1996). From data mining to knowledge discovery in databases. *AI Magazine*, *17*(3), 37–54. doi:10.1609/aimag.v17i3.1230

Ferreira Maia Neves, J. C. (1984, January). A logic interpreter to handle time and negation in logic databases.*Proceedings of the 1984 annual conference of the ACM on The fifth generation challenge* (pp. 50-54). ACM. doi:10.1145/800171.809603

Compilation of References

Ferreira, J., & Queiroz, S. (2010). Avaliação da aceitação de um ambiente virtual de aprendizagem em uma disciplina de comunicação científica. *Revista Latinoamericana de Tecnología Educativa RELATEC, 9*(2), 187205.

Foshay, N., & Kuziemsky, C. (2014). Towards an implementation framework for business intelligence in healthcare. *International Journal of Information Management, 34*(1), 20–27. doi:10.1016/j.ijinfomgt.2013.09.003"ttp://

Foshay, N., & Kuziemsky, C. (2014). Towards an implementation framework for business intelligence in healthcare. *International Journal of Information Management, 34*(1), 20–27. doi:10.1016/j.ijinfomgt.2013.09.003

Foundation, K. F. (2006). *Comparing Projected Growth in Health Care Expenditures and the Economy, Snapshots: Health Care Costs.* Retrieved from http://www.kff.org/insurance/snapshot/chcm050206oth2.cfm

Fry, J. (1993). *General practice: the facts.* Radcliffe Medical Press.

Gamble, J. E., Savage, G. T., & Icenogle, M. L. (2004). Value-chain analysis of a rural health program: Toward understanding the cost benefit of telemedicine applications. *Hospital Topics, 82*(1), 10–17. PMID:15490956

Gearing, R. E., & Mian, I. a, Barber, J., & Ickowicz, A. (2006). A methodology for conducting retrospective chart review research in child and adolescent psychiatry. *Journal de l'Académie Canadienne de Psychiatrie de L'enfant et de L'adolescent* [Journal of the Canadian Academy of Child and Adolescent Psychiatry], *15*, 126–34. Retrieved from http://www.pubmedcentral.nih.gov/articlerender.fcgi?artid=2277255&tool=pmcentrez&rendertype=abstract

Gelfond, M., & Lifschitz, V. (1988). The stable model semantics for logic programming. In R. Kowalski, & K. Bowen (Eds.), *Logic Programming – Proceedings of the Fifth International Conference and Symposium* (pp. 1070-1080).

Gelfond, M., & Lifschitz, V. (1988, August). *The stable model semantics for logic programming* (Vol. 88, pp. 1070–1080). ICLP/SLP.

Ghazanfari, M., Jafari, M., & Rouhani, S. (2011). A tool to evaluate the business intelligence of enterprise systems. *Scientia Iranica, 18*(6), 1579–1590. doi:10.1016/j.scient.2011.11.011

Gibb, J., & Haar, J. (2009). e-business connections in the health sector: IT challenges and the effects of practice size. *Journal of Management & Organization, 15*(4), 500–513. doi:10.5172/jmo.15.4.500

Glaser, J., & Stone, J. (2008). Effective use of business intelligence. *Healthcare Financial Management : Journal of the Healthcare Financial Management Association, 62*, 68–72. PMID:18309596

Glaser, J., & Stone, J. (2008). Effective use of business intelligence. *Healthcare Financial Management, 62*(2), 68–72. PMID:18309596

Goebel, R. Siekmann. J., Wahlster, W. (Eds), (2010). Advances in Knowledge Discovery and Data Mining, Lecture Notes in Computer Science (Vol. 6118). Springer.

Golfarelli, M., & Rizzi, S. (2010). WAND: A CASE Tool for Data Warehouse Design. *Proceedings of 17th International Conference on Data Engineering (ICDE)* (pp. 7-9).

Golfarelli, M., & Rizzi, S. (2009). *Data Warehouse Design: Modern Principles and Methodologies*. McGraw-Hill Osborne Media.

Gonçalves, J., Portela, F., Santos, M. F., Silva, Á., Machado, J., Abelha, A., & Rua, F. (2013). *Real-time Predictive Analytics for Sepsis Level and Therapeutic Plans in Intensive Care Medicine*. International Information Institute.

Graybeal, J. (2009). *Achieving semantic interoperability*.

Gregory, K. E., & Radovinsky, L. (2012). Research strategies that result in optimal data collection from the patient medical record. *Applied Nursing Research*, *25*(2), 108–116. doi:10.1016/j.apnr.2010.02.004 PMID:20974093

Gritzalis, D. A. (1998). Enhancing security and improving interoperability in healthcare information systems. *Informatics for Health & Social Care*, *23*(4), 309–323. doi:10.3109/14639239809025367 PMID:9922951

Grupo Português de Triagem. (2002). *Triagem no serviço de Urgência – Manual do Formador* (2nd ed.). Lisboa: BMJ Publishing Group.

Grupo Português de Triagem. (2014). Grupo Português de Triagem. Retrieved from http://www.grupoportuguestriagem.pt/jm/

Gyssens, M., & Lakshmanan, L. V. S. (1997). A Foundation for Multi-dimensional Databases. *Proceedings of 23rd International Conference on Very Large Data Bases (VLDB)* (pp. 106-111).

Halley, E., Sensmeier, J., & Brokel, J. (2009). Nurses exchanging information: Understanding electronic health record standards and interoperability. *Urologic Nursing*, *29*(5), 305–313. PMID:19863037

Halpern, J. a. (2003). *Reasoning about uncertainty*. MIT press Cambridge.

Halpern, J. Y. (2003). *Reasoning about uncertainty* (Vol. 21). Cambridge: MIT press.

Hammond, W. E., Jaffe, C., Cimino, J. J., & Huff, S. M. (2014). Standards in Biomedical Informatics. In E. H. Shortliffe & J. J. Cimino (Eds.), *Biomedical Informatics: Computer Applications in Health Care and Biomedicine* (4th ed., pp. 211–253). New York: Springer-Verlag; doi:10.1007/978-1-4471-4474-8_7

Hardin, J. M., & Chhieng, D. C. (2007). Data mining and clinical decision support systems. In E. S. Berner (Ed.), *Clinical Decision Support Systems* (pp. 44–63). New York, USA: Springer; doi:10.1007/978-0-387-38319-4_3

Compilation of References

Harrison, J. P., & McDowell, G. M. (2008). The role of laboratory information systems in healthcare quality improvement. *International Journal of Health Care Quality Assurance, 21*(7), 679–691. doi:10.1108/09526860810910159 PMID:19055276

Hasman, A. (1998). Education and health informatics. International Journal of Medical Informatics, 52(1-3), 209–216. doi:10.1016/S1386-5056(98)90133-3

Haux, R. (2006). Health information systems–past, present, future. *International Journal of Medical Informatics, 75*(3-4), 268–281. doi:10.1016/j.ijmedinf.2005.08.002 PMID:16169771

Health Information Systems, Toolkit on monitoring health systems strengthening. (2008). *World Health Organization.* Retrieved from http://www.who.int/healthinfo/statistics/toolkit_hss/EN_PDF_Toolkit_HSS_InformationSystems.pdf

Healthcare Information and Management Systems Society. (n. d.). *Clinical Decision Support.* Retrieved from http://www.himss.org/library/clinical-decision-support

HealthIT.gov. (n. d.). *Clinical Decision Support (CDS).* Retrieved from http://www.healthit.gov/policy-researchers-implementers/clinical-decision-support-cds

Heeks, R. (2006). Health information systems: Failure, success and improvisation. *International Journal of Medical Informatics, 75*(2), 125–137. doi:10.1016/j.ijmedinf.2005.07.024 PMID:16112893

Heinrichs, J. H., & Lim, J. S. (2003). Integrating web-based data mining tools with business models for knowledge management. *Decision Support Systems, 35*(1), 103–112. doi:10.1016/S0167-9236(02)00098-2

Helfenbein, S. (1987). *Technologies for management information systems in primary health care.*

Helferich, A., Schmid, K., & Herzwurm, G. (2006). Product management for software product lines: An unsolved problem? *Communications of the ACM, 49*(12), 66–67. doi:10.1145/1183236.1183268

Hema, R., & Malik, N. (2011). *Data Mining and Business Intelligence.* Bvicamacin.

Hersh, W. (2002). Medical informatics: Improving health care through information. *Journal of the American Medical Association, 288*(16), 1955–1958. doi:10.1001/jama.288.16.1955 PMID:12387634

HIMSS. (n. d.). *Transforming healthcare through IT.* Retrieved from http://www.himss.org/library/interoperability-standards/what-is

Hurtubise, R. (1984). *Managing information systems: concepts and tools.*

Hüsemann, B., Lechtenbörger, J., & Vossen, G. (2000). Conceptual data warehouse design.*Proceedings International Workshop on Design and Management of Data Warehouses, Stockholm,* (pp. 3-9).

Inmon, W. H. (2005). *Building the Data Warehouse.* John Wiley & Sons Inc.

International Health Terminology Standards Development Organization. (2014). *International Health Terminology Standards Development Organization*. Retrieved from http://www.ihtsdo. org/snomed-ct/snomed-ct0/

Inweregbu, K., Dave, J., & Pittard, A. (2005). Nosocomial infection. *Continuing Education in Anaesthesia, Critical Care and Pain, 5*, 14–17.

Inweregbu, K., Dave, J., & Pittard, A. (2005). Nosocomial infections. *Continuing Education in Anaesthesia. Critical Care & Pain, 5*(1), 14–17. doi:10.1093/bjaceaccp/mki006

Jamal, A., McKenzie, K., & Clark, M. (2009). The impact of health information technology on the quality of medical and health care: A systematic review. *Health Information Management Journal, 38*(3), 26–37. PMID:19875852

Jeffery, M., & Leliveld, I. (2004). Best practices in IT portfolio management. *MIT Sloan Management Review, 45*(3), 41–49.

Kahn, J., Aulakh, V., & Bosworth, A. (2009). What it takes: Characteristics of the ideal personal health record. *Health Affairs, 28*(2), 369–376. doi:10.1377/hlthaff.28.2.369 PMID:19275992

Kakas, A. C., Kowalski, R. A., & Toni, F. (1998). The role of abduction in logic programming. Handbook of logic in artificial intelligence and logic programming, 5, 235-324.

Kakas, A., Kowalski, R., & Toni, F. (1998). The Role of Abduction in Logic Programming. Handbook of logic in artificial intelligence and logic programming (pp. 235-324).

Kakas, A., Kowalski, R., & Toni, F. (1998). The role of abduction in logic programming. In D. Gabbay, C. Hogger, & I. Robinson (Eds.), *Handbook of Logic in Artificial Intelligence and Logic Programming* (Vol. 5, pp. 235–324). Oxford, United Kingdom: Oxford University Press.

Kaushal, R., Bates, D., Landrigan, C., McKenna, K., Clapp, M., Frederico, F., & Goldmann, D. (2001). Medication errors and adverse drug events in pediatric inpatients. *Journal of the American Medical Association, 285*(16), 2114–2120. doi:10.1001/jama.285.16.2114 PMID:11311101

Kawado, M., Hinotsu, S., Matsuyama, Y., Yamaguchi, T., Hashimoto, S., & Ohashi, Y. (2003). A comparison of error detection rates between the reading aloud method and the double data entry method. *Controlled Clinical Trials, 24*(5), 560–569. doi:10.1016/S0197-2456(03)00089-8 PMID:14500053

Khodambashi, S. (2013). Business Process Re-engineering Application in Healthcare in a Relation to Health Information Systems. *Procedia Technology, 9*, 949–957. doi:10.1016/j.protcy.2013.12.106

Kimball, R., & Ross, M. (2002). *The Data Warehouse Toolkit*. John Wiley and Sons, Inc.

Kimball, R., & Ross, M. (2002). *The data warehouse toolkit: the complete guide to dimensional modelling*. New York: Wiley. doi:10.1145/945721.945741

Kivinena, T., & Lammintakanen, J. (2012). The success of a management information system in health care - a case study from Finland. *International Journal of Medical Informatics*.

Compilation of References

Kohavi, R., & Provost, F. (1998). Glossary of terms. *Machine Learning - Special Issue on Applications of Machine Learning and the Knowledge Discovery Process, 30*(2-3), 271-274

Koh, H. C., & Tan, G. (2005). Data mining applications in healthcare. *Journal of Healthcare Information Management, 19*(2), 64–72. PMID:15869215

Kovalerchuk, B., & Resconi, G. (2010, July). Agent-based uncertainty logic network. *Proceedings of the 2010 IEEE International Conference on Fuzzy Systems (FUZZ)* (pp. 1-8). IEEE. doi:10.1109/FUZZY.2010.5584836

Krenker, A., Bešter, J., & Kos, A. (2011). *Artificial Neural Networks - Methodological Advances and Biomedical Applications*. InTech.

Kumar, S. (2012). *Semantic Web Agents-Based Semantic Web Service Composition*. doi:10.1007/978-1-4614-4663-7

Langefors, B. (1975). *Information Systems Architecture.*

Lee, D., Cornet, R., Lau, F., & Keizer, N. (2012). A survey of SNOMED CT implementations. *Journal of Biomedical Informatics, 46(1), 87-96*. PMID:23041717

Lee, M. L., & Ling, T. W. (1997). Resolving Constraint Conflicts in the Integration of Entity-Relationship Schemas. *Proceedings of the 16th International Conference on Conceptual Modeling,* Los Angeles, California, USA (pp. 394-407). doi:10.1007/3-540-63699-4_32

Legris, P., Ingham, J., & Collerette, P. (2003, January). Why Do People Use Information Technology?: A Critical Review of the Technology Acceptance Model. Inf. & Manage., 40(3), 191-204.

LeRouge, C., Mantzana, V., & Wilson, E. (2007). Healthcare information systems research, revelations and visions. *European Journal of Information Systems, 16*(6), 669–671. doi:10.1057/palgrave.ejis.3000712

Levene, M., & Loizou, G. (2003). Why is the Snowflake Schema a Good Data Warehouse Design? *Information Systems Journal, 28*(3), 225–240. doi:10.1016/S0306-4379(02)00021-2

Lippeveld, T., Sauerborn, R., & Bodart, C. (2000). *Design and implementation of health information systems*. Geneva: World Health Organization.

Littlejohns, P., Wyatt, J. C., & Garvican, L. (2003). Evaluating computerised health information systems: Hard lessons still to be learnt. *BMJ (Clinical Research Ed.), 326*(7394), 860–863. doi:10.1136/bmj.326.7394.860 PMID:12702622

Liu, W., Lian, Z., & Liu, Y. (2008). Heart rate variability at different thermal comfort levels. *European Journal of Applied Physiology, 103*(3), 361–366. doi:10.1007/s00421-008-0718-6 PMID:18351379

Liu, Y., & Sun, M. (2007, November). Fuzzy optimization BP neural network model for pavement performance assessment. *Proceedings of the IEEE International Conference on Grey Systems and Intelligent Services GSIS '07* (pp. 1031-1034). IEEE.

Locatelli, P., Restifo, N., Gastaldi, L., & Corso, M. (2012). Health care information systems: Architectural models and governance. *Innovative information systems modelling techniques* (Ch. 4, pp. 73-98). Intech.

Longstreth, W. T. Jr, Bernick, C., Fitzpatrick, A., Cushman, M., Knepper, L., Lima, J., & Furberg, C. (2001, February). Frequency and predictors of stroke death in 5,888 participants in the Cardiovascular Health Study. *Neurology, 56*(3), 368–375. doi:10.1212/WNL.56.3.368 PMID:11171903

Loshin, D. (2013). Business Intelligence: The Savvy Manager's Guide. Morgan Kaufmann. Retrieved from http://scholar.google.com/scholar?hl=en&btnG=Search&q=intitle:Business+Intelligence:+The+Savvy+Manager's+Guide#4

Lucas, P. (2004). Quality checking of medical guidelines through logical abduction. In F. Coenen, A. Preece, & A. Mackintosh (Eds.), *Research and Developments in Intelligent Systems XX* (pp. 309–321). London, United Kingdom: Springer. doi:10.1007/978-0-85729-412-8_23

Ludwick, D. A., & Doucette, J. (2009). Adopting electronic medical records in primary care: Lessons learned from health information systems implementation experience in seven countries. *International Journal of Medical Informatics, 78*(1), 22–31. doi:10.1016/j.ijmedinf.2008.06.005 PMID:18644745

Luftman, J. (2003). Assessing IT/business alignment. *Information Systems Management, 20*(4), 9–15. doi:10.1201/1078/43647.20.4.20030901/77287.2

Lumley, T., Kronmal, R. A., Cushman, M., Manolio, T. A., & Goldstein, S. (2002, February). A stroke prediction score in the elderly: Validation and web-based application. *Journal of Clinical Epidemiology, 55*(2), 129–136. doi:10.1016/S0895-4356(01)00434-6 PMID:11809350

Machado, J. M., Abelha, A., Santos, M., Portela, F., Pereira, E., & Brandão, A. (2015). Predicting the risk associated to pregnancy using data mining.

Machado, J., Alves, V., Abelha, A., & Neves, J. (2007). Ambient intelligence via multiagent systems in the medical arena. *Engineering Intelligent Systems for Electrical Engineering and Communications, 15*(3), 151–157. Retrieved from http://www.refdoc.fr/Detailnotice?idarticle=696527

Machado, J. (2002). *Agentes Inteligentes como Objectos dum Sistema Distribuído de Realidade Virtual*. Braga.

Machado, J., Abelha, A., Novais, P., Neves, J., & Neves, J. (2010). Quality of service in healthcare units. *International Journal of Computer Aided Engineering and Technology, 2*(4), 436–449. doi:10.1504/IJCAET.2010.035396

Mackway-Jones, K., M. J. & W. J. (1997). Emergency triage: Manchester triage group. *BMJ (Clinical Research Ed.)*.

Malinowski, E., & Zimanyi, E. (2008). *Advanced Data Warehouse Design, From Conventional to Spatial and Temporal Applications*. Springer Verlag Berlin Heidelberg.

Compilation of References

Mantzana, V., Themistocleous, M., Irani, Z., & Morabito, V. (2007). Identifying healthcare actors involved in the adoption of information systems. *European Journal of Information Systems*, *16*(1), 91–102. doi:10.1057/palgrave.ejis.3000660

Marins, F., Cardoso, L., Portela, F., Santos, M. F., Abelha, A., & Machado, J. (2014). Improving High Availability and Reliability of Health Interoperability Systems. *New Perspectives in Information Systems and Technologies* (Vol. 2, pp. 207–216). Springer. doi:10.1007/978-3-319-05948-8_20

Martney, S. A., Warren, J. J., Evans, J. L., Kim, T. Y., Coenen, A., & Auld, V. A. (2012, August). Development of the nursing problem list subset of SNOMED. *Journal of Biomedical Informatics*, *45*(4), 683–688. doi:10.1016/j.jbi.2011.12.003 PMID:22202620

Matinez-Costa, C., Menárguez-Tortosa, M., & Fernández-Breis, J. (2011). Clinical data interoperability based on archetype transformation. *Journal of Biomedical Informatics*, *44*(5), 869–880. doi:10.1016/j.jbi.2011.05.006 PMID:21645637

Medicity. (n. d.). *Medicity: Semantic Interoperability in HIE's*. Retrieved from www.medicity.com

Mei, H., Chen, F., Feng, Y. D., & Yang, J. (2003). ABC: An architecture based, component oriented approach to software development. *Journal of Software*, *14*(4), 721–732.

Mei, H., & Shen, J. R. (2006). Progress of research on software architecture. *Ruan Jian Xue Bao* [Journal of Software], *17*(6), 1257–1275.

Mendes, R., Kennedy, J., & Neves, J. (2004). The fully informed particle swarm: Simpler, maybe better. *IEEE Transactions on Evolutionary Computation*, *8*(3), 204–210. doi:10.1109/TEVC.2004.826074

MeSH. (1987). *Medical subject headings - health information systems*. Retrieved from Medical subject headings - health information systems. Retrieved from http://www.ncbi.nlm.nih.gov/mesh/68006751

Mettler, T., & Vimarlund, V. (2009). Understanding Business Intelligence in the Context of Healthcare. *Health Informatics Journal*, *15*(3), 254–264. doi:10.1177/1460458209337446 PMID:19713399

Mike, D. (2014). *Clinical Data Warehouse: Why You Really Need One*. Retrieved from http://www.healthcatalyst.com/clinical-data-warehouse-why-you-need-one

Miller, R., Gardner, R., Johnson, K., & Hripcsak, G. (2005, July). Clinical Decision Support and Electronic Prescribing Systems: A Time for Responsible Thought and Action. *Journal of the American Medical Informatics Association*, *12*(4), 403–409. doi:10.1197/jamia.M1830 PMID:15905481

Miranda, M., Duarte, J., Abelha, A., Machado, J., & Neves, J. (2009). Interoperability and healthcare. *Proceedings of the European Simulation and Modelling Conference* (pp. 205-212). EUROSIS.

Mitchell, M. (1999). *An Introduction to Genetic Algorithms*. MIT Press.

Moher, D., Liberati, A., Tetzlaff, J., & Altman, D. G.The PRISMA Group. (2009). Preferred Reporting *I*tems for *S*ystematic Reviews and *M*eta-Analyses: The PRISMA Statement. *PLoS Medicine, 6*(6), e1000097. doi:10.1371/journal.pmed.1000097 PMID:19621072

Moody, D. L., & Kortink, M. A. R. (2000). From Enterprise Models to Dimensional Models: a Methodology for Data Warehouse and Data Mart Design.*Proceedings of the Second International Workshop on Design and Management of Data Warehouses (DMDW)* (pp.1-12).

Mul, M. D., Alons, P., Velde, P. V. D., Konings, I., Bakker, J., & Hazelzet, J. (2012). Development of a Clinical Data Warehouse from an Intensive Care Clinical Information System. *Computer Methods and Programs in Biomedicine, 105*(1), 22–30. doi:10.1016/j.cmpb.2010.07.002 PMID:20728956

Munyisia, E. N., Yu, P., & Hailey, D. (2011). The changes in caregivers' perceptions about the quality of information and benefits of nursing documentation associated with the introduction of an electronic documentation system in a nursing home. *International Journal of Medical Informatics, 80*(2), 116–126. doi:10.1016/j.ijmedinf.2010.10.011 PMID:21242104

Murray, M., Bullard, M., & Grafstein, E. (2004). Revisions to the Canadian Emergency Department Triage and Acuity Scale implementation guidelines. *Cjem, 6*(6), 421–7. Retrieved from http://www.ncbi.nlm.nih.gov/pubmed/17378961

Murray, P., Wright, G., Karopka, T., Betts, H., & Orel, A. (2009). Open source and healthcare in europe - time to put leading edge ideas into practice. Medical Informatics in a United and Healthy Europe (pp. 963-967).

Murray, M. D., Smith, F. E., Fox, J., Teal, E. Y., Kesterson, J. G., Stiffler, T. A., & McDonald, C. J. et al. (2003). Structure, functions, and activities of a research support informatics section. *Journal of the American Medical Informatics Association, 10*(4), 389–398. doi:10.1197/jamia. M1252 PMID:12668695

Negash, S. (2004). Business Intelligence. *Communications of the Association for Information Systems, 13*, 54.

Neves, J., Machado, J., Analide, C., Abelha, A., & Brito, L. (2007, December 3-7). The halt condition in genetic programming. In J. Neves, M. F. Santos, & J. Machado (Eds.), *Progress in Artificial Intelligence: Proceedings of the 13th Portuguese Conference on Artificial Intelligence EPIA 2007*, Guimarães, Portugal, *LNAI* (Vol. 4874, pp. 160-169). Berlin, Germany: Springer. doi:10.1007/978-3-540-77002-2_14

Neves, J., Ribeiro, J., Pereira, P., Alves, V., Machado, J., Abelha, A., . . . Fernández-Delgado, M. (2012). Evolutionary intelligence in asphalt pavement modeling and quality-of-information. *Progress in Artificial Intelligence* (pp. 119-135).

Neves, J., Ribeiro, J., Pereira, P., Alves, V., Machado, J., Abelha, A., Novais, P., Analide, C., Santos, M., Fernández-Delgado, M. (2012). Evolutionary intelligence in asphalt pavement modeling and quality-of- information. Progress in Artificial Intelligence. *Progress in Artificial Intelligence, 1*(1), 119-135.

Compilation of References

Neves, J. (1984). A logic interpreter to handle time and negation in logic databases. In R. L. Muller, & J. J. Pottmyer (Eds.), *Proceedings of the Annual Conference of the ACM on the Fifth Generation Challenge* (pp. 50-54). New York, NY: Association for Computing Machinery.

Neves, J., & Analide, C. (1996). *Representação de Informação Incompleta*. Braga, Portugal.

Neves, J., Guimarães, T., Gomes, S., Vicente, H., Santos, M., Neves, J., & Novais, P. et al. (2015). Logic Programming and Artificial Neural Networks in Breast Cancer Detection. In I. Rojas, G. Joya, & A. Catala (Eds.), *Advances in Computational Intelligence – Part II,*LNCS (Vol. 9095, pp. 211–224). Cham, Switzerland: Springer International Publishing. doi:10.1007/978-3-319-19222-2_18

Neves, J., Martins, M. R., Vilhena, J., Neves, J., Gomes, S., Abelha, A., & Vicente, H. et al. (2015). A Soft Computing Approach to Kidney Diseases Evaluation. *Journal of Medical Systems*, *39*(10), 131. doi:10.1007/s10916-015-0313-4 PMID:26310948

Novo, A., Duarte, J., Portela, F., Abelha, A., Santos, M., & Machado, J. (2015). *Information systems assessment in pathologic anatomy service*. In A. Rocha, A. M. Correia, S. Costanzo, & L. P. Reis (Eds.), New Contributions in Information Systems and Technologies (Vol. 2, pp. 199–209). doi:10.1007/978-3-319-16528-8_19

Obenshain, M. (2004). Application of data mining techniques to healthcare data. *Infection Control and Hospital Epidemiology*, *25*(8), 690–695. http://www.jstor.org/stable/10.1086/502460 doi:10.1086/502460 PMID:15357163

OpenEHR. (2007). *OpenEHR Fundation*. Retrieved from http://www.openehr.org/

Oracle (2008). Oracle data mining concepts. Retrieved from http://docs.oracle.com/cd/B28359_01/datamine.111/b28129/toc.htm

Palaniappan, S., & Awang, R. (2008). Intelligent Heart Disease Prediction System Using Data Mining Techniques.*Proceedings of the 2008 IEEE/ACS International Conference on Computer Systems and Applications* (pp. 108–115). Washington, DC, USA: IEEE Computer Society. doi:10.1109/AICCSA.2008.4493524

Pan, L., Fergusson, D., Schweitzer, I., & Hebert, P. C. (2005). Ensuring high accuracy of data abstracted from patient charts: The use of a standardized medical record as a training tool. *Journal of Clinical Epidemiology*, *58*(9), 918–923. doi:10.1016/j.jclinepi.2005.02.004 PMID:16085195

Paramasivam, V., Yee, T. S., Dhillon, S. K., & Sidhu, A. S. (2014). A methodological review of data mining techniques in predictive medicine: An application in hemodynamic prediction for abdominal aortic aneurysm disease. *Biocybernetics and Biomedical Engineering*, *34*(3), 139–145. doi:10.1016/j.bbe.2014.03.003

Pardillo, J., Mazón, J. N., & Trujillo, J. (2010). Extending OCL for OLAP querying on conceptual multidimensional models of data warehouses. *Information Sciences*, *180*(5), 584–601. doi:10.1016/j.ins.2009.11.006

Park, H., Suh, W., & Lee, H. (2004). A role-driven component-oriented methodology for developing collaborative commerce systems. *Information and Software Technology, 46*(12), 819–837. doi:10.1016/j.infsof.2004.02.002

Park, T., & Kim, H. (2013). A data warehouse-based decision support system for sewer infrastructure management. *Automation in Construction, 30,* 37–49. doi:10.1016/j.autcon.2012.11.017

Parsons, K. (2010). *Human thermal environments: the effects of hot, moderate, and cold environments on human health, comfort and performance.* Taylor & Francis. Retrieved from http://books.google.pt/books?id=4oxA6W_Os50C

Parsons, K. C. (2000). Environmental ergonomics: A review of principles, methods and models. *Applied Ergonomics, 31*(6), 581–594. doi:10.1016/S0003-6870(00)00044-2 PMID:11132043

Paul, J., Seib, R., & Prescott, T. (2005). The internet and clinical trials: Background, online resources, examples and issues. *Journal of Medical Internet Research, 7*(1), e5. doi:10.2196/jmir.7.1.e5 PMID:15829477

Pavlović, I., Kern, T., & Miklavčič, D. (2009). Comparison of paper-based and electronic data collection process in clinical trials: Costs simulation study. *Contemporary Clinical Trials, 30*(4), 300–316. doi:10.1016/j.cct.2009.03.008 PMID:19345286

Peixoto, H., Machado, J., Abelha, A., & Neves, J. (2010). Semantic Interoperability and Health Records. Em S. Boston, IFIP Advances in Information and Communication Technology (pp. 236-237). Springer Boston. doi:10.1007/978-3-642-15515-4_30

Peixoto, H., Santos, M., Abelha, A., & Machado, J. (2012). Intelligence in Interoperability with AIDA. In L. Chen, A. Felfernig, J. Liu, & Z. Ras, (Eds.), Foundations of Intelligent Systems SE (Vol. 7661, pp. 264-273).

Peixoto, H., Machado, J., Abelha, A., & Santos, M. (2012). *Intelligence in interoperability with AIDA.* Springer. doi:10.1007/978-3-642-34624-8_31

Peralta, V., Illarze, A., & Ruggia, R. (2003). On the Applicability of Rules to Automate Data Warehouse Logical Design.*Proceedings of the 15th Conference on Advanced Information Systems Engineering* (pp. 329-340).

Pereira, E., Brandão, A., Portela, C. F., Santos, M. F., Machado, J., & Abelha, A. (2014). Business intelligence in maternity care. *Proceedings of IDEAS 2014 - International Database Engineering & Applications Symposium,* Porto, Portugal. ACM. doi:10.1145/2628194.2628248

Pereira, E., Brandão, A., Salazar, M., Portela, C. F., Santos, M. F., & Machado, J. … Jorge, B. (2014). Pre-Triage Decision Support Improvement in Maternity Care by means of Data Mining. In A. Azevedo, & M. F. Santos (Eds.), Integration of Data Mining in Business Intelligence Systems. Hershey, PA, USA: IGI Global Book.

Pereira, E., Portela, F., & Abelha, A. (n. d.). A Clinical Recommendation System to Maternity Care.

Compilation of References

Pereira, L. M., & Anh, H. T. (2009). Evolution prospection. In K. Nakamatsu (Ed.), *New Advances in Intelligent Decision Technologies: Results of the First KES International Symposium IDT 2009 (Studies in Computational Intelligence)* (Vol. 199, pp. 51-64). Berlin, Germany: Springer. doi:10.1007/978-3-642-00909-9_6

Pereira, L., & Lopes, G. (2007). Prospective logic agents. In J. Neves, M.F. Santos, & J.M. Machado (Eds.), Progress in Artificial Intelligence (pp. 73–86). Springer. doi:10.1007/978-3-540-77002-2_7

Pereira, R., Duarte, J., Salazar, M., Santos, M., Abelha, A., & Machado, J. (2012). Usability of an electronic health record. *Proceedings of the4th IEEE International Conference on Industrial Engineering and Engineering Management.* Hong Kong.

Pereira, E., Portela, F., & Abelha, A. (n. d.). A Clinical Recommendation System to Maternity Care. In *Applying Business Intelligence to Clinical and Healthcare Organizations.* IGI Global.

PhridviRaj, M. S. B., & GuruRao, C. V. (2014). Data Mining – Past, Present and Future – A Typical Survey on Data Streams. *Procedia Technology, 12,* 255–263. doi:10.1016/j.protcy.2013.12.483

Pinto, L. F. B. (2009). *Sistemas de Informação e Profissionais de Enfermagem.* Universidade de Trás-os-Montes e Alto Douro.

Pinto, M., Fuentes, L., Fayad, M. E., & Troya, J. M. (2002). Separation of coordination in a dynamic aspect oriented framework.*Proceedings of the 1st international conference on Aspect-oriented software development* (pp. 134-140). New York, NY: ACM. doi:10.1145/508386.508403

Piro, G., Cianci, I., Grieco, L., Boggia, G., & Camarda, P. (2014). Information centric services in Smart Cities. *Journal of Systems and Software, 88,* 169–188. doi:10.1016/j.jss.2013.10.029

Popovič, A., Hackney, R., Coelho, P. S., & Jaklič, J. (2012). Towards business intelligence systems success: Effects of maturity and culture on analytical decision making. *Decision Support Systems, 54*(1), 729–739. doi:10.1016/j.dss.2012.08.017

Portela, F., Aguiar, J., Santos, M. F., Silva, Á., & Rua, F. (2013). Pervasive Intelligent Decision Support System - Technology Acceptance in Intensive Care Units. In Á Roch, A.M. Correia, T. Wilson, & K.A. Stroetmann (Ed.), Advances in Intelligent Systems and Computing. Springer.

Portela, F., Aguiar, J., Santos, M. F., Silva, Á., & Rua, F. (2013). Pervasive Intelligent Decision Support System - Technology Acceptance in Intensive Care Units. In Á. Rocha, A.M. Correia, T. Wilson, & K.A. Stroetmann (Ed.), Advances in Intelligent Systems and Computing, CCIS (Vol. 206, pp. 279-292). Springer.

Portela, F., Cabral, A., Abelha, A., Salazar, M., Quintas, C., Machado, J., & Santos, M. (2014). Knowledge Acquisition Process for Intelligent Decision Support in Critical Health Care. *In Healthcare Administration: Concepts, Methodologies, Tools, and Applications: Concepts, Methodologies, Tools, and Applications.* Hershey, PA, USA: IGI Global.

Portela, F., Cabral, A., Abelha, A., Salazar, M., Quintas, C., Machado, J., Neves, J., & Santos, M. F. (2013). Knowledge Acquisition Process for Intelligent Decision Support in Critical Health Care. In R. Martinho, R. Rijo, M.M. Cruz-Cunha, & J. Verajao (Eds.), Information Systems and Technologies for Enhancing Health and Social Care (Ch. 4, pp. 55-68). Hershey, PA, USA: IGI Global.

Portela, F., Gago, P., Santos, M. F., Silva, A., Rua, F., Machado, J., ... (2011). Knowledge Discovery for Pervasive and Real-Time Intelligent Decision Support in Intensive Care Medicine. *Proceedings of KMIS 2011- International Conference on Knowledge Management and Information Sharing*, Paris, France.

Portela, F., Santos, M. F., & Vilas-Boas, M. (2012). A Pervasive Approach to a Real-Time Intelligent Decision Support System in Intensive Medicine. In A. Fred, J.L.G. Dietz, K. Liu, & J. Filipe (Ed.), Communications in Computer and Information Science, LNCS (Vol. 272, 368-381).

Portela, F., Santos, M. F., Gago, P., Silva, Á., Rua, F., Abelha, A., ... (2011). Enabling real-time intelligent decision support in intensive care. *Paper presented at the 25th European Simulation and Modelling Conference ESM'2011*, Guimarães, Portugal.

Portela, F., Santos, M. F., Silva, A., Machado, J., & Abelha, A. (2011). Enabling a Pervasive Approach for Intelligent Decision Support in Critical Health Care. In M. M. Cruz Cunha, J. Varajao, P. Powell & R. Martinho (Eds.), Enterprise Information Systems, Pt 3 (Vol. 221, pp. 233-243).

Portela, F., Santos, M.F., & Abelha, A., Machado, J. (2015). A Real-Time Intelligent System for tracking patient condition.

Portela, F., Vilas-Boas, M., Santos, M. F., Abelha, A., Machado, J., Cabral, A., & Aragão, I. (2010). Electronic Health Records in the Emergency Room. *Proceedings of the 2010 IEEE/ACIS 9th International Conference on Computer and Information Science (ICIS)*. doi:10.1109/ICIS.2010.98

Portela, F., Pinto, F., & Santos, M. F. (2012). Data Mining Predictive Models For Pervasive Intelligent Decision Support. *Intensive Care Medicine*.

Portela, F., Santos, M., Silva, Á., Machado, J., Abelha, A., & Rua, F. (2014). *Pervasive and Intelligent Decision Support in Intensive Medicine – The Complete Picture*. Springer. doi:10.1007/978-3-319-10265-8_9

Porter, M. E. (1985). *Competitive advantage: Creating and sustaining superior performance*. New York, NY: Free Press.

Power, D. J. (2008). Understanding data-driven decision support systems. *Information Systems Management*, 25(8), 149–154. doi:10.1080/10580530801941124

Powsner, S. M., Wyatt, J. C., & Wright, P. (1998). Opportunities for and challenges of computerisation. *Lancet*, 352(9140), 1617–1622. doi:10.1016/S0140-6736(98)08309-3 PMID:9843122

Compilation of References

Prevedello, L. M., Andriole, K. P., Hanson, R., Kelly, P., & Khorasani, R. (2010). Business intelligence tools for radiology: Creating a prototype model using open-source tools. *Journal of Digital Imaging*, *23*(2), 133–141. doi:10.1007/s10278-008-9167-3 PMID:19011943

Pritchard, P. M. (1981). *Manual of primary health care: its nature and organization*. Oxford University Press.

Rada, R. (2008). *Information Systems and Healthcare Enterprises*. Hershey, PA: IGI Publishing. doi:10.4018/978-1-59904-651-8

Ramnarayan, P., & Britto, J. (2002). Paediatric clinical decision support systems. *Archives of Disease in Childhood*, *87*(5), 361–362. doi:10.1136/adc.87.5.361 PMID:12390900

Rana, R., Kusy, B., Jurdak, R., Wall, J., & Hu, W. (2013). Feasibility analysis of using humidex as an indoor thermal comfort predictor. *Energy and Building*, *64*, 17–25. doi:10.1016/j.enbuild.2013.04.019

Raquel, O., & Oliveira, F. (2012). *Extração de Conhecimento nas Listas de Espera para Consulta e Cirurgia*. Universidade do Minho.

Rayport, J., & Sviokla, J. (1995). Exploiting the virtual value chain. *Harvard Business Review*, *73*(6), 75–85.

RedHat. (2007). *RedHAT*. Retrieved from Open-Source and Healthcare IT: http://www.redhat.com/f/pdf/OSHealthcareWhitepaper web.pdf

Reinschmidt, J., & Francoise, A. (2000). *Business intelligence certification guide*. IBM International Technical Support Organisation.

Reinschmidt, J., & Francoise, A. (2000). *Business Intelligence Certification Guide*. IBM.

Reti, S. R., Feldman, H. J., & Safran, C. (2009). Governance for personal health records. *Journal of the American Medical Informatics Association*, *16*(1), 14–17. doi:10.1197/jamia.M2854 PMID:18952939

Rigor, H., Machado, J., Abelha, A., Neves, J., & Alberto, C. (2008). A web-based system to reduce the nosocomial infection impact in healthcare units. *Proceedings of the International Conference on Web Information Systems – WEBIST 2008* (pp. 264-268). Funchal, Portugal: Scitepress.

Rigor, H., Machado, J., Abelha, A., Neves, J., & Alberto, C. (2008). A web-based system to reduce the nosocomial infection impact in healthcare units.*Proceedings of the WEBIST 2008 - International Conference on Web Information Systems*, Madeira, Portugal.

Rodrigues, J. J. P. C. (2010). Preface. In J. J. P. C. Rodrigues (Ed.), *Health Information Systems: Concepts, Methodologies, Tools, and Applications* (pp. i–vi). Hershey, PA: Medical Information Science Reference. doi:10.4018/978-1-60566-988-5

Root, R. W., & Draper, S. (1983). Questionnaires as a software evaluation tool.

Rossi, M., Campbell, K. L., & Ferguson, M. (2014). Implementation of the nutrition care process and international dietetics and nutrition terminology in a single-center hemodialysis unit: Comparing paper vs electronic records. *Journal of the Academy of Nutrition and Dietetics, 114*(1), 124–130. doi:10.1016/j.jand.2013.07.033 PMID:24161368

Rowlands, B. H. (2006). The user as social actor: A focus on systems development methodology enactment. *Paper presented at theSAC '06: Proceedings of the 2006 ACM Symposium on Applied Computing*, Dijon, France (pp. 1540-1545). doi:10.1145/1141277.1141634

Russel, S., & Norvig, P. (1995). *Artificial Intelligence: A Modern Approach*. New Jersey: Prentice-Hall, Inc.

Sahama, T. R., & Croll, P. R. (2007). A Data Warehouse Architecture for Clinical Data Warehousing.*Proceedings of the fifth Australasian symposium on ACSW frontiers* (vol. 68, pp. 227-232).

Salazar, M., Duarte, J., Pereira, R., Portela, F., Santos, M., Abelha, A., & Machado, J. (2013). Step towards Paper Free Hospital through Electronic Health Record. In Á. Rocha, A. M. Correia, T. Wilson, & K. A. Stroetmann (Eds.), *Advances in Information Systems and Technologies, Advances in Intelligent Systems and Computing* (Vol. 206, pp. 685–694). Springer. doi:10.1007/978-3-642-36981-0_63

Saleem, J. J., Russ, A. L., Justice, C. F., Hagg, H., Ebright, P. R., Woodbridge, P. A., & Doebbeling, B. N. (2009). Exploring the persistence of paper with the electronic health record. *International Journal of Medical Informatics, 78*(9), 618–628. doi:10.1016/j.ijmedinf.2009.04.001 PMID:19464231

Saleem, N., Jones, D. R., Van Tran, H., & Moses, B. (2006). Forming design teams to develop healthcare information systems. *Hospital Topics, 84*(1), 22–30. doi:10.3200/HTPS.84.1.22-31 PMID:16573013

Santos, M. F., & Portela, F. (2011). Enabling Ubiquitous Data Mining in Intensive Care - Features selection and data pre-processing. *Proceedings of the 13th International Conference on Enterprise Information Systems*, Beijing, China.

Santos, P. (2008, October). *Content Addressable Multimedia Database Server for Medicine: Registro Eletrónico de Saúde "PANORAMIX"* [Content Addressable Multimedia Database Server for Medicine: Registro Eletrónico de Saúde "PANORAMIX"] [Master's Thesis]. Instituto Superior Técnico.

Schulz, S., Suntisrivaraporn, B., Baader, F., & Boeker, M. (2009). SNOMED reaching its adolescence: Ontologists and logicians health check. *International Journal of Medical Informatics, 78*(Suppl. 1), S86–S94.

Semantic Web. (n. d.). *Semantic Web*. Retrieved from http://semanticweb.org/wiki/Main_Page

Sen, A., & Jacob, V. S. (1998). Industrial Strength Data Warehousing. *Communications of the ACM, 41*(9), 28–31. doi:10.1145/285070.285076

Sharma, S., Osei-Bryson, K.-M., & Kasper, G. M. (2012). Evaluation of an integrated Knowledge Discovery and Data Mining process model. *Expert Systems with Applications*, *39*(13), 11335–11348. doi:10.1016/j.eswa.2012.02.044

Sheta, O. E., & Eldeen, A. N. (2012). Building a Health Care Data Warehouse for Cancer Diseases. *International Journal of Database Management Systems*, *4*(5), 39–46. doi:10.5121/ijdms.2012.4503

Silva, E., Cardoso, L., Marins, F., Abelha, A., & Machado, J. (n). *Business intelligence platform for nosocomial infection incidence.*

Silva, E., Alpuim, A., Cardoso, L., Marins, F., Quintas, C., Portela, C. F., & Abelha, A. et al. (2014). Business intelligence and nosocomial infection decision making. In A. Azevedo & M. Santos (Eds.), *Integration of Data Mining in Business Intelligence Systems* (pp. 193–215). Hershey, PA: IGI Global; doi:10.4018/978-1-4666-6477-7.ch010

Silva, F., Olivares, T., Royo, F., Vergara, M. A., & Analide, C. (2013). Experimental Study of the Stress Level at the Workplace Using an Smart Testbed of Wireless Sensor Networks and Ambient Intelligence Techniques. In J. Ferrández Vicente, J. Álvarez Sánchez, F. de la Paz López, & F. J. Toledo Moreo (Eds.), *Natural and Artificial Computation in Engineering and Medical Applications SE - 21* (Vol. 7931, pp. 200–209). Springer Berlin Heidelberg; doi:10.1007/978-3-642-38622-0_21

Silverstein, S. (1999). *What is medical informatics, and why is it an important specialty?* Retrieved from http://www.ischool.drexel.edu/faculty/ssilverstein/informaticsmd/infordef1.htm

Smithson, D. S., Twohey, R., Rice, T., Watts, N., Fernandes, C. M., & Gratton, R. J. (2013). Implementing an obstetric triage acuity scale: Interrater reliability and patient flow analysis. *American Journal of Obstetrics and Gynecology*, *209*(4), 287–293. doi:10.1016/j.ajog.2013.03.031 PMID:23535239

Snyder, L., Mcewen Dean, L., Davidson, A., Thrun, M., Mccormick, E., & Mettenbrink, J. C. (2014). Integrating Data into Meaningful HIV Indicators Using Business Intelligence. *2014 Council of State and Territorial Epidemiologists Annual Conference.*

Solanas, A., Patsakis, C., Conti, M., Vlachos, I., Ramos, V., Falcone, F., & Martinez-Balleste, A. et al. (2014). Smart health: A context-aware health paradigm within smart cities. *IEEE Communications Magazine*, *52*(8), 74–81. doi:10.1109/MCOM.2014.6871673

Soler, E., Trujillo, J., Fernández-Medina, E., & Piattini, M. (2008). Building a secure star schema in data warehouses by an extension of the relational package from CWM. *Computer Standards & Interfaces*, *30*(6), 341–350. doi:10.1016/j.csi.2008.03.002

Spackman, K. A., Campbell, K. E., & Côte, R. A. (1997). SNOMED RT: A reference terminology for health care.Proceedings of the AMIA annual Fall symposium (pp. 640–644). PMID:9357704

Steele, R., & Clarke, A. (2013). The Internet of Things and Next-generation Public Health Information Systems. *Communications and Network*, *05*(03), 4–9. doi:10.4236/cn.2013.53B1002

Steiner, M., Soma, N., & Shimizu, T. (2006). Abordagem de um problema médico por meio do processo de KDD com ênfase à análise exploratória dos dados. *Gest Prod*. Retrieved from http://www.scielo.br/pdf/gp/v13n2/31177.pdf

Stroetmann, N., Kalra, D., Lewalle, P., Rector, A., Rodrigues, M., & Stroetmann, A. (2009). *Semantic Interoperability for better health and safer healthcare*. Deployment and Research for Europe.

Strong, D. M., Volkoff, O., Johnson, S. A., Bar-On, I., & Pelletier, L. (2009). Electronic health records and the changing roles of health care professionals: A social informatics perspective. *Proceedings of AMCIS 2009 Paper 560*. Retrieved from http://aisel.aisnet.org/amcis2009/560

Subrahmanian, V. (2001). Probabilistic databases and logic programming. In P. Codognet (Ed.), Logic Programming (p. 10). Springer. doi:10.1007/3-540-45635-X_8

Sullivan. (2009). *Overview of global economy*.

Tauseef, M. (2012). *Human Emotion Recognition Using Smart Sensors*. Massey University.

Tavakoli, N., Jahanbakhsh, M., Mokhtari, H., & Tadayon, H. R. (2011). Opportunities of electronic health record implementation in Isfahan. Procedia Computer Science (Vol. 3, pp. 1195–1198). doi:10.1016/j.procs.2010.12.193

The International Health Terminology Standards Development Organisation. (2012, July 31). *The International Health Terminology Standards Development Organisation: SNOMED CT Technical Implementation Guide*. Retrieved from http://ihtsdo.org/fileadmin/userupload/doc/download/docTechnicalImplementationGuideCurrent-en-USINT20120731.pdf

The International Health Terminology Standards Development Organization. (2014, July). SNOMED Clinical Terms User Guide.

The International Health Terminology Standards Development Organization. (n. d.). *SNOMED-CT-Supporting Meaningful User*.

The R Foundation. (n. d.). *What is R?* Retrieved from https://www.r-project.org/about.html

U.S. National Library of Medicine. (n. d.). *NIH*. Retrieved from http://www.nlm.nih.gov/research/umls/mapping projects/snomedcttoicd10cm.html

Valente, C., Cristina, T., Rosário, F., & Alcina, B. (2012). *Acompanhamento de enfermagem na interrupção da gravidez por opção da mulher*. Porto: I.G.O.

Van Akkeren, J., & Rowlands, B. (2007). An epidemic of pain in an Australian radiology practice. *European Journal of Information Systems*, *16*(6), 695–711. doi:10.1057/palgrave.ejis.3000715

van Rosse, F., Maat, B., Rademaker, C. M. A., van Vught, A. J., Egberts, A. C. G., & Bollen, C. W. (2009). The Effect of Computerized Physician Order Entry on Medication Prescription Errors and Clinical Outcome in Pediatric and Intensive Care: A Systematic Review. *Pediatrics*, *123*(4), 1184–1190. doi:10.1542/peds.2008-1494 PMID:19336379

Compilation of References

Vicente, H., Couto, C., Machado, J., Abelha, A., & Neves, J. (2012). Prediction of Water Quality Parameters in a Reservoir using Artificial Neural Networks. *International Journal of Design & Nature and Ecodynamics*, *7*(3), 309–318. doi:10.2495/DNE-V7-N3-309-318

Vicente, H., Dias, S., Fernandes, A., Abelha, A., Machado, J., & Neves, J. (2012). Prediction of the Quality of Public Water Supply using Artificial Neural Networks. *Journal of Water Supply: Research & Technology - Aqua*, *61*(7), 446–459. doi:10.2166/aqua.2012.014

Vicente, H., Roseiro, J., Arteiro, J., Neves, J., & Caldeira, A. T. (2013). Prediction of bioactive compound activity against wood contaminant fungi using artificial neural networks. *Canadian Journal of Forest Research*, *43*(11), 985–992. doi:10.1139/cjfr-2013-0142

von Krogh, G., & vonHippel, E. (2006). The promise of research on open source software. *Management Science*, *52*(7), 975–983. doi:10.1287/mnsc.1060.0560

W3C. (2010). *World Wide Web Consortium*. Retrieved from World Wide Web Consortium. Retrieved from http://www.w3.org/

Waegemann, C. (2003). EHR vs. CPR vs. EMR. *Healthcare Informatics Online*.

Walker, J., Pan, E., Johnston, D., Adler-Milstein, J., Bates, D. W., & Middleton, B. (2005). The Value of Health Care Information Exchange and Interoperability. *Health Affairs*. doi:10.1377/hlthaff.w5.10 PMID:15659453

Wang, F., & Hannafin, M. J. (2005). Design-based research and technology-enhanced learning environments. *Educational Technology Research and Development*, *53*(4), 5–23. doi:10.1007/BF02504682

Ward, J., & Peppard, J. (2002). *Strategic planning for information systems* (3rd ed.). New York, NY: Wiley.

Watkins, T. J., Haskell, R. E., Lundberg, C. B., Brokel, J. M., Wilson, M. L., & Hardiker, N. (2009). Terminology use in electronic health records: Basic principles. *Urologic Nursing*, *29*(5), 321–326. PMID:19863039

Watson, H., & Wixom, B. (2007, September). The Current State of Business Intelligence. *Computer*, *40*(9), 96–99. doi:10.1109/MC.2007.331

Weiser, M. (1991). The Computer for the Twenty-First Century. *Scientific American*, *264*(3), 94–103. doi:10.1038/scientificamerican0991-94 PMID:1675486

World Health Organization, & Unicef. (1978). Primary health care: a joint report.

World Health Organization. (2011). *Report on the burden of endemic health care associated infection worldwide: A systematic review of the literature*. Geneva, Switzerland: WHO Press.

World Health Organization. (2014). *International Classifications of Diseases*.

Worster, A., & Haines, T. (2004). Advanced Statistics: Understanding Medical Record Review (MRR) Studies. *Academic Emergency Medicine, 11*(2), 187–192. doi:10.1111/j.1553-2712.2004. tb01433.x PMID:14759964

Yoo, I., Alafaireet, P., Marinov, M., Pena-Hernandez, K., Gopidi, R., Chang, J.-F., & Hua, L. (2012). Data mining in healthcare and biomedicine: A survey of the literature. *Journal of Medical Systems, 36*(4), 2431–2448. doi:10.1007/s10916-011-9710-5 PMID:21537851

Zhang, X.-F., Attia, J., D'este, C., Yu, X.-H., & Wu, X.-G. (2005). A risk score predicted coronary heart disease and stroke in a Chinese cohort. *Journal of Clinical Epidemiology, 58*(9), 951–958. doi:10.1016/j.jclinepi.2005.01.013 PMID:16085199

Zheng, K. (2010). Clinical Decision-Support Systems. In Encyclopedia of Library and Information Sciences (Vol. 3).

Zokaei, A. K., & Simons, D. W. (2006). Value chain analysis in consumer focus improvement. *International Journal of Logistics Management, 17*(2), 141–162. doi:10.1108/09574090610689934

About the Contributors

José Machado is an Associate Professor with Habilitation at the Department of Informatics of the University of Minho, in Braga, Portugal, where he has been since 1988. He got his PhD in Informatics, in 2002, and Habilitation in 2011, and he is now the Director of the Computer Science and Technology Centre (in Portuguese CCTC) and the header of the Computer Science and Technology Group of Centro ALGORITMI. His research interests span the domain of Knowledge and Data Engineering, Health Informatics and Artificial Intelligence. He is the author of over 200 papers in international books, journals and conference proceedings.

António Abelha is an Assistant Professor at the Department of Informatics of the University of Minho, in Braga, Portugal. He got his PhD in 2004. He is a member of ALGORITMI research centre and co-founder of the Knowledge and Data Engineering Lab. His research interests span the domain of Knowledge and Data Engineering, Health Informatics and Artificial Intelligence. He is the author of over 150 papers in international books, journals and conference proceedings.

* * *

Vasco Abelha is an MsC student in Informatics Engineering from the University of Minho, in Braga, Portugal.

Jalel Akaichi received his PhD in Computer Science from the University of Sciences and Technologies of Lille (France) and then his Habilitation degree from the University of Tunis (Tunisia) where he is currently a Professor in the Computer Science Department. He has published in international journals and conferences, and has served on the program committees of several international conferences and journals. He is currently the Chair of the Master Science in Business Intelligence. He visited and taught in many institutions such as the State University of New York, Worcester Polytechnic Institute, INSA-Lyon, University of Blaise Pascal, University of Lille 1, just to refer a few.

Ana Alpuim obtained an MSc degree in Biomedical Engineering (Medical Informatics) in 2014 from the University of Minho in Braga, Portugal.

Magda Amorim obtained an MSc degree in Biomedical Engineering (Medical Informatics) in 2014 from the University of Minho in Braga, Portugal.

Cesar Analide is an Assistant Professor at the Department of Informatics of the School of Engineering of the University of Minho, and a researcher of the group Computer Science and Technology (CST) of Centro ALGORITMI. Also, he is founder member of the ISLab - Intelligent Systems Laboratory, a branch of the CST group of ALGORITMI. His main interests are in the areas of knowledge representation, intelligent agents and multi-agent systems, sensorization and computational sustainability.

Nouha Arfaoui received her master degree in management computing from High Institute of Management, Tunis, Tunisia. She is currently a Ph.D. student under the supervision of Prof. Jalel Akaichi and assistant in Faculty of Sciences Gabes. Her research is centered on the design of data warehouse schema and she has published in international journals and conferences.

Luis Barreiro is an MsC student in Informatics Engineering from the University of Minho, in Braga, Portugal.

Wilfred Bonney is currently working as a Health Informatics Specialist at the University of Dundee, Scotland, United Kingdom. He holds a Doctor of Philosophy (Ph.D.) degree in Information Technology from Capella University; a Master of Health Informatics (MHI) degree from Dalhousie University; and a Bachelor of Science (B.Sc.) degree in Information Technology from the International University in Germany. His research interests include health data standards, business intelligence, data mining, knowledge management, algorithms, research methods, survey design, scientific and statistical computing. He has published and presented research papers at major conferences in Health Informatics and Information Systems. He is also fluent in seven spoken languages including German, Russian, and Lithuanian.

Andreia Brandão obtained an MSc degree in Biomedical Engineering (Medical Informatics) in 2014 from the University of Minho in Braga, Portugal.

Luciana Cardoso obtained an MSc degree in Biomedical Engineering (Medical Informatics) in 2013 from the University of Minho in Braga, Portugal. Currently, she is working towards her Ph.D. in Biomedical Engineering at the University of Minho in Portugal under the topic of "Semantic Interoperability Issues with openEHR archetypes."

Ana Coimbra is an MsC student in Biomedical Engineering (Medical Informatics) from the University of Minho, in Braga, Portugal. She is a researcher of ALGORITMI research centre.

Andrea Domingues is an MsC student in Biomedical Engineering (Medical Informatics) from the University of Minho, in Braga, Portugal. She is a researcher of ALGORITMI research centre.

Julio Duarte holds a PHD in Biomedical Informatics since 2015. He is a teacher of the Polytechnic Institute of Cavado and Ave and a Pos-Doc researcher of the ALGORITMI research Centre, in the Computer Science and Technology Group and the Knowledge and Data Engineering Lab.

Marisa Esteves is an MsC student in Biomedical Engineering (Medical Informatics) from the University of Minho, in Braga, Portugal. She is a researcher of ALGORITMI Centre.

Ricardo Faria is an MsC student in Biomedical Engineering (Medical Informatics) from the University of Minho, in Braga, Portugal.

Bruno Fernandes is an MsC student in Biomedical Engineering (Medical Informatics) from the University of Minho, in Braga, Portugal. He is a researcher of ALGORITMI Centre.

Simão Frutuoso holds a degree in Medicine in 1985, at the Faculty of Medicine of the University of Oporto. He specialized in Paediatrics in 1993. His areas of interests are Neonatology, Intensive Cares and Transfontanellar ultrasound. He is a physician in Hospital Santo Antonio in Centro Hospitalar of Oporto.

Nuno Gonçalves is an MsC student in Informatics Engineering from the University of Minho, in Braga, Portugal.

Tiago Guimarães obtained an MSc degree in Biomedical Engineering (Medical Informatics) in 2015 from the University of Minho in Braga, Portugal.

Fernando Marins obtained an MSc degree in Biomedical Engineering (Medical Informatics) in 2013 from the University of Minho in Braga, Portugal. Currently, he is working towards his Ph.D. in Biomedical Engineering at the University of Minho in Portugal under the topic of "An intelligent recommender system for organ transplantation."

Filipe Miranda is an MsC student in Biomedical Engineering (Medical Informatics) from the University of Minho, in Braga, Portugal.

José Neves is a Full Professor at the Department of Informatics of the University of Minho, in Braga, Portugal. He got his PhD in 1982, and habilitation in 1999, and he is now the Director of the Doctoral Program in Biomedical Engineering. He is a member of ALGORITMI research centre and the header of the Knowledge and Data Engineering Lab. His research interests span the domain of Knowledge and Data Engineering and Artificial Intelligence. He is the author of over 300 papers in international books, journals and conference proceedings.

Lucas Oliveira is an MsC student in Informatics Engineering from the University of Minho, in Braga, Portugal.

Hugo Peixoto holds a PHD in Biomedical Informatics since 2014. He is a member of the Department of Information Systems of Centro Hospitalar of Tamega and Sousa.

Ana Pereira obtained an MSc degree in Biomedical Engineering (Medical Informatics) in 2014 from the University of Minho in Braga, Portugal.

Eliana Pereira obtained an MSc degree in Biomedical Engineering (Medical Informatics) in 2014 from the University of Minho in Braga, Portugal.

Sónia Pereira obtained an MSc degree in Biomedical Engineering (Medical Informatics) in 2015 from the University of Minho in Braga, Portugal.

Serafim Pinto is an MsC student in Informatics Engineering from the University of Minho, in Braga, Portugal.

Filipe Portela was born in Trofa, Portugal and went to the University of Minho in Guimarães, where he studied Information Systems and obtained his degree in 2007 (Lic), 2009 (MSc) and 2013 (PhD). He belongs to the Research Centre ALGORITMI where he is developing his post-doctoral research work in the topic "Pervasive Intelligent Decision Support Systems". His research was started in the INTCare R&D project (Intensive Medicine area) being then extended to education and public administration areas. He already has relevant indexed publications in the main research topics: Intelligent Decision Support Systems, Intelligent Systems, Pervasive Data, Business Intelligence, Data Mining and Knowledge Discovery. He has also been co-organizer of several workshops and reviewer of many indexed journals and conferences in these topics. Currently he also is an Invited Assistant Professor of the Information Systems Department, School of Engineering, University of Minho, Portugal, where he has been supervising several master students in the areas above mentioned. He is always in a continuing looking for opportunities to research and innovation in the society. He is now teaching in the Polytechnic Institute of Oporto.

Cesar Quintas is a PhD student in Biomedical Engineering (Medical Informatics). He is a member of the Department of Information System of the Centro Hospitalar of Oporto, one of the main hospital centre of Portugal.

Maria Salazar is a PhD student in Biomedical Engineering (Medical Informatics). She is the header of the Department of Information System of the Centro Hospitalar of Oporto, one of the main hospital centre of Portugal.

Manuel Santos holds a PhD in Computer Science – Artificial Intelligence. Actually he is an Associate Professor in the Department of Information Systems, School of Engineering, University of Minho, Portugal. He is the Investigator Responsible in research projects (grid data mining and intelligent decision support systems for intensive care). He is the head of the Intelligent Data Systems group in the R&D Centre Algoritmi. He has around 200 publications in conference proceedings, chapter books and journals. His main interests are: Knowledge Discovery from Databases and Data Mining, Intelligent Decision Support Systems, Machine Learning.

Eva Silva obtained an MSc degree in Biomedical Engineering (Medical Informatics) in 2014 from the University of Minho in Braga, Portugal.

Fábio Silva obtained an MSc degree in Informatics Engineering in 2011 from the University of Minho in Braga, Portugal. Currently, he is working towards his Ph.D. in Informatics at the University of Minho in Portugal. Also, he is a member of the ISLab - Intelligent Systems Laboratory, a branch of the Computer Science and Technology (CST) group of ALGORITMI. His current research interests include, computational sustainability, energetic efficient systems and multi-agent support systems.

Henrique Vicente holds a PhD in Chemistry from the University of Évora in 2005. He is currently Assistant Professor at the Chemistry Department of the University of Évora. He is a member of the Évora Chemistry Centre, and its research activities concentrated in the scientific areas of Chemical Environment; Quality Control of Lakes and Reservoirs of Water; Decision Support Systems; Multi-Agent Systems; Genetic and Evolutionary Programming; Logic Programming and Knowledge Discovery in Databases and Data Mining.

Index

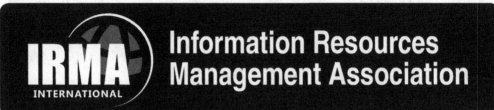
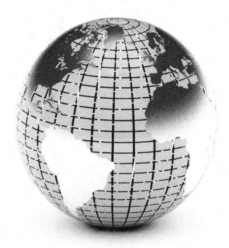